"This is a wonderful in-depth case study of Rhode Island's Medicaid Waiver debate. Every few years the debate about block granting Medicaid remerges. It is only with details found within that we can enter into those debates with a clear idea of its implications. We should thank Miller for such an insightful analysis."

—Colleen Grogan, *University of Chicago*

"In this book, one of the nation's foremost experts on Medicaid and state health policy dissects the challenging process of translating a bold idea into a workable new system of care for Rhode Island's most vulnerable citizens. It delivers bad news for those who would reflexively put all states on fixed block grants for their Medicaid programs. It reminds reformers of all persuasions of how important leadership, expertise, and outreach to community stakeholders are to producing even modest improvements in vital services and system efficiency."

—Tom Oliver, *University of Wisconsin-Madison*

Block Granting Medicaid

Medicaid is the largest grant-in-aid program in the United States. As such, reform in this area provides a unique opportunity to study the intersection between federal and state policy making in an area characterized by substantial uncertainty deriving from the lingering effects of the Great Recession, ongoing debate over the federal budget, and implementation of the Patient Protection and Affordable Care Act. Invariably, states reform the way health care is delivered, regulated, and financed within broader parameters established by federal statutes and regulations. It is critical that effective strategies be put into place at each level of government if both current and future health and long-term care reform efforts are to have their greatest chances at success. Rhode Island is the first state to receive permission to operate its entire Medicaid program under a global cap. As a consequence, it has entered the national consciousness as a key data point potentially supporting the block grant approach to Medicaid reform.

In this book, Edward Alan Miller draws on Rhode Island's experiences to assess conservatives' claims that the state's Global Consumer Choice Compact Medicaid Waiver represents a national model for Medicaid reform. Evidence gathered from archival sources and in-depth interviews with key stakeholders exposes factors that facilitated and impeded the design and implementation of Rhode Island's Global Waiver. These factors, in turn, suggest broader lessons for the Medicaid block grant debate and health and long-term care reform more generally; that, for example, Rhode Island's experience does not support block granting Medicaid while highlighting the role of stakeholder engagement, provider capacity, and federal fiscal support in the implementation process.

By providing a sophisticated understanding of factors enhancing or hindering state health reform, this book will contribute to improvements in the development and administration of policy development at both the state and federal levels.

Edward Alan Miller is associate professor in the Departments of Gerontology and Public Policy and Fellow in the Gerontology Institute at the University of Massachusetts Boston, and adjunct associate professor in the Departments of Political Science and Health Services, Policy and Practice at Brown University. He is a Fellow of the Social Research, Policy and Practice Section of the Gerontological Society of America.

Routledge Research in Public Administration and Public Policy

1 **A Complexity Theory for Public Policy**
Göktuğ Morçöl

2 **Network Governance in Response to Acts of Terrorism**
Comparative Analyses
Naim Kapucu

3 **Leadership and Policy Innovations—From Clinton to Bush**
Countering the Proliferation of Weapons of Mass Destruction
Joseph R. Cerami

4 **Disaster Resiliency**
Interdisciplinary Perspectives
Edited by Naim Kapucu, Christopher V. Hawkins, and Fernando I. Rivera

5 **Paying Our High Public Officials**
Evaluating the Political Justifications of Top Wages in the Public Sector
Teun J. Dekker

6 **The Politics of Regulatory Reform**
Stuart Shapiro and Debra Borie-Holtz

7 **Block Granting Medicaid**
A Model for 21st-Century Health Reform?
Edward Alan Miller

Block Granting Medicaid

A Model for 21st Century Health Reform?

Edward Alan Miller

Routledge
Taylor & Francis Group
NEW YORK AND LONDON

First published 2014
by Routledge
605 Third Avenue, New York, NY 10017

and by Routledge
2 Park Square, Milton Park, Abingdon, Oxon OX14 4RN

Routledge is an imprint of the Taylor & Francis Group, an informa business

Library of Congress Cataloging-in-Publication Data

Miller, Edward Alan.
Block granting Medicaid : a model for 21st century health reform? / Edward Alan Miller.
pages cm — (Routledge research in public administration and public policy ; volume 7)
1. Medicaid—Finance—Mathematical models. 2. Health care reform—United States—21st century. 3. Medical care, Cost of—United States—Mathematical models. 4. Medicaid—Rhode Island. I. Title.
RA412.4.M55 2013
368.4'200973—dc23
2013022304

ISBN: 978-0-415-72062-5 (hbk)
ISBN: 978-1-315-86688-8 (ebk)

Typeset in Sabon
by Apex CoVantage, LLC

This book is dedicated to my wife Jessica and daughters Anabelle and Dina, without whom this or anything else would not be possible.

Contents

Tables

Acknowledgements

The author would like to thank the Robert Wood Johnson Foundation for invaluable financial support (grant #64214). The author would also like to thank the staff at the State Health Access Data Assistance Center (SHADAC), but especially Caroline Au-Yeung, Elizabeth Lukanen, and Lynn Blewett for their efforts administering the grant. The author would further like to thank the students and colleagues at the University of Massachusetts Boston and Brown University who contributed to the research that informed this work. These individuals include Divya Samuel, Susan Allen, Amal Trivedi, Vincent Mor, Corina Ronneberg, Emily Gadbois, and Pamela Nadash. Views expressed belong to the author only. No other entity or individual is responsible for the content contained herein.

Acknowledgements

[illegible]

1 Rhode Island as Policy Laboratory

Medicaid is the jointly-funded federal-state health insurance program for the poor and disabled. Although administered by the states, the federal government matches state Medicaid spending at a rate determined by the Federal Medical Assistance Percentage (FMAP), which currently ranges from 50% to 73.4% and is dependent on state per capita income (Snyder et al. November 2012). Concomitant with provisions in the Patient Protection and Affordable Care Act of 2010 expanding Medicaid coverage to millions more Americans[1] and a U.S. Supreme Court decision making this expansion a state option, conservative opinion leaders and Republicans officials have sought program retrenchment. This policy priority is most prominently reflected in revival of the block grant approach to Medicaid reform by Republican Congressman, House Budget Committee Chair and former Vice Presidential candidate Paul Ryan's Fiscal Year (FY) 2012, 2013, and 2014 House budget proposals (Ryan 2011, 2012, 2013). In exchange for virtually unlimited flexibility administering Medicaid, the block grant approach would provide states with a fixed, upfront federal allotment or block grant that would no longer require a state match. All three House budget proposals which, in addition to block granting Medicaid would repeal the Affordable Care Act, passed the Republican controlled House of Representatives along a party line vote. Indeed, the Republican House has voted to repeal the Affordable Care Act 40 times and counting, with, for example, a 229 to 195 vote on May 16, 2013, drawing just two Democrats (Fahrenthold May 16, 2013).

Former Massachusetts Governor and unsuccessful Republican Presidential candidate Mitt Romney drew from his Vice Presidential candidate's proposals to adopt the block grant approach for Medicaid reform, with his economic plan claiming that "block grants have huge potential to generate both superior results and cost savings by establishing local control and promoting innovation" (Romney 2012). Romney even mentioned the potential of the block grant concept on October 22, 2012, during the last Presidential debate, arguing that "states like Arizona, Rhode Island have taken these, these Medicaid dollars, [and] have shown they can run these programs more cost-effectively" (Millman October 24, 2012). Romney also famously promised to repeal "ObamaCare" on day one.

These and other recent proposals to block grant Medicaid come less than 10 years after the George W. Bush Administration's 2003 proposal to do so (Guyer May 2003; Thompson 2012). Moreover, the Bush Administration's proposal came less than 10 years after the House Republican majority's 1995 Medigrant proposal to block grant Medicaid, which, in turn, came 15 years after the block grant proposal put forth by the Reagan administration in 1981 (Lambrew 2005; Holahan and Liska 1995; Thompson 2012). There are several reasons proponents cite to support both the block grant strategy and further devolution of responsibility for Medicaid program design and administration to the states more generally (Davidson 1997; Lambrew 2005; Anonymous February 4, 2003; Holahan and Weil May 27, 2003; Leichter 2008; Miller 2004; Office of U.S. Senator Tom Coburn May 19, 2011; Rivlin and Ryan November 17, 2010; Ryan 2011, 2012, 2013). Most obviously, it would provide the federal government with fiscal certainty regarding the amount it would need to pay out for Medicaid in any given year. Additionally, it theoretically offers those government officials "closest to the people" greater freedom to appropriate funds where they might have the most beneficial impact. This is both because doing so takes advantage of experience state and local officials have in managing day-to-day program operations and because state and locally run programs tend to be less rigid and bureaucratic than their nationally administered counterparts. It is also because state and locally administered programs best account for local norms, circumstances, values, and standards with regard to, say, the amount of funding allocated and service delivery options made available. Proponents further believe that the additional flexibility provided by a block grant would enable states to reshape Medicaid to promote greater personal responsibility, thereby mirroring trends visible in the private health insurance market. For example, greater cost sharing could be imposed and benefit packages made to more closely resemble private insurance benefits to better preclude crowd-out of the private market. Fundamentally, block grant enthusiasts express confidence in the capacities of state and local officials to experiment, innovate, and ultimately develop policy approaches that best meet people's needs and preferences when freed from policymaking constraints otherwise placed on them by the federal government.

There are several reasons opponents cite to oppose both the block grant strategy and greater state control over health policy (Davidson 1997; Anonymous February 4, 2003; Holahan and Weil May 27, 2003; Lambrew 2005; Park January 6, 2011; Holahan, et al. October 2012). Those opposing block granting Medicaid fear marked reductions in federal fiscal support for the vulnerable populations Medicaid serves. It is feared that growth in state allotments would fail to keep pace with increases in health and medical costs over time. It is also feared that state allotments would fail to keep pace with growth in Medicaid enrollment, particularly during economic downturns. The result would be a gradual shifting of costs from the federal to state and local governments, providers, and programs beneficiaries over time. Opponents of block grants also fear a race-to-the bottom dynamic if national standards are loosened or lifted and as a growing proportion of the financial burden falls to the states. States already exhibit considerable discretion when administering Medicaid, resulting in substantial cross-state variation in program spending, eligibility, benefits, provider payments, and service delivery system characteristics nationally (Miller 2002; Snyder, et al. November 2012). This variation would likely increase dramatically as state political, economic, programmatic, and cultural characteristics became even more determinative of state policymaking in this area. Fundamentally, opponents believe that it is the responsibility of the federal government to reduce interstate variation, or to bring it within a reasonable or acceptable range, so that the locus of one's birth or residency does not influence one's ability to receive health and medical care as a result of states' varying commitments and willingness to act.

EXPERIMENTATION IN THE OCEAN STATE

Under former Republican Governor Donald L. Carcieri, Rhode Island became the first state to receive permission to operate its entire Medicaid program under a single global cap through its Global Consumer Choice Compact Medicaid Waiver. As a consequence, Rhode Island has entered the national consciousness as a key data point potentially supporting the block grant approach to Medicaid reform. In a January 2011 report, Carcieri's former Secretary of the Executive Office of Health and Human Services (EOHHS), Gary Alexander, argued that the Global Waiver represented a model for entitlement reform throughout the nation (Alexander January 28, 2011). He claimed that in exchange for the aggregate cap agreed upon with the federal government, the state received "unprecedented flexibility and some relief from onerous federal rules" to "tailor its program to meet the needs of its population." He also claimed that the Waiver enabled the state to achieve $100 million in savings during the first 18 months, a figure he projected to reach $146 million over two years. Soon after Alexander's report was issued, Rhode Island's Medicaid Director, Elena Nicolella, indicated that it was not accurate nor authorized by the state (Hall January 20, 2011); a spokesman for the newly elected Governor, Lincoln Chafee, an independent and former Republican Senator, stated that it was "difficult to offer a comment on the veracity of the statements contained" therein (Levy February 1, 2011); and current EOHHS Secretary, former Democratic Chairmen of the House Finance Committee, Steven Costantino indicated that the state "can't substantiate any of those numbers" (Pugh June 12, 2011). Indeed, the results of an independent evaluation later conducted by The Lewin Group (December 6, 2011) would demonstrate substantially lower Medicaid savings. This is reflected in a subsequent article in the *Providence Journal*, which noted that while "Alexander claimed $100 million in savings from the 'global waiver' that gives Rhode Island some flexibility in managing its Medicaid program. . . [his] replacement, Steven Costantino [a Democratic appointed by Chafee], has put the figure at $23 million" (Edgar December 13, 2012).

Despite doubts raised within Rhode Island about the veracity of Alexander's conclusions, conservative politicians and commentators have since held up the Global Waiver as a successful example of what might be achieved nationally if all states received block grants to run their Medicaid programs (Anonymous March 28, 2011; Howard September 2012; Lawless and Ferrier June 15, 2011; Pugh June 12, 2011; Roberts May 15, 2011; Senate Finance Committee July 14, 2011; Volsky March 30, 2011). Thus, at a February 15, 2011, Senate Finance Committee hearing, Senator Tom Coburn, Republican from Oklahoma, asked U.S. Department of Health and Human Services Secretary Kathleen Sebelius "if Rhode Island can save 15.8%, why don't we just block grant every state . . . and take rules off and let them do these strategies that you're outlining rather than spending money in [ways] Washington is [telling] them what to do" (Volsky March 30, 2011). Similarly, at a July 14, 2011, Senate Finance Committee hearing, Haley Barbour, then a Republican Governor from Mississippi, pointed out that

> Rhode Island, in 2009, started a historic program that the Bush administration had approved. . . . Rhode Island said, 'We will take the same amount of money for 5 years if, in return, you will give us essentially total flexibility. Give us a block grant.' They collapsed 11 waivers together, and they saved a hundred million dollars a year in this program in the first 2-year period. . . . Our point is, they should never have had to go to Washington to ask for that. They should have the authority to do that themselves. And it would save the Federal Government money.

At an event sponsored by the Heritage Foundation, a conservative think tank, Senator Orin Hatch, Republican from Utah, held up Rhode Island as an example of conservative health care reform, noting that "Rhode Island implemented a global cap on Medicaid expenditures back in 2009. The Waiver gave the state flexibility from Washington's bureaucracy. Not only did the state improve patient care . . . but the state saved [a] significant amount of money by making its program more competitive and efficient" (Lawless and Ferrier June 15, 2011). According to a spokesman for Congressman Ryan, "Rhode Island's experience underscores the positive gains from loosening Washington's misguided one-size-fits-all approach that ties the hands of too many state governments. . . . Governors across the country continue to demand less onerous restrictions from Washington so they can better deliver quality, affordable health care to their Medicaid populations" (Roberts May 15, 2011).

Conservative commentators and analysts have been just as complimentary as Republican politicians about Rhode Island's Global Waiver. "If

Congress and the White House are serious about reducing the cost of entitlements," asserted an editorial in *The Wall Street Journal,* "they'll grant a Rhode Island-style Waiver to any state that requests one" (Anonymous March 28, 2011). "At the tail end of the George W. Bush administration," explained Avik Roy (September 30, 2012), a contributor to Forbes' *The Apothecary* blog,

> Rhode Island was granted a waiver by the federal government that, in effect, was a block grant: the state was assigned a five-year cap on Medicaid spending of $12.075 billion, in exchange for substantial flexibility to make changes to the program. The program was a smashing success. Rhode Island was able to save $100 million, and slow the growth of Medicaid from 8 percent per year to 3 percent, by making a few tweaks to their program that they couldn't before. . . . The best part is that, under a block-grant system, states can identify ways to save money while improving care, and other states can adopt best practices.

John R. Graham (January 2011), Deputy Director of the Pacific Research Institute, a conservative think tank, further explained that although the "Rhode Island waiver is not a block grant . . . it appears to have had the results one would expect from a block grant: Spending has plummeted from what was anticipated. Remarkably, through the first six quarters of the waiver . . . actual spending was $2.7 billion versus $3.8 billion budgeted—savings of almost one-third. . . . Governors and state legislators who wish to reform Medicaid in the best interests of taxpayers and beneficiaries should look to Rhode Island's success as they craft ways to push back against federal overreach in the delivery of medical care."

Block grant advocates' believe that the basic concepts underlying the Global Waiver should spread from Rhode Island to other states, consistent with the general finding that policy innovations often begin in one or a handful of states before being adopted nationally (Balla 2001; Berry and Berry 2007; Miller and Banaszak-Holl 2005; Walker 1969). Block grant advocates also believe that the basic concepts underlying the Waiver should spread to other states from Rhode Island consistent with Justice Louis Brandeis famous conclusion that "it is one of the happy incidents of the federal system that a single courageous state may, if its citizens choose, serve as a laboratory; and try novel social and economic experiments without risk to the rest of the country."[2] The purpose of this book is therefore twofold. First, it draws on Rhode Island's actual experiences to assess conservatives' claims that the state's Global Consumer Choice Compact Medicaid Waiver represents a national model for Medicaid reform. Second, it identifies factors that either facilitated or impeded the design and implementation of the Global Waiver in order to draw broader lessons, not only for the debate over Medicaid blocks grants and retrenchment but health and long-term care reform more generally.

AN INTRODUCTION TO THE GLOBAL WAIVER

States administer their Medicaid programs under specific authorities provided in Title XIX of the Social Security Act, which is consolidated into an agreement states enter into with the federal government, called the state plan. This authority includes certain requirements that states must adhere to if they are to receive federal funds. States must cover certain services and populations that meet the program's minimum income and categorical requirements for mandatory coverage. Although states cannot cap funding or enrollment for mandatory populations, they can alter eligibility criteria and benefit packages as long as such changes are within the bounds of federal mandates. Most Medicaid spending, however, is on optional populations or services that states are not required to cover but choose to do so anyway, both because it is politically desirable and because the federal government picks up at least 50% of the tab. Thus, although representing only 30% of enrollees nationally, optional coverage groups constitute 65% of total Medicaid program spending (Lambrew 2005). Core Medicaid program requirements also include: comparability of benefits—states generally cannot provide services that differ in type or amount across beneficiary groups; free choice of providers by recipients; limits on cost-sharing; and bars on service rationing due to funding shortfalls—a state may alter eligibility or benefits as specified in the state plan, but cannot impose caps or waitlists for core populations.

States may also obtain federal waivers which, according to Thompson and Burke (2009), "are congressional delegation of authority to the executive branch to permit selective deviations from the law." States seek out waivers so that they may gain the freedom to customize their Medicaid programs, including under sections 1115 and 1915 of the Social Security Act. In 1962, Congress enacted Section 1115, which permits the federal government to offer states "research and demonstration" waivers, including, subsequently, general authority to make extensive changes that go beyond traditional Medicaid program rules. Although ostensibly requiring rigorous formal assessment to further policy learning, the evaluation function of these waivers have largely been neglected; instead, they have been used primarily for purposes of permitting states to engage in large-scale program restructuring (Thompson and Burke 2007). In 1981, Congress promulgated Section 1915, which authorizes the federal government to provide states with additional waivers, though not subject to evaluation and much more limited in scope than their Section 1115 counterparts. There are two types of 1915 waivers: 1915(b) and 1915(c). In allowing states to limit beneficiary freedom of choice and to use payment approaches other than fee-for-service, 1915(b) waivers permit states to enter into contracts with Medicaid-managed care organizations. By contrast, 1915(c) waivers allow states to provide home- and community-based services not otherwise authorized in the state plan.

Specific reasons why states apply for federal waivers include obtaining increased flexibility to innovate, expand coverage, control costs, and provide consumer-driven care. The pace with which the federal government granted both 1115 and 1915(b) and (c) waivers increased considerably under the Presidential administrations of Bill Clinton and George W. Bush, both of whom, as former governors, proved sympathetic to state calls for increased flexibility in administering Medicaid. Previously, for example, federal officials required states to demonstrate that one nursing home bed was emptied for each 1915(c) home- and community-based waiver recipient served. This "cold-bed" rule was rescinded by the Clinton administration in 1994, making it substantially easier for states to meet requirements for cost neutrality; now all they had to show was that the average cost of home- and community-based care received would be less than or equal to the amount otherwise paid the pertinent institutional providers (e.g., nursing homes, intermediate care facilities for the mentally retarded) (Wiener and Tilly 2003). Subsequent to the 1999 U.S. Supreme Court decision in *Olmstead v. L.C.*, which reaffirmed the legal right of individuals with disabilities to choose to receive care in community-based settings as opposed to institutions, approval of 1915(c) waivers further accelerated. This was largely due to the Bush administration's New Freedom Initiative, which outlined the federal government's approach to assisting state and local governments in implementing the *Olmstead* ruling and overcoming barriers to rebalancing long-term care (Miller, Allen, and Mor 2009).

Under the Clinton administration, 1115 waivers were more likely to focus on shifting Medicaid beneficiaries into managed care (typically with eligibility expansions), increasing health coverage for pregnant women and children, and restructuring long-term care service delivery and financing. Under the Bush administration, 1115 waivers were more likely to focus on expanding eligibility, though with fewer benefits and increased beneficiary cost-sharing, improving access to pharmaceutical benefits, and subsidizing private health insurance coverage, say, through premium assistance for employer-based plans. Although not required by law, the federal government requires states to demonstrate budget neutrality with their 1115 "research and demonstration" applications, that the federal government would not spend more than it would have spent without the waiver. It is important to note that these projections provide for a per capita cap, but *not* an overall cap on federal spending (Artiga March 2009; Shirk August 26, 2009). Federal spending per enrollee may be fixed under such a waiver, but the number of enrollees served is unrestricted; as such, the federal government must continue to match spending increases caused by enrollment growth.

On July 29, 2008, Republican Governor Donald Carcieri made his administration's Global Consumer Choice Compact Medicaid Waiver application public; on August 8, 2008, it was submitted to the Centers for Medicaid and Medicare Services (CMS), the federal agency responsible for administering Medicaid. The state originally requested substantially more flexibility administering Medicaid than it would ultimately receive in exchange for accepting a limit on the federal contribution. In particular, it asked for the provision of a fixed, upfront federal allotment or block grant that would no longer require a state match. It instead proposed a state maintenance of effort provision where Rhode Island would continue to allocate 23% of its general revenue budget to the Medicaid program every year. On December 19, 2008, CMS gave provisional approval to Rhode Island's Global Consumer Choice Compact Waiver, subject to a 30 day review period by Rhode Island's Democratic party-dominated General Assembly, as previously stipulated in the state's 2008 Medicaid Reform Act. If the General Assembly had wished, it could have voted to block implementation of the Global Waiver; since it chose not to do so, CMS gave its official approval on January 16, 2009, the Waiver's official start date. Rhode Island became the first state granted permission from the federal government to operate its entire Medicaid program—excepting Disproportionate Share Hospital payments and local education agency funding—under the state plan and a single 1115 Waiver. Prior to the Global Waiver, Rhode Island's Medicaid program operated under the state plan and multiple waiver authorities, including an 1115 RIte Care waiver, a 1915(b) Dental waiver, and nine 1915(c) home- and community-based services waivers.

The final version of the Wavier did not include the block grant structure. It instead set a cap whereby the state agreed to limit federal fiscal participation to a level no higher than the federal share of total state and federal spending of $12.075 billion over a five year demonstration period

Table 1.1 Timeline of Key Events for Rhode Island Global Waiver

January 2008: Governor announces plan to pursue the Global Waiver.
February 2008: Legislation authorizing pursuit of the Global Waiver introduced as part of FY 2009 budget.
June 26, 2008: Legislation authorizing pursuit of Global Waiver signed into law as part of FY 2009 budget.
July 29, 2008: Global Waiver application released to the public.
August 8, 2008: Global Waiver application submitted to the Centers for Medicare and Medicaid Services.
December 19, 2008: State receives initial federal approval of the Global Waiver; General Assembly had 30 days to review the waiver and if desired, vote to block it, but it chose not to do so.
January 16, 2009: Global Waiver receives official federal approval and takes effect.
July 1, 2009: State begins implementing Global Waiver's provisions; General Assembly establishes legislative oversight and process for community input.
December 31, 2013: Global Waiver is set to expire unless renewed for another five years.

in exchange for the ability to make certain program changes. This five-year budget was based on historical caseload and health utilization trends, accounting for a 7.8% program growth rate. This structure kept Medicaid's traditional funding structure intact, with the state having to spend a dollar first in order to receive the federal match. Rhode Island began implementing the Global Waiver on July 1, 2009, the same day that the state legislature amended the 2008 Medicaid Reform Act to legally require legislative oversight, to establish a process for community input, and to make other program changes. The Global Waiver is set to expire December 31, 2013, unless it is renewed. Table 1.1 provides a timeline of key Global Waiver-related events.

METHODS

The study relies on two primary sources of data: archival documents and in-depth open-ended interviews with key stakeholders. The interviews were undertaken with people chosen through a combination of purposive and snowball sampling (Patton 2002). Thus, selection of subjects was initially based on our own knowledge about Rhode Island and the Medicaid program but later on information provided by our respondents regarding additional actors who should be interviewed about the design and implementation of the Global Waiver.

Twenty-six semi-structured interviews were conducted with 30 individuals from March 17, 2010, through May 28, 2010. Two interviews included two subjects each (two consumer advocates; two executive branch officials); one interview included three subjects (three state officials). Interviews were about one hour long. Interview subjects included: legislative staff (two individuals); current and former officials within the pertinent executive/administrative agencies (seven individuals); consumer advocates representing different populations (e.g., the elderly, the developmentally disabled, the mentally ill, the physically disabled, and children and families) (10 individuals); provider representatives representing different service modalities (e.g., nursing homes, home care, managed care, shared living, and community providers) (eight individuals); and three others (i.e., a consultant and other executive branch officials).

Stakeholders representing different backgrounds were recruited as interview subjects to ensure representation of varying points of view about Medicaid and the Global Waiver (Glaser and Strauss 1967). Use of a diverse sample is important because the greater the degree to which the perceptions of people about a particular phenomenon converge, the more likely that they provide a reasonably accurate portrayal of the process studied (Jick 1979). Use of a diverse sample also is important because employing multiple types of informants minimizes the threat of single-source information bias while maximizing the breadth of the information consulted (Pothas and de Wet 2000).

Through our interviews, we sought to identify what factors contributed to the design of the Global Waiver. This includes the purpose of the Waiver, the contours of the drafting process, and the reactions and/or involvement of government officials and other interested actors. We also sought to understand factors influencing subsequent approval and oversight of the Global Waiver by the federal government and state legislature. This includes negotiations between the state and the federal governments and changes to the state's Waiver application resulting from those negotiations. It also includes the timing of legislative approval and the enactment of legislation formalizing the legislature's oversight role. The reactions and/or involvement of key stakeholders in each of these areas were examined as well.

We further sought to understand factors facilitating and/or impeding implementation of the Global Waiver by EOHSS and its constituent agencies. This includes identifying and exploring the effectiveness of processes put into place to implement the Global Waiver (e.g., the Global Waiver Implementation Task Force, internal state work groups) and the involvement and/or reactions of key stakeholders to these endeavors. It also includes identifying how much progress had been made in implementing the Global Waiver and the role of the economic recession, state budget crisis, federal stimulus package, state administrative capacity, provider capacity, and other factors in this regard.

All interviews were recorded and transcribed. Each transcript was subsequently coded to identify recurring themes and patterns in responses (Miles and Huberman 1994). This was an emergent process to the extent that we formulated new categories and revised old ones as we read through the transcripts. Once a full set of codes was developed, we went back and recoded all transcripts using the common set of themes developed. Quotes illustrative of each theme were excerpted.

In addition to analyzing interview transcripts, more than 375 archival sources published between 2007 and 2013 were reviewed. Pertinent statutes and regulations about Medicaid and the Global Waiver were identified and collected; so too were relevant government reports, press releases, letters, and other documents. Information was collected from consumer advocacy groups, provider organizations, and other nongovernmental entities, in addition to articles published in the *Providence Journal* and other news sources. This information was used to cross-validate the descriptions and perspectives of key informants (Jick 1979), corroborating accounts given by interviewees through independent verification in alternative sources. They also provided historical background on Rhode Island's Medicaid program and the Global Waiver.

OVERVIEW

Chapter 2 analyzes the development of the Global Waiver. This includes identifying factors motivating state officials to pursue the waiver. It also includes examination of key administrative personnel, community input, and stakeholder concerns. Results indicate that the Global Waiver was largely motivated by state fiscal pressures deriving from the rapidly deteriorating economy and disproportionate amount of the state budget devoted to Medicaid. Results also indicate that the Global Waiver was motivated by specific programmatic goals, both with the aim of improving patient care and reducing program costs. Uncertainty associated with the Global Waiver stemmed, in part, from the fact that no state had ever operated its Medicaid program in this way. It was also unclear why the state needed to pursue the Global Waiver in light of the disproportionate programmatic focus on rebalancing long-term care services away from nursing homes towards home- and community-based settings; other strategies could have been pursued to achieve this goal without involving other program dimensions. Community stakeholders were particularly concerned about the uncertain implications of the Waiver for certain populations, including the developmentally disabled, the mentally ill, and children and families. In light of the proposed block grant structure, most believed that the Global Waiver would not have been pursued without political and ideological alignment between Rhode Island's Republican governor and the Republican George W. Bush administration.

The Global Waiver was largely designed by high-level state officials and consultants. There was little to no opportunity for provider representatives, consumer advocates, and the general public to inform its development, though prior discussions about rebalancing long-term care away from institutions and toward home- and community-based services influenced the final product. Few details were made available to community stakeholders during the Waiver development process. This was, in part, a conscious decision on the part of state officials who felt that what was being proposed was a general framework with which to achieve greater administrative flexibility with specific details to be worked out once the Waiver had been approved. The absence of specifics, however, made it difficult for outside observers to provide feedback on what was being proposed. It also exacerbated stakeholder distrust and concern about the Waiver and its implications for affected populations. There was fear that the state might run out of federal money before the five-year demonstration period expired, particularly given the state of the economy and likely increase in Medicaid rolls.

Chapter 3 reviews the federal approval process; in particular, how it unfolded and what changes were made to the Global Waiver as a result of the state's negotiations with the federal government. State legislative approval and oversight and stakeholder views of the final Waiver agreement were examined as well. Findings suggests that fears about state officials' intentions in pursuing the Global Waiver were exacerbated by the lack of transparency and community input in its negotiations with the federal government. Several major changes were made during the negotiation process. Rather than block grant Medicaid, the state accepted a capped federal match whereby a limit was placed on combined federal and state spending over five years with the state being still required to expend its own resources before it could receive federal money. Rather than gaining nearly unlimited flexibility, state discretion was limited to specific proposals outlined in the Waiver's "Special Terms and Conditions," with additional changes subject to varying degrees of federal oversight. Although more acceptable than a block grant, stakeholders were concerned about the adequacy of the expenditure cap. A clause permitting the state to opt out of the Global Waiver, basically at any time, raised fears that if the state ended the Global Waiver, populations previously served by separate waiver programs would no longer be eligible for needed services.

The state legislature permitted the Global Waiver to go into effect, largely because millions of dollars in promised savings were deemed critical in light of the state's growing budget deficit. Once approved, the General Assembly used both existing and newly established mechanisms to oversee implementation. Existing mechanisms include the state budget process, periodic hearings, and routine communications. Waiver-specific mechanisms include a Global Waiver Implementation Task Force and Joint House-Senate oversight committee, though the letter never seems to have been implemented. They also include a requirement that all but simple administrative changes be approved by the state legislature before being submitted for federal approval. Overall, the larger role reserved by the state legislature in Medicaid since the Global Waiver has gone into effect has made it more difficult for administrators to adopt changes that previously garnered little if any legislative interest.

Chapter 4 provides an overview of the Global Waiver's provisions as authorized and approved by the federal government and state legislature. Under the Global Waiver, Rhode Island gained permission to implement specific changes targeted at achieving three major programmatic goals: (1) Rebalancing the publicly funded long-term care system to increase access to home- and community-based services and supports and to decrease reliance on institutional stays; (2) Ensuring all Medicaid beneficiaries have access to care management whereby primary and acute care is managed and coordinated with other services and supports; and (3) Procuring Medicaid-funded services through cost-effective payment and purchasing strategies that align with programmatic goals. The federal government also authorized the state to receive federal matching funds for populations and services previously covered by state-only funded programs through the Global Waiver's Costs Not Otherwise Matchable, or CNOM, provision. The level of federal and state legislative scrutiny was made more commensurate with the scope of future program changes as well through the inclusion of a three-tier system of federal oversight.

Chapter 5 examines external (to EOHHS) factors that have influenced implementation of the Global Waiver on the part of program administrators. This is with respect to efforts to promote involvement on the part of community stakeholders, including a Global Waiver Implementation Task

Force authorized by the General Assembly. It is also with respect to collaboration across key stakeholders representing different patient populations and service delivery sectors. The role of the state's fiscal and budgetary environment on implementation of the Global Waiver is examined as well.

Most stakeholders have not been satisfied with the way the Task Force has been administered. Because the Task Force has not served as a useful conduit for public input, it has not had much influence on implementation of the Global Waiver's provisions. Greater support by state administrative personnel and greater integration with ongoing implementation efforts within the pertinent state administrative agencies were deemed critical for increasing the effectiveness of the Task Force's role. Whereas some believe that silos across population sectors have remained largely intact, others observe increased cross-sector cooperation since the Global Waiver was designed and implemented. This has been driven, in part, by the changing needs of the populations served and the program-wide scope of the Global Waiver.

There is general agreement that decisions made under the Global Waiver have been driven largely by the adverse fiscal and budgetary environment facing the state. Thus, the emphasis has largely been weighted toward controlling costs rather achieving savings and improving care through programmatic changes. The provision of hundreds of millions of dollars in federal stimulus money, however, helped the state support caseload increases resulting from rising unemployment levels while softening the emphasis on reducing spending. That the state had to maintain eligibility levels at July 1, 2008, levels to qualify for federal stimulus support, a provision since extended by the federal health reform law, has also helped to ameliorate stakeholder concern. So too has been recognition that the state would not come close to losing its federal match as a result of exceeding the funding cap agreed upon with the federal government. This was both because of the generosity of the funding cap itself and because the level of state appropriations and spending were simply not high enough in the prevailing fiscal climate to draw in sufficient federal dollars to exceed the cap.

Chapter 6 examines internal factors that have influenced the implementation of the Global Waiver. This is both with respect to state administrative personnel and the data and informational architecture. It is also with respect to collaboration across state administrative agencies. Due to changes to the state's retirement system, there was widespread concern that it did not have sufficient numbers of administrative personnel to properly implement the Global Waiver. This concern was exacerbated both by heavy reliance on outside consultants and by prevailing fiscal and budgetary conditions, which increased demands on the Medicaid program while slowing down the rate of new hires. The result was significant levels of stress among program administrators. A particular worry was a dearth of experienced leadership with a history of working collaboratively with providers and advocates. Although significant barriers remain, some detect greater communication, collaboration, and understanding across the health and human services departments responsible for administering Medicaid since implementation of the Global Waiver began.

Although the state tracks a variety of key data elements across a number of different information systems, it has traditionally relied on antiquated technology that requires considerable resources to maintain and prevents timely access to the data needed to track and evaluate progress. The state has thus sought to modernize its information technology architecture as part of its Global Waiver implementation strategy and in preparation for health care reform. Moreover, several additional data elements were identified that should be collected and reported, both routinely and as part of the state's evaluation plan for the federal government. Quarterly progress reports to the federal government and the Rhode Island General Assembly have subsequently provided some of the additional data requested.

Chapter 7 examines the impact of the Global Waiver on service provision within Rhode Island. This includes the role that provider capacity has played in the implementation process. It also includes the state's new authority to obtain federal matching dollars for previously state-only funded programs. Doubt was expressed about the ability of providers to serve significantly greater numbers of long-term care recipients within the community. This has served, in part, to impede the state's long-term care rebalancing efforts. It was felt that reimbursement levels were still too low to stimulate sufficient levels of market growth. There was also concern that even if the number of providers increased significantly, the state would be unable to monitor the quality of care provided in light of recent staff reductions within the pertinent administrative agencies. Nursing home providers generally recognized the need to increase use of home- and community-based service options within the state. Although overall spending was reduced slightly, the state began to reimburse facilities, in part, on the needs of residents served in recognition of the growing complexity and severity of the nursing home population due to the transition and diversion of lower care beneficiaries to home- and community-based settings.

Perhaps the most popular aspect of the Global Waiver has been the state's ability to use its Costs Not Otherwise Matchable (CNOM) authority to draw in additional federal matching funds to help finance programs previously paid for entirely out of the general treasury. This provision was particularly appreciated as the state's budget situation would have resulted in significant reductions in these efforts. Although desirable, "CNOMing" previously state-only funded programs has resulted in additional administrative burdens being placed on state agencies and provider organizations. The general consensus, however, was that the benefits of doing so far outweighed the costs and, as such, both state officials and provide representatives reported looking out for additional opportunities in this area.

Chapter 8 examines whether the Global Waiver lived up to the expectations of its proponents, both overall and with respect to each of the three major programmatic areas impacted: long-term care rebalancing, care coordination, and "smart purchasing." It also draws lessons and recommendations from Rhode Island's experience with the Global Waiver, both regarding the design and administration of state health reform and long-term care rebalancing. As a capped federal match, the Global Waiver is not a model that supports the block grant approach to Medicaid reform. Moreover, the state did not receive unlimited discretion to administer the Global Waiver nor achieved nearly as much savings as has been claimed. Indeed, most of the savings obtained by Rhode Island during this time period derive not from the Global Waiver but from increased spending on the part of the federal government and from measures the state could have implemented independently of the state's Global Waiver authority. Although limited progress has been made coordinating care and rebalancing long-term services and supports, efforts in both areas have largely stagnated. Moreover, the state made little use of "smart purchasing" strategies during the Waiver's first four years. The desire to make further progress in achieving the Waiver's cost and programmatic goals has resulted in the inclusion of additional initiatives in the state's application to renew the Global Waiver for another five years.

Independent of summative impact, the Global Waiver suggests several lessons for health and long-term care reform. When pursuing reform, it is important to ensure adequate levels of stakeholder input and transparency. This includes providing sufficient detail on proposed changes and adopting mechanisms for public participation during the design, approval, and implementation processes. Ultimately, the familiarity and trust that consultation and collaboration promotes should contribute to the creation of a less challenging environment both politically, when new programs or initiatives are being designed, and administratively, when they are being implemented.

When undertaking major reform, it is critical that states ensure the presence of sufficient numbers of experienced administrative personnel. This includes not undertaking significant endeavors at the same time as other policy changes are being putting into place to markedly reduce the size of the state's workforce. It also includes not undertaking significant endeavors when the ability to fill key positions is in doubt, as occurs during major fiscal crises. Especially important is a state's ability to retain or seek out agency leaders with both the management and communications skills necessary to oversee comprehensive reform and to work productively with community stakeholders. It is also crucial that the requisite technology systems be put into place to undertake all major programmatic tasks and to meet most reasonable data requests, including timely access to the key data elements necessary to track and evaluate progress.

The combination of economic and political conditions that facilitate adoption of major Medicaid reform can, in turn, make the implementation environment especially challenging. In Rhode Island, for example, reform adopted, in part, due to conservative ideological alignment contributed to concern on the part of community stakeholders regarding the state's commitment to the program, distrust that extended into implementation stages of the policy process. Furthermore, moving forward with significant program change during an economic downturn adversely impacted state administrative capacity and funding levels, thereby compromising implementation and contributing to weaker-than-expected results. The scope of reform matters as well. While reforms that touch on most aspects of the Medicaid program can make it difficult for critics to foment a clear and coherent opposition, thereby contributing to ultimate adoption, the breadth of such reform can make implementation far more challenging than if it was more limited. This is because the large number of populations impacted may pose challenges to shorthanded state bureaucracies charged with incorporating feedback from multiple stakeholder groups. It is also because the imposition of organizational barriers may preclude effective cooperation across the multiple state departments affected.

That overall spending on home- and community-based services has largely remained stagnant suggests just how difficult it can be for laggard states that have historically spent substantially more on nursing homes to make more than marginal progress even with the provision of options and incentives that otherwise should promote increased reliance on the home- and community-based sector. Because expanding reliance on home- and community-based services tends to entail short-term increases in spending before subsequent longer-term savings can be achieved, states need to recognize that eventual savings take time to materialize, but only with continued investments that promote both the supply and demand for services. Clearly, prospectively documenting provider capacity is important because if the plan is to rely more on home- and community-based resources, it is critical that the extent to which those resources are able to meet the complex care needs of an increasingly larger service clientele be assessed. Increased reimbursement is especially important for attracting participating providers. Adjusting payment for client acuity should help promote buy-in on the part of both institutional and non-institutional providers given that rebalancing increases complexity among clients served in both locations.

Chapter 9 looks beyond Rhode Island to examine the implications of Medicaid blocking granting and retrenchment more generally. Rhode Island's Global Waiver is in marked contrast to most block grant proposals that would substantially reduce the level of federal fiscal support nor permit states to back out via a Global Waiver-like escape clause should the fiscal situation become untenable due to emergent conditions. Such a marked reduction in federal spending would have devastating consequences, not only for state budgets but for provider reimbursement, beneficiary access and quality, and program benefits and eligibility. How exactly would particular states respond if the Medicaid program was block granted? The answer will depend largely on a combination of political and economic considerations. Traditionally, states of all types—rich and poor, conservative and liberal—have responded reliably to financial incentives promulgated by the federal government under Medicaid. This bipartisan consensus has broken down, however, during periods of intense, partisan polarization when Republican leaders at the state level view themselves as part of a broader ideological movement to vitiate government programs such as Medicaid. Ironically, today's hyper-partisan political environment suggests that those Republican-led states that might be most adversely impacted if the program were block granted may, in fact, be most supportive if the federal government pursued this approach to Medicaid reform. Of course, neither block granting Medicaid nor repealing health care reform is going to happen anytime soon in light of President Barack Obama's electoral triumph. Still, Democrats and Republicans may nonetheless include Medicaid in a deal to reduce the long-term budget deficit. Furthermore, it is likely that the block grants and other forms of Medicaid retrenchment will continue to be proposed by Republican officials, both in future budget proposals and presidential party platforms.

NOTES

1. Passed by the Democratic majority in Congress and signed into law by Democratic President Barack Obama on March 23, 2010. It was subsequently modified with enactment of the Health Care and Education Reconciliation Act on March 30, 2010.
2. New State Ice Co. v. Liebmann, 285 U.S. 262, 311 (1932) (Dissenting).

2 Waiver Genesis

Medicaid provides coverage for more than 62 million low income individuals or approximately one in five Americans, including 31 million children, 16 million adults in low income families, and 16 million elderly and persons with disabilities (Kaiser Family Foundation March 1, 2013). As the largest federal grant-in-aid program, total Medicaid expenditures reached $413.9 billion in 2011. It is also the largest fiscal item in state budgets, accounting for 23.7% of total state spending (National Association of State Budget Officers 2011). At 2.5%, average annual growth in per capita Medicaid spending has been lower than average annual growth in both national health expenditures per capita (3.3%) and private health insurance per enrollee (5.5%) (Kaiser Family Foundation March 1, 2013). Still, annual growth in states' Medicaid expenditures has exceeded growth in general revenues, thereby causing Medicaid to consume increasingly larger proportions of state budgets. This has forced a tradeoff with other priorities such as education and highways since all states but Vermont must balance their budgets.

Elderly and disabled beneficiaries consume a disproportionate share of Medicaid program costs. Although constituting just 10% and 15% of total Medicaid enrollees, respectively, in 2009, for example, the elderly and disabled consumed 23% and 42% of program expenditures (Kaiser Family Foundation March 1, 2013). This is as compared to children and non-elderly adults who, while representing 49% and 26% of program enrollees, respectively, consumed just 20% and 15% of program spending. Not surprisingly, per capita costs vary considerably, ranging from $2,305 for children and $2,900 for non-elderly adults, to $15,840 for disabled adults and $13,149 for the elderly. The top 5% of program spenders alone account for more than half (54%) of program spending. A large proportion of those excess costs pay for long-term services and supports.

Indeed, long-term care is particularly salient where Medicaid is concerned. On the one hand, 62.2% of the nation's $207.9 billion long-term care bill in 2010 was paid for by Medicaid, as compared to 21.9% out-of-pocket, 11.6% through long-term care insurance and other private sources, and 4.4% by other public programs (The Scan Foundation January 2013). On the other hand, long-term care constituted 34.5% of total Medicaid spending in 2009, with 56% of all Medicaid long-term care spending being directed toward institutional care and 44% toward noninstitutional services, up from 18% in 1995 (Eiken et al. October 31, 2011). However, a much smaller proportion of long-term care spending for older adults and people with physical disabilities is spent on noninstitutional care, 36%, up from 17% in 1995, than for people with developmental disabilities, 66%, up from 30% in 1995. Indeed, in 2009, only six states[1] expended more than 50% of Medicaid long-term care expenditures on noninstitutional services for the aged and physically disabled, while just another six states[2] spent more than 50% on institutional care for the developmentally disabled.

Like other states, Rhode Island has faced considerable pressure to restrain Medicaid spending. In state FY 2006, for example, more than one-fifth of the state's population obtained health insurance coverage from Medicaid (EOHHS October 2007). This includes 15% of the state's elderly residents and 40% of its school-aged children. That year, the program constituted about $800 million or approximately one-quarter of the state's budget (EOHHS October 2007). Given that the state projected a structural deficit of more than $350 million over five years and that Medicaid spending growth had far exceeded general revenue growth, Medicaid stood at the forefront of state budget discussions (EOHHS October 2007).

While Rhode Island has been a leader in some areas—for example, providing access to high quality care for low-income children and parents up to 250% and 175% of the Federal Poverty Level (FPL), respectively, since the 1990s (Holahan and Rifkin February 2012), it is ranked near the bottom in others; most conspicuously, in the provision of long-term care in home and community settings. Thus, despite several ongoing initiatives to improve the distribution in spending, just 11% of Medicaid long-term care expenditures in 2006 were directed toward home- and community-based services and 89% toward nursing homes, far below national totals (AARP 2009).

This chapter examines economic and programmatic factors motivating the Governor and administration officials in Rhode Island to pursue the Global Waiver. It also examines key personnel involved in the design of the Waiver while reviewing the extent of community input in this area. Stakeholder concerns about the Global Waiver and its development are discussed as well. It begins, however, with a brief overview of Rhode Island's political and administrative environment.

SETTING THE STAGE FOR REFORM

Rhode Island politics has been dominated by the Democratic Party since the early 1930s, with, for example, the Democratic Party's presidential ticket winning all of the state's electoral votes since 1988, and the state's Congressional delegation consisting entirely of Democrats since 2007, including Senators Jack Reed (1997–present) and Sheldon Whitehouse (2007–present) and Congressmen James Langevin (2001–present), Patrick Kennedy (1995–2010), and David Cicilline (2011–present). Moreover, few Republicans have been elected to the Rhode Island General Assembly. During the 2009–2010 biennium, for example, Rhode Island's 38 State Senate seats were held by 33 Democrats, 4 Republicans, and 1 independent, and Rhode Island's 75 State House of Representatives seats were held by 69 Democrats and 6 Republicans. Similarly, during the 2011–2012 biennium, Rhode Island's 38 State Senate seats were held by 29 Democrats, 8 Republicans, and 1 independent, and Rhode Island's 75 House of Representatives seats were held by 65 Democrats, 9 Republicans, and 1 former Republican who switched to the Libertarian party during the middle of the term.

The state, however, has elected moderate Republicans to Congress, including the father and son duo of John Chafee (1977–1999) and Lincoln Chafee (1999–2006), the latter being appointed to the Senate after his father's death in 1999 before winning election in his own right in 2000. The state has also experienced divided government in all but four years since 1985. Thus, outside of Democrat Governor Bruce Sundlun (1991–1994), Republicans have dominated the governor's office, including Edward DiPete (1985–1990), Lincoln Almond (1995–2002), and Donald Carcieri (2003–2010). The present governor is Republican turned Independent Lincoln Chafee, who recently announced plans to switch parties and run for reelection as a Democrat (2011–present). "The governor [who championed the Global Waiver], Donald Carcieri," explained Kevin P. Donnelly (January 1, 2009), "is widely considered to be a conservative Republican, indicating that . . . despite its Democrat leanings Rhode Island is not a one-party state. The imbalance in the legislative branch sets the stage for strong ideological differences with the governor, creating a hostile environment that nearly guarantees a legislative impasse whenever issues concerning the size and scope of government are being considered." The scene was therefore set for a contentious debate over the future of Medicaid, including the Global Consumer Choice Compact Waiver.

Rhode Island's Medicaid program has traditionally been administered with minimal coordination across multiple state agencies. In 2006, the General Assembly included a provision in the state's FY 2007 budget approving a December 2005 executive order by then Republican Governor Donald Carcieri establishing the state's Executive Office of Health and Human Services within which Rhode Island's Medicaid program is now housed. The 2006 legislation consolidated all five health and human service departments within the secretariat, including the Department of Human Services (designated the single state Medicaid agency); the Department of Health; the Department of Children, Youth and Families; the Department of Elderly Affairs; and the Department of Behavioral Healthcare, Developmental Disabilities, and Hospitals, then known as the Department of Mental Health, Retardation, and Hospitals. Medicaid spending was divided across these departments, with the vast majority of expenditures in state FY 2010 being managed by the Departments of Human Services (75%) and Behavioral Healthcare, Developmental Disabilities, and Hospitals (22%) (EOHHS June 2011). Beginning July 1, 2011, single state Medicaid agency designation was transferred from the Department of Human Services to EOHHS, while the Department of Elderly Affairs has been incorporated into the Department of Human Services as the Division of Elderly Affairs.

The FY 2007 budget legislation creating EOHHS also authorized the Governor to "conduct a study of the Medicaid programs administered by the state to review and analyze the options available for reducing or stabilizing the level of uninsured Rhode Islanders and containing Medicaid spending" (EOHHS October 2007). The resulting report entitled *The Future of Medicaid* contained recommendations on how to better coordinate Medicaid's financing and administration, make the program more consumer-centered, and contain costs (EOHHS October 2007). Another significant focus of the report was rebalancing and improving the long-term care system.

Building on earlier calls for reform, Governor Carcieri made a January 2008 announcement during his annual State of the State address that he planned to pursue a Global Waiver from traditional Medicaid program rules, claiming $67 million in potential first-year budgetary savings, an intended submission date of July 11, 2009, and an intended start date of October 1, 2008 (Peoples May 23, 2008). A month later, the Governor included the "The Medicaid Reform Act of 2008," or Budget Article 17, in his FY 2008 budget proposal. The stated intent of Article 17, which was approved on June 26, 2008, by the General Assembly as part of the state budget, was to ensure that "Medicaid shall be a sustainable, cost-effective, person-centered and opportunity-driven program," by authorizing the Department of Human Services/EOHHS to pursue "any necessary waiver(s) and/or state plan amendments" from the federal government with which to achieve this goal.

STATE MOTIVATION

Waiver Driven Largely by State Budgetary Pressures

Almost all states have seen budget shortfalls since 2000, most for several years in a row. An economic recession in the first half of the decade had created combined state budget deficits of $240 billion between 2002 and 2005 (Oliff, Mai, and Palacios June 27, 2012). This had also been true of the most recent downturn where shortfalls were much higher than those of the last recession, with nationwide deficits totaling $538 billion between 2009 and 2012. Trends seen at the national level played out in full force in Rhode Island. The early 2000s saw comparatively high Medicaid expenditure growth in the state—an average of 11.6% per year—higher than the national average of 9.4% (Carceri February 5, 2007; EOHHS October

2007). Cost control measures were instituted at that time to curb enrollment, contain costs, and improve efficiency. These included reductions in provider payments, cuts in program benefits and eligibility, and institution of co-payments for certain beneficiary groups. Despite such measures, Medicaid's contribution to the state's budget crisis was expected to intensify. Already, Medicaid made up 26% of total spending even before the recent recession hit; estimates forecasted as much as fifty cents or more of every general revenue dollar being directed toward the program by 2011 (EOHHS October 2007). Moreover, the state projected a budget shortfall of $425 million in state FY 2009 (Peoples and Needham June 19, 2008). Without reform, the Governor and EOHHS asserted, Medicaid spending would prove unsustainable, necessitating drastic reductions such as the removal of tens of thousands of beneficiaries from the program's rolls (Donnelly January 1, 2009; EOHHS October 2007, August 7, 2008; Peoples May 23, 2008).

Although there was recognition that the Global Waiver was motivated, in part, by a desire for programmatic improvement, particularly in the area of long-term care rebalancing, most interviewees believed it was mainly a response to ongoing fiscal and programmatic pressures to reduce Medicaid expenditures, particularly during a worsening economy and increasingly adverse state budgetary climate. Thus, according to interviewees, the Waiver was "mostly cost-driven," "absolutely and positively, no question, budget driven," an attempt to "ratchet down [the state's] investment," a way of "reducing costs," "weighted more toward the cost side rather than the care improvement side," a strategy to "generate a lot of savings," was "more of a budget exercise," and "a way to reconfigure the program . . . to decrease real costs," "to show . . . that [state officials] were doing something to reign-in costs," and to make the program "cheaper for the state."

Several interviewees reported that Governor Carcieri had sought to restrain Medicaid program spending since the very beginning of his administration, believing the program, as the largest component of the state budget, to be too expensive and inefficient and a drain on state resources. Prior policy initiatives in this vein contributed to distrust on the part of providers and consumers (Donnelly January 1, 2012). "Because of the cuts that the Governor had proposed to Medicaid over the years," explained one consumer advocate, "people didn't believe that this was really coming from a good place of wanting people to get what they needed. . . . Advocates felt like it had to be coming from a cost perspective, so there was sort of this initial feeling of, 'I don't believe you.'" That the Governor proposed the Global Waiver in the midst of the state's worst budget crisis in decades only served to reinforce such concerns.

Consistent with other reports, state officials admitted that the intention to restrain Medicaid spending had been around for many years, particularly since the rate of growth in program expenditures had routinely outpaced the rate of growth in state revenues, a dynamic exacerbated by the rising unemployment rate, which increased the demand for Medicaid while causing state revenues to plummet. In a November 11, 2008, *Providence Journal* article, for example, then Department of Human Services Director Gary Alexander noted that "we all understand the problems with the budget. That's why we're trying to redesign the program" (Davis November 11, 2008). In a December 19, 2008, press release touting agreement with the federal government on the Waiver's provisions, Governor Carcieri observed that "Medicaid spending has increased drastically and the current funding structure is forcing states to cut other critical programs. . . . This agreement will put us on a sustainable path for growth in Medicaid, while also maintaining services for those most in need" (Office of the Governor December 19, 2008). "Like most states," recalled one of the state officials interviewed, "the economy . . . has not been flourishing and revenues were growing at 2 to 3 percent, while we were seeing Medicaid expenditures grow at 7 or 8 percent. . . . There was this notion that we could not afford business as usual."

Traditionally, state officials would reduce benefits, restrict eligibility, and/or tighten provider payments to achieve their cost containment goals. The depth of the prevailing fiscal crisis, however, limited the perceived effectiveness of these approaches in reaching the state's desired budget targets. Furthermore, there was some trepidation associated with cutting thousands of beneficiaries off the state's Medicaid rolls. The Global Waiver and its focus on granting the state the additional administrative flexibility necessary to undertake broader system restructuring proved to be the alternative pathway chosen in the context of the state's rapidly deteriorating fiscal environment. "[The Governor] wanted to know how we could save money on the Medicaid program," reported one provider representative. "And he had his people there in Medicaid . . . who kept telling him, 'Look, our hands are tied. Our hands are tied. Our hands are tied.' 'Well, what would it take to untie our hands?' 'Well, see, if we had a waiver that would let us manage this program, and free us from a lot of these ridiculous things . . . We could probably do it cheaper.' 'Go for it.' "

Waiver Driven in Part by Programmatic Concerns Affecting Patient Care and Costs

The 2007 EOHHS study, *The Future of Medicaid,* identified both positive and negative aspects of Rhode Island's Medicaid program (EOHHS October 2007). On the positive side, Rhode Island ranked well in overall access and quality of programs for children, families, and pregnant women, especially through RIte Care, its managed care program for this population that began enrollment as a Section 1115 waiver during August 1994. On the negative side, Rhode Island had low provider reimbursement rates, high program costs, and slow or inadequate reform in long-term care, particularly in providing services in the least restrictive settings possible. Thus, in addition to cost containment, state officials concluded that Medicaid reform needed to target program improvement, namely ensuring that beneficiaries were "provided the right level and kind of services in the most appropriate setting" (EOHHS October 2007). This dual perspective on reform is reflected in the view of one state official who reported that the state sought greater administrative flexibility under the Global Waiver because existing regulatory burdens led to "decisions that were both costly and not necessarily the best for patients, so having some flexibility would hopefully either deliver both or one: better patient care or better costs." It is also reflected in the underlying principles of reform laid out in the state's Waiver application: consumer empowerment and choice; personal responsibility; community-based care solutions; prevention, wellness, and independence; competition; pay-for-performance; and improved technology (EOHHS August 7, 2008). These, in turn, inform the Waiver's basic provisions which include: 1) "rebalancing the state's long-term care system"; 2) "integrating care across all Medicaid populations"; and 3) "completing the transition from a payer to purchaser for all Medicaid populations" (EOHHS August 7, 2008).

Long-term Care Rebalancing

Due to a lack of investment in the home- and community-based sector in states such as Rhode Island, a large proportion of prevailing need goes unmet, including one in five community-dwelling adults with limitations in activities of daily living, according to one estimate (Komisar, Feder, and Kasper 2005). Moreover, up to 19.0% of long-stay nursing home residents and 24.9% of new admissions in Rhode Island can be categorized as low care, as compared to 11.8% and 13.5% nationally, suggesting that a particularly large proportion of nursing home residents in Rhode Island could be transferred back to the community, or prevented from going into a nursing home in the first place, if sufficient services and supports were made available (Mor et al. 2007).

Widespread support exists for rebalancing long-term care away from institutions toward home- and community-based settings, not just in especially unbalanced states such as Rhode Island but nationally (Grabowski et al. 2010; Miller, Mor, and Clark, 2010). Nursing home care is a mandatory service that all states must provide under Medicaid. States also have three main home- and community-based service benefits that they can provide: mandatory home health services, optional personal care services, and optional home- and community-based waiver services provided under Section 1915(c) of the Social Security Act (Eiken et al. October 31, 2011; Harrington et al. 2012; Howard, Ng, and Harrington December 2011; Ng and Harrington October 2011; Ng et al. December 2012).[3] The program's home health care benefit encompasses nursing and home health aide services and medical supplies, equipment, and appliances. If a state chooses, it may cover physical and occupational therapy, speech pathology, and audiology services as well. Home health services must be offered to all clinically eligible Medicaid recipients on a statewide basis. Personal care services, by contrast, is an optional service offered by 34 states. It provides assistance with both basic activities of daily living (e.g., bathing, dressing, toileting) and instrumental activities of daily living (e.g., meal preparation, medication administration). Like home health, states choosing to offer this service must do so statewide to all clinically eligible Medicaid recipients.

The program's 1915(c) home- and community-based waiver service benefit may also pay for home health and personal care, in addition to case management, homemaker services, adult day care, habilitation, respite care, and other service options. It occasionally pays for services provided in assisted-living facilities as well, though not room and board. Unlike home health and personal care, states may restrict participation in its 1915(c) waiver programs to selected populations of Medicaid recipients and particular localities and regions. They may also limit the number of participants served and choose to offer services not typically covered by the Medicaid program. In order to participate, prospective waiver participants must be deemed nursing facility eligible. The total costs of each waiver program must not be more than what the federal government would have otherwise paid for institutional care. In 2009, approximately two-thirds (62.9%) of Medicaid home- and community-based spending derived from 1915(c) waiver services, about a quarter (24.6%) from the personal care option, and only 8.7% from the mandatory home health care benefit (Eiken et al. October 31, 2011).

Driven, in part, by the disproportionately high level of spending on nursing homes and the 1999 U.S. Supreme Court decision in *Olmstead v. L.C.*, Rhode Island had long sought to rebalance long-term care spending from institutional to noninstitutional settings (Donnelly January 1, 2009). In 2002, a joint resolution by the Rhode Island House and Senate called for a "multi-year approach to regulatory and financial reform" in long-term care. A subsequent 2005 resolution called for a study to examine the need and financing options for a variety of community-based long-term care services. Together, these resolutions led to the passage of the Long-Term Care Service and Finance Reform Act of 2006, more widely known as the Perry-Sullivan legislation in honor of its two primary sponsors, Democratic State Senator Rhoda Perry and then Democratic State Representative Raymond Sullivan. Perry-Sullivan established a mandate to rebalance Medicaid long-term care, prevent inappropriate institutionalization, and reinvest savings from reduced nursing home use into home- and community-based care. It also directed the state to pursue any necessary waivers or state plan amendments needed to achieve a 50–50 spending split between Medicaid institutional and home- and community-based services, and to establish a single budget for long-term care whereby savings resulting from reduced institutional service use would be reinvested in home- and community-based care. In addition, Rhode Island applied for and received a Federal Real Choices System Change Grant in 2002 to help rebalance long-term care. This was followed by receipt of a five-year Real Choices System Change Transformation Grant in 2006. It was subsequently decided that strategic planning effort required under Real Choices would be combined with that required under Perry-Sullivan given that both initiatives sought to promote the state's rebalancing efforts (Senior Agenda Coalition February 2007).

In light of this history, a genuine desire to bolster state efforts to rebalance long-term care away from institutions and toward home- and community-based services was foremost among the Global Waiver's goals. This desire is part of a broader national trend to save money by meeting people's needs in the least costly settings possible. Government officials recognized the desirability of aligning Medicaid long-term care with consumer preferences for noninstitutional options to nursing home placement (EOHHS October 2007, August 7, 2008), with, for example, 84% of people 50 or older desiring to "age in place" and 87% of disabled individuals preferring to live at home (Gibson April 2003; Kochera, Straight, and Guterbock May 2005). They also recognized that on a per-unit basis, home- and community-based care is significantly less expensive to provide than institutional care. The national average cost for a semi-private nursing home room in 2008 was $191 per day, compared with the $64 per day for adult day care and about $72 per day ($18/hour*4 hours) for home health aide or homemaker services (MetLife Mature Market Institute October 2009). In 2012, the costs of nursing home care averaged $81,030 a year for a semiprivate room and $90,520 for a private room versus $42,600 annually, on average, for assisted living, $18,200 for five days of adult day services, and $29,120 to $30,576 for four hours of homemaker, companion, and/or home health services, seven days per week (MetLife Mature Market Institute November 2012). Shifting the locus of service provision to favor more home- and community-based services thus represents a potential source of savings for the federal and state governments, as well as taxpayers.

Moreover, over the long term, Rhode Island, like other states, faces growing budgetary pressures due to the aging of the baby boom generation. It is estimated that by 2025 there will be 224,507 Rhode Islanders aged 65 years or older, up from 150,891 in 2005 (Proximity 2012). This will increase the demand for high quality, cost effective services, particularly since the aged and disabled, though only 24% of beneficiaries, account for 66% of program expenditures, with spending on providers that deliver long-term care constituting nearly 55% of program spending (EOHHS October 2007). Thus, restructuring Medicaid long-term care will be critical in the coming years, and the Global Waiver was seen as one method to create much needed change in this area. According to then Department of Human Services Director Gary Alexander, "rebalancing will give beneficiaries the care they prefer while saving the tax payers millions" (Office of the Governor December 19, 2008).

Consistent with this discussion, state officials hoped to achieve both cost savings and a more consumer-responsive long-term care system by keeping care recipients out of nursing homes and other institutions. Thus, according to one legislative staffer, the Global Waiver was sought "because of the large share of the costs . . . and the large share of people [in nursing homes and because] nobody was completely satisfied with that part of the delivery [system]." "Clearly we need to save money," confirmed a state official, "because . . . nursing home care is one of the big cost drivers in Medicaid. . . . So there's a reality to need to do that but as a benefit of that reality we were able to look at innovative ways to use home and community care services, which is really a good thing."

Several interviewees highlighted the lack of progress made toward rebalancing despite Perry-Sullivan and other ongoing initiatives in this area, including the state's Real Choices grants. "On the long-term care side," explained one state official, "the state was really quite far behind, despite whatever efforts had been put in over the years. . . . It was another one of those things which I term all talk and no action. . . . A lot of work, a lot of talk, a lot of planning, but not a lot of doing." Thus, in announcing the intent to pursue the Global Waiver in his January 2008 annual State of the State address, Governor Carcieri argued that older people should have a choice of where to receive long-term care services and that they should not have to go into a nursing home if they do not want to. State officials also felt that having the authority to provide a limited package of services to otherwise non-Medicaid eligible individuals early on in the trajectory of their disability through the Waiver's Costs Not Otherwise Matchable, or CNOM, programs would contribute to better care management within the community, thereby reducing the eventual likelihood of full Medicaid eligibility and long-term institutional placement. If successful, this, of course, would have the added benefit of saving money, certainly for the state but possibly the federal government as well. Each time someone is kept at or moved down to a lower level of care, average per member per month costs declines.

Care Coordination and "Smart" Purchasing

Several other programmatic goals were noted in addition to long-term care rebalancing. State officials expressed a desire to extend the efficiencies and benefits of care coordination beyond RIte Care's children and families to other populations. It was felt that greater care management could help control costs and improve quality of care for high-cost aged and disabled individuals (EOHHS October 2007, August 7, 2008). It was also felt that care management enrollment would ensure that aged and disabled beneficiaries received services in the most appropriate settings possible, especially since they have been excluded from care management initiatives in the past.

State officials expressed a desire to implement alternative purchasing strategies to better enable the state to "get the best price on the value," including "reimburse[ing] providers based on quality rather than just [on the] units of service that they perform." Indeed, the 2007 *Future of Medicaid* report concluded that Rhode Island could benefit from updating its provider payment methodologies (EOHHS October 2007). It was felt that further reductions in provider reimbursement were unlikely to generate significant additional savings given the state's already low reimbursement rates. What could be done, however, according to state officials, was the creation of "smarter" payment methodologies and purchasing mechanisms that better ensured value for money (EOHHS October 2007, August 7, 2008). It was believed that both care management and "smart" purchasing would serve the overall Waiver goal of controlling costs while incentivizing the provision of more appropriate and cost-effective care.

Coordination Across State Agencies and Stakeholders

Prior to the creation of EOHHS, there was little to no policy connection between the state's five health and human services departments, resulting in, for example, conflicting budget requests over which the Department of Human Services, as the single state Medicaid agency, may or may not have been aware or have any sort of oversight over. Indeed, a "fiscal fitness" audit conducted in 2003–2004 found Medicaid's programmatic and operational responsibilities were highly fragmented and prone to inefficiency in both organization and financing (Carcieri February 5, 2004). The purpose of the subsequent consolidation, therefore, was to facilitate cooperation across the five departments that administer the state's health and human services programs, including streamlining administration, in part, by centralizing common functions such as finance, human resources, and legal services. Still, responsibility for administering Medicaid-funded services continued to be distributed across the separate departments, each with its own priorities, constituencies, policies and staff, and director who reports independently to the Governor rather than to the state's EOHHS Secretary.

Through the Global Waiver, state officials wished to improve coordination even further (EOHHS August 7, 2008; Alexander January 28, 2011). Although the state had a Medicaid agency, the program was "spread out amongst five agencies with five separate directors," according to one state official, "[each of whom] is a king in his or her own kingdom. My funding is my funding. My population is my population. . . . The program was not coordinated. . . . Funds were not evenly distributed. Care packages were not carefully planned. . . . [The goal was] to come up with a plan that would address those administrative problems but more importantly, serve the beneficiary in a better way." By reducing the number of silos under which the Medicaid program operated, the intention was for beneficiaries to receive services based on their level of function, not label, with their needs being met more seamlessly, though in different ways at different times in their disability or aging.

It was also expected that the Global Waiver would reduce competition among advocacy organizations representing different beneficiary populations. "We've always had a silo between the long-term care system, and children and families," explained one state official, "and one of the results is that the different advocacy organizations were always fighting against each other, and there was always the sense that one population was being more favorably treated than the other, so we really wanted to address that, and think about the Medicaid program as an overall approach that the state is taking to provide needed health care services and support services for eligible populations."

State officials also hoped to improve coordination and efficiency by consolidating the state's existing waivers program into a single Global Waiver (EOHHS August 7, 2008; Alexander January 28, 2011). Having multiple 1915(c) waivers, for example, can be confusing, both for providers and for consumers. "We have three different waivers associated with assisted living," reported one legislative staffer, "all paying different amounts of money or with different eligibility criteria. Something we've been asking like for years, can we consolidate those?. . . . It's confusing. You can't even imagine how people negotiate the system." Having multiple waivers can also lead to fragmentation within the state bureaucracy. "If everybody's pots of money are kept separate," explained one provider representative, "we're always just going to keep passing the buck to the other system, and that's what happens now between this waiver and that waiver, and Medicaid versus waiver money, and [the Department of Human Services versus the Department of Mental Health, Retardation, and Hospitals]. If everybody's pot of money [is] separate, then you're not going to see true rebalancing." Having multiple waivers can also lead to additional administration burdens for the state while complicating its relationship with the federal government. "The more waivers you have," explained one state official, "the more coordination you need to do with CMS. . . . [Each waiver had] different timeframes, different approval and re-approval times, and we had to collect admin costs associated with each, so from an administrative process, it was much easier [operating on the state plan and the single Global Waiver]."

Despite the potential benefits of consolidation, a number of provider representatives and consumer advocates felt that the state could have accomplished its goals either through existing processes and initiatives such as Perry-Sullivan, Real Choices, the states Aging and Disability Resource Center, and/or through more limited changes to the Medicaid program framework (Bryant August 5, 2008; The Poverty Institute August 15, 2008; Coffey January 2009; Solomon January 2009; Reed et al. August 5, 2009; Freyer April 11, 2011). One consultant, for example, believed that state officials "could have actually done 90 percent" of what they sought to achieve through the state's "existing waivers and state plan amendment." A state official believed that the state "could have rebalanced the long-term care system without the Global Waiver." Indeed, it was estimated at the time the Waiver was first submitted that the state could have obtained $22 million in savings from rebalancing long-term care under its existing waiver authorities simply by implementing activities that it planned to undertake already (The Poverty Institute August 15, 2008). Alternative strategies suggested ranged from relying on or modifying the state's existing 1915(c) waiver authorities, or adopting a separate 1115 waiver targeted specifically at long-term care, thereby keeping the state's RIte Care waiver separate and intact. "We . . . noted at the time," reported one consumer advocate, "that rebalancing long-term care could be done without this comprehensive Global Waiver that had a lot of unknowns to it; for example, it could possibly be done by a separate 1115 waiver or some changes to the 1915(c) waiver process."

That the Global Waiver may not have been necessary for rebalancing is reflected in the continuing use of 1915(c)-related terminology in policy and budget making discussions. "It's still a little bit murky," as one consumer advocate explained, "because even though they've consolidated all of the home and community care waivers, or almost all of them, they still talk, for example, about the [developmental disability]," assisted living, and home care waivers. That the Global Waiver has indeed helped to promote progress on rebalancing is reflected in the numerous activities that have been undertaken in this area after years of stagnation. "The good thing about having a bigger long-term care waiver is it pushes the conversation," explained one executive branch official. "The people who have been having this conversation for 20 years all of a sudden have an actual way to make it work and a financial incentive to make it work, which they'd never had before." "While rebalancing long-term care has been on the table for years and years," explained a consumer advocate, "it wasn't really moving forward and quickly. . . . Since that was sort of the cornerstone of the Waiver, it has really put the department on the hook to move that forward. So, I see that as another value of the Waiver, even though it could have happened without the Waiver." Said Steven Costantino, current EOHHS Secretary and former Democratic House Finance Committee Chair, the Global Waiver "changed the mindset . . . creating a strong impetus to move forward toward rebalancing the long-term care system" (Freyer April 11, 2011).

Uncertain Implications of the Global Waiver for Certain Populations

Uncertainty associated with the Global Waiver stemmed, in part, from the fact that no state had ever operated its Medicaid program in this way. Consequently, it was unclear why state officials needed to place the state's entire Medicaid program under the Global Waiver if the primary goal was to rebalance long-term care for elderly people. Indeed, the added value of the Global Waiver was particularly difficult to discern for certain populations. It was widely acknowledged, for example, that the system for caring for developmentally disabled people was working well, with most of that population already being served in the community under the state's Intermediate Care Facilities for the Mentally Retarded (ICF-MR) waiver. Thus, "it's been a little bit frustrating from the [Developmental Disability] perspective," reported one provider representative, "to be kind of grouped into this rebalancing initiative, when in fact, we do provide community-based services and have for years." The same was true for the state's mental health system. The Department of Human Services/EOHHS said " 'we're going to go to more community-based care,' " reported one consumer representative. "The community mental health system's been about the community-based care since the beginning and we're like, 'how are you going to get another couple million out of us doing that?' " It was also largely true for the state's system for caring for people with physical disabilities where, according to one consumer advocate, "most of [the state's] Medicaid services have been community based. . . . We really don't have large institutions here, so in some respects Rhode Island is a little ahead of the curve . . . in terms of the kinds of supports it provides to people with disabilities."

The implication of the Global Waiver for the state's RIte Care population was especially worrisome for providers and advocates (Donnelly January 1, 2009; Peoples May 23, 2008; Byrant August 5, 2008; The Poverty Institute August 15, 2008). Prior to implementation, Rhode Island was already reducing RIte Care eligibility. As of June 1, 2008, for example, 2,800 children who had been U.S. residents for less than five years, 225 self-employed family child-care providers and their children, and 600 adults participating in the Starting Right Health Care Insurance Assistance Program for Child Care Providers were dropped or disenrolled from the Medicaid program (Department of Human Services January 2010–February 2012). "My biggest concern," reported one knowledgeable observer, "is that you end up with population warfare rather than system reform, because if in fact you're not successful in long-term care . . . which is where a huge proportion of the dollars are . . . it can actually come back to impact areas that may have been very successful in reform like RIte care."

Interviewees feared that state officials would use its additional freedom under the Global Waiver to redesign benefit packages to eliminate optional services for certain groups or to tighten eligibility and expand cost-sharing for expansion populations such as children and families under RIte Care. A particular concern was the Waiver's proposed increase in cost sharing up to the maximum levels allowed by law (The Poverty Institute August 15, 2008). Advocates in Rhode Island were particularly sensitive to this issue as a prior increase in the state's RIte Care premiums for individuals above 150% of FPL to 3 to 4% of income (depending on income) led nearly one in five families to disenroll from the program (Artiga and O'Malley May 2005). Under the Global Waiver, it was proposed that these premiums be raised even further, and instated for previously excluded populations (i.e., those with incomes between 133% and 150% of the FPL).

Waiver Politically and Ideologically Motivated

In light of perceived challenges, Rhode Island would have been unlikely to propose its plan for Medicaid restructuring in the absence of federal encouragement. On January 31, 2003, the Bush administration unveiled a proposal through which states could volunteer to block grant Medicaid (Lambrew 2005; Holahan and Weil May 27, 2003; Guyer May 2003; Thompson 2012). Under this proposal, states that chose to participate would no longer have to apply for waivers to modify federal standards for Medicaid design. While participating states would still be required to provide comprehensive benefits for low-income beneficiaries whose coverage is federally mandated, they would have significantly more flexibility to change service delivery, eligibility, and benefits for optional beneficiaries without going through the labor-intensive waiver process each time. Instead of receiving matching funds based on actual needs and costs, state would have received a fixed amount of money per year from the federal government, with responsibility for expenditures beyond this cap falling solely on the states. Under this proposal, spending levels in FY 2002 would have been used as the base from which federal allotments would be determined. These would have then been increased by 8.5% per year, the average Medicaid growth rate at the time. As an incentive for states to participate, federal contributions would have increased by an additional 2% in 2004 to fund new programs and an additional 1% between 2004 and 2010 but subsequently reduced for three years so that the total amount would have been budget neutral to the federal government over 10 years. States, however, would have been obligated to show maintenance of effort, requiring them to devote, at a minimum, an amount equal to their FY 2002 spending, increased each year by the medical inflation portion of the Consumer Price Index (CPI).

Not able to convince Congress to give them the authority to block grant the program, however, the Bush administration sought to demonstrate the effectiveness of the general approach by recruiting states willing to place an overall cap on federal contributions. This is consistent with the view articulated by Thompson and Burke (2007) that during this period, "CMS acted more as a teacher of the states than as a student of them. The Bush administration held strong views on how to improve Medicaid. . . . The administration invited states to submit waivers targeted toward these ends less because it thought it could learn from the demonstrations than because it wanted states to adopt its approach. 'Try it, you'll like it' might as well have been the motto." The only states that considered the administration's proposal were states with Republican governors, including Connecticut, California, Colorado, New Hampshire, and Florida (Anonymous February 4, 2003; Gold August 2004). Ultimately, the governors in these states either chose not to pursue this policy, or were blocked in doing so by Democratic-controlled state legislatures. Thus, Rhode Island proved to be the only volunteer, though Vermont had previously received two such 1115 waivers with separate caps for acute and long-term care.[4]

Because of its small size, state officials believed that Rhode Island was in an excellent position to test Medicaid reform models, which could then be transferred to other states (EOHHS August 7, 2008). "One of the things we really wanted . . . was . . . to test the financial model," reported one state official. You pick up a newspaper in this country once a week and you find out some state is talking about [how] it can't sustain Medicaid. We actually wanted to say, 'Well, try us. Rhode Island is a small state; we've got some good budget projections. Give us a bag of money; give us the rules you want us to run by, and let us see what we can do.'" Like other states, however, the political alignment of the state's Republican governor and Bush administration proved to be the key reason why the state first considered and then opted to pursue the Global Waiver. Thus, explained one provider representative, "this governor being the Republican that he is wanted to do something that was more along the lines of good Republican politics." Indeed, respondents felt that the Waiver was ideologically motivated, spurred on by federal and state Republican administrations focused more on restraining spending and delegating further responsibilities to the states than on improving beneficiary access and quality. Recalled another provider representative: "There were conversations with CMS in the waning days of the Bush administration. . . . There appeared to be a fair amount of interest . . . both on the part of the Bush administration, as well as the local administration in attaining a waiver that had a cap on expenditures. That turned out . . . to be a driving force in getting that approved."

The delayed Waiver application—it was not submitted until August 8, 2008, although it was first proposed in January of that year—made it uncertain whether it would be approved before the coming change in federal administration. It also made it clear that an October 1, 2008, start date, as originally proposed, would not be met. Still, lacking confidence that the Waiver would be approved by the next administration, subsequent negotiations between the state and federal governments were ultimately accelerated so approval would take place before President Bush left office, with, in fact, the state receiving final approval January 16, 2009, just days before Democratic President Barack Obama was inaugurated. Indeed, in early December, Gary Alexander, then Director of the Department of Human Services, was quoted as saying that the "Bush Administration has a number of waivers that they want to take care of before they leave and this is one of them" (Davis November 11, 2008). This accelerated process received considerable criticism, particularly given expectations of federal financial relief in light of the rapidly deteriorating fiscal situation. In view of the cratering economy, there was little reason to rush the federal review process except that approval of the Global Waiver would have been less likely under the new administration (Solomon January 2009).

WAIVER DESIGN

Developed by a Few High-Level State Officials and Consultants

Development of the Global Waiver was dominated by senior government officials within the state's Department of Human Services, including its then

Director, Gary Alexander, who was relieved of day-to-day duties at the Department to focus on the state's Waiver negotiations with the federal government and was subsequently appointed as EOHHS Secretary. Also playing a significant role was Acting State Medicaid Director Frank Spinelli, who was formerly in charge of services for elders and people with disabilities within Department of Human Services. Although Spinelli retired during the fall of 2008, he continued to work voluntarily on the Global Waiver as the state negotiated terms with the federal government. Soon thereafter, he was hired by a consulting firm, ACS State Health Care, which also worked voluntarily as the state negotiated terms (Peoples March 3, 2009).

Through interagency meetings, state officials in other EOHHS departments informed the general conceptual outlines of the Waiver although most state officials interviewed agreed that it was high-level staff within the Department of Human Services who drafted the state's Waiver application and led subsequent negotiations with the federal government. In addition to ACS, there was heavy reliance on at least one additional outside consultancy—the Boston-based Lucas Group Partners, although their role was initially downplayed or denied to the chagrin of outside observers who were told that their services were voluntary but ultimately were not. Governor Carcieri initially insisted that the company had offered its services pro bono. It became clear over time that this assistance was not provided on a voluntary basis (Gregg January 9, 2009; Peoples March 3, 2009). Indeed, it was revealed that the Lucas Group was promised payment (and subsequently received) $370,000 for its services (Gregg June 13, 2009). Moreover, the company took credit for negotiating federal approval of the Global Waiver, thereby undermining the Carcieri administration's contention that Department of Human Services Director Alexander and his team of senior-level staffers were primarily responsible for this success (Rhode Island Government February 26, 2009; Gregg June 9, 2009).

The friendship between Director Alexander and John Stephen, a Lucas Group employee, former Commissioner of New Hampshire's Department of Health and Human Services, and subsequent unsuccessful Republican nominee for New Hampshire Governor in 2010, led Senate leaders to temporarily postpone Alexander's ultimately successful confirmation as the state's EOHHS Secretary (Gregg May 21, 2009, June 10, 2009). It also led Democratic Lieutenant Governor Elizabeth Roberts, Democratic Attorney General Patrick Lynch, and others to request a Senate inquiry into the administrations seemingly no bid $370,000 agreement with Lucas for which no state funds had been appropriated (Gregg June 16, 2009). It was reported that uncertainty about Lucas' role reinforced prevailing distrust regarding the administration's intentions, making general acceptance of the Global Waiver even more challenging than it may have been otherwise. "They were saying that [these consultants] were doing this voluntarily," explained one consumer advocate, "and then [it] became clear . . . that they were, in fact, paid. . . . It doesn't make any sense to say that a consulting firm is working for free; that's just not something that makes any sense; cognitive dissonance, like you're telling me that I just need to believe you? And so I don't believe you, but now I have to work with you, and you've lied to me on this, but you won't admit that you lied. It just created a very negative atmosphere."

Developed with Little to No Community Input

Lack of public input into the Waiver development process has been an ongoing concern among both elected officials and community stakeholders (Alker March 2012; Donnelly January 1, 2009; U.S. General Accountability Office 2007, 2012). Consistent with this concern, most stakeholders in Rhode Island reported few, if any opportunities for provider representatives, consumer advocates, and the general public to comment on and influence the Waiver's design and direction (Reichard September 15, 2008; Reed and Whitehouse September 23, 2008; Katz November 4, 2008; Trapp November 17, 2008), thereby helping to sow the seeds of distrust between the administration and other parties. "[Because] the stakeholder community, in general, had felt really sort of shut out of the drafting process," explained one provider representative, "and not included in the original design and discussions around how this might work . . . we [were] not confident that our constituents' best interests [were] being weighed in this process." Indeed, most felt that there wasn't any real attempt to reach out and have sustained conversations with communities of interest, either from the advocacy or provider perspective, even though some meetings with state officials did in fact take place. This is because while Department of Human Services/EOHHS held some public forums, met with certain provider associations and consumer groups, and made reports to the Lieutenant Governor's Long-Term Care Coordinating Council and the state's Real Choice Systems Change Grant team, such interactions were less about acquiring public input than about reporting what that state had done. "To my knowledge," reported a consumer advocate, "there were no meetings where [the Department of Human Services] or EOHHS sat with stakeholders and said, 'What would you like to see in the Waiver? What are your concerns about the Waiver?' It was all these public hearings where they presented and then people commented." Said a provider representative, "when they submitted the proposal to CMS . . . they listed all these community forums . . . [and] you'd see your name on the list and you'd think, 'Wow, that was considered a community forum' . . . [because] it was a lot of reporting at you; it wasn't necessarily opportunity for dialogue."

There was also limited opportunity for stakeholders to review the final Waiver application before it was submitted to the federal government. After several delays, the draft of the Waiver application was submitted to the state legislature on July 29, 2008, less than two weeks before its August 8 submission date to the federal government (Peoples July 21, 2008, July 30, 2008). When the General Assembly passed the FY 2009 state budget, it included a provision indicating its willingness to consider the state's Waiver application as long as it received the Waiver 10 days before it was sent to CMS. While this did provide state legislators and other interested parties an opportunity to review and provide feedback on the application, including at a joint House and Senate hearing held on August 5, it did not provide the Department of Human Services/EOHHS sufficient time to make modifications in light of the feedback received. One consumer advocate reported that "it sort of perpetuated the whole sort of 'public process' . . . where there wasn't a whole lot of opportunity for input. I don't think [the Department of Human Services] was viewing the public hearing up there as an opportunity to get ideas on how to make it better, certainly not from the community."

Some of the state personnel interviewed "would have preferred a more open kind of engagement," recognizing that "the lack of . . . active engagement . . . caused a lot of problems," including stakeholder resentment that the process was "basically being done behind closed doors." The need to develop the Waiver quickly in light of prevailing fiscal imperatives and the timing of the state's budget process were the primary reasons given for the lack of preliminary discussions and openness. That the approach taken in this instance contrasted so markedly with the much more collaborative approach that normally characterized the way the state did business with respect to RIte Care and other programs further contributed to stakeholder anxiety and distrust regarding Department of Human Services/EOHHS' intentions. Thus, "for somebody like me," explained one consumer advocate, "who had done years of work in partnership with the state, for this to kind of come out of nowhere, it was such a violation of trust. . . . I know a lot of people share that concern. 'Why weren't we consulted?. . . . This was kind of something literally dropped out of the sky on us.' "

Community Input More Prevalent in Some Areas

Although there was a general absence of community engagement, some interviewees felt that prior discussions around the state's Perry-Sullivan Legislation and Real Choices System Transformation Grants influenced important dimensions of the Waiver and the political dynamic surrounding it. That there had been at least some previous communication about certain aspects of the Waiver's is one reason why there may have been less concern about the Waiver from some provider/advocacy communities than others. "Groups concerned about long-term care for seniors," explained one consumer advocate, "may have had a different initial reaction than the children's groups and groups in mental health and developmental [disabilities] because of the fact that there had been ongoing stakeholder meetings with [the Department of Human Services] about how to achieve rebalancing." Several interviewees, for example, pointed to a series of meetings where a small work group developed the Waiver's provision for leveling long-term care applicants, possibly under the auspices of Real Choices. In addition to state staff, membership on that work group consisted of consumer advocates, nursing home industry representatives, and a director of nursing at a local Rhode Island nursing home. Participating in this work group helped to ameliorate at least one advocate's concerns because "I had confidence in that process that we used and in the people who were in that small group that we would do what we could do to—I'm going to use the word, [to] 'protect' consumers."

Limited Details During Development of the Global Waiver

A number of interviewees reported that for a long time all the Global Waiver seemed to consist of were a series of short PowerPoint presentations with uncontroversial generalities that no one could disagree with; for example, ensuring that beneficiaries receive "the right services at the right time in the right setting." Although advocates and policymakers had been rallying around such goals for years, there was little specificity about how the Global Waiver would, in fact, enable the state to get from point A to point B, say, with respect to making long-term care more home- and community-based. As one executive official explained, "this general statement of principles on slides was great, but there was literally no information when you drove down in terms of how that would be implemented, what the details were. And it often wasn't because they were holding back information . . . it simply was it was not yet designed. . . . They were designing the airplane as they were flying it." It was felt that even at well over 100 pages the final Waiver application lacked specifics—it proposed giving state officials the power to make changes but offered few details about the particular changes they intended to make (Peoples July 30, 2008).

The lack of specifics regarding the state's intentions made it difficult for outside observers to provide feedback on what was being proposed. "There were meetings scheduled by the Department around the state," recalled one consumer advocate. "[Attendees] felt like the state was certainly telling them that they were going to do stuff, but it didn't feel like people's ideas were being solicited, nor was it clear how you would provide input into the design, because you couldn't really figure out what the design was." More fundamentally, lack of information made it difficult to understand why the Global Waiver should be preferred over other potential strategies for achieving the same goals. "They presented it as there would be economy and efficiency of having all of the Medicaid programs in one bucket so to speak," recalled one citizen advocate, "but I don't think they ever clearly were able to document how those efficiencies and economies would take place."

State officials generally admitted that the Global Waiver lacked details because what they were proposing was an overall framework more than anything else; that in exchange for limiting the federal government's fiscal contributions, the state would receive greater administrative flexibility with which to achieve the general goals outlined in the Waiver application. Thus, explained one state official, "a lot of the reason why we were seeking the Waiver was for new authority and flexibility but we did not have established programs in mind, per se. We had this idea that, well, let's get authority first, develop it [later]." The result was there were few, if any, definitive answers to stakeholders' questions about what was going to happen once the federal government approved the state's Waiver application. Consequently, state officials could not inform stakeholders about the future of specific populations and programs because that had not been worked out yet. Indeed, when the Department of Human Services/EOHHS submitted the draft Waiver application to the state legislature, the *Providence Journal* quoted Adelita Orefice, then the Deputy EOHHS Secretary, as saying that "[you're] going to see some of the larger concepts in here about the direction and the values and that sort of thing, but not a whole lot of detail about programs specifically, in part because we want to be able to preserve that flexibility. . . . If we propose right now the details then we're going to be wedded to that. And if in a year that doesn't work, and that kind of program makes no sense, we're stuck" (Peoples July 30, 2008). The absence of specifics, however, only fed stakeholder suspicion that there were details being worked out behind closed doors without their consultation.

Absence of Specifics and Block Grant Structure Heightened Stakeholder Concern

The absence of specifics, combined with the proposed block grant structure of the proposed Global Waiver, contributed to considerable distrust and concern on the part of outside groups (Donnelly January 1, 2009; Peoples July 30, 2008; Alker August 5, 2008; Byrant August 5, 2008; Solomon September 4, 2008; Reed and Whitehouse September 23, 2008; Katz November 4, 2008; Davis December 1, 2008). What was clear was that the state could acquire additional flexibility to shape Medicaid, possibly under more limited state and federal funding authority than existed before. What was unclear was what the state would use that additional flexibility for an era of increasing fiscal scarcity. In the midst of the worst state budget crisis since the Great Depression, providers, consumers, and their representatives assumed that the Global Waiver would be used by the Governor to cut back on the state's commitment to the program and the vulnerable populations it serves, particularly since official pronouncements emphasized protecting mandatory populations and services but not optional benefits and eligibility groups to which most program funding has traditionally been devoted (Alker August 15, 2008; Bryant August 5, 2008; The Poverty Institute August 15, 2008; Beckwith September 15, 2008; Davis December 1, 2008). "There were lots of concerns that the state was getting some blanket waiver of federal laws," recalled one consumer advocate, "without them really having to be specific about what they would do. They were given flexibility to carve out different populations and offer them different benefit packages but we didn't know who those populations were, or what the benefit packages were, that kind of thing. "

As noted, concerns ranged from the future of RIte Care to the treatment of physically disabled adults and children. There was even concern about the state's intentions with respect to long-term care rebalancing, an area over which there seemed to be greater levels of agreement (Peoples May 23, 2008; Peoples July 21, 2008; The Poverty Institute August 15, 2008; Beckwith September 15, 2008; Katz November 4, 2008). Take the state's long-term care diversion strategy, for example. Previously, anyone deemed eligible for institutional placement was eligible for nursing home care or 1915(c) home- and community-based waiver services. Under a new three-level care system proposed by the Global Waiver, only those deemed "highest" would be entitled to coverage; those deemed "high" and "preventive" would only be eligible for home- and community-based care, funding permitting. What criteria would be used to allocate individuals across these three different groups? How many of those who would have been deemed eligible for nursing home care under the old standards would no longer be so? How extensive would the waitlists be for those given a "high" or "preventive" designation? To the chagrin of many providers and consumer advocates, answers to questions such these were not forthcoming.

Key stakeholders were especially fearful that the state might have underestimated the amount of funding needed and, as such, run out of federal block grant money during the second or third year of the five-year Waiver period, particularly given the state of the economy and likely increase in Medicaid rolls (Peoples July 21, 2008; Alker August 15, 2008; Lillis September 10, 2008; Reichard September 15, 2008; Katz November 4, 2008). This, in turn, would leave state officials with no choice but to fund the program entirely with state dollars or, more likely, to severely ratchet back its commitment to the populations served. "The idea was the state was saying to the feds," explained one consumer advocate, " 'you give us X amount of federal dollars over the course of five years, and which we could access at any time we want,' and we will agree to a maintenance of effort amount, where we'll put in a state amount [equal to] I think 23 percent of the budget. . . . That really locked Rhode Island into a capped amount of money, which potentially they could have used more up front, leaving us with nothing towards the end of the five years." This concern stemmed largely from doubts about the baseline figures and trend rates chosen to estimate the federal and state allocations requested.

SUMMARY

The Global Waiver was largely motivated by state fiscal pressures deriving from the rapidly deteriorating economy and disproportionate proportion of the state budget devoted to Medicaid. It was also motivated by specific programmatic goals, both with the aim of improving patient care and reducing program costs. Specific areas included long-term care rebalancing, care coordination, "smart purchasing," and interagency coordination. Uncertainty associated with the Global Waiver stemmed, in part, from the fact that no state had ever operated its Medicaid program in this way. It was also unclear why the state needed to pursue the Global Waiver in light of the disproportionate programmatic focus on rebalancing. Community stakeholders were particularly concerned about the uncertain implications of the Waiver for certain populations, including the developmentally disabled, mentally ill, and children and families served by RIte Care. In light of the proposed block grant structure, most believed that the Global Waiver would not have been pursued without the political and ideological alignment between Rhode Island's Republican governor and the Bush administration.

The Global Waiver was largely designed by high-level state officials and consultants. There was little to no opportunity for provider representatives, consumer advocates, and the general public to inform its development, though prior discussions about long-term care rebalancing influenced the final product. Few details were made available to community stakeholders during the Waiver development process. This was, in part, a conscious decision on the part of state officials who felt that what was being proposed was a general framework with which to achieve greater administrative flexibility with specific details to be worked out once the Waiver had been approved. The absence of specifics, however, made it difficult for outside observers to provide feedback on what was being proposed. It also exacerbated stakeholder distrust and concern about the Waiver and its implications for affected populations. There was fear that the state might run out of federal money before the five-year demonstration period expired, particularly given the state of the economy and likely increase in Medicaid rolls.

NOTES

1. The few states with more than 50% of Medicaid long-term care expenditures directed toward noninstitutional care for the aged and physically disabled include: New Mexico, Washington, Minnesota, Oregon, Alaska, and California.
2. The few states with more than 50% of Medicaid long-term care expenditures directed toward institutional care for the developmentally disabled include: Mississippi, Texas, Illinois, Louisiana, Texas, and Arkansas.
3. Other less-used Medicaid home- and community-based options include the Program for Inclusive Care for the Elderly (PACE), home- and community-based services authorized under Section 1115 or Section 1915(a) of the Social Security Act, self-directed personal assistance services provided under Section 1915(j) of the Social Security Act, and state plan authorized home- and community-based services under Section 1915(i) of the Social Security Act. Just 3.9% of total Medicaid home- and community-based spending derived from these options combined (Eiken et al. October 31, 2011).

4. Although Rhode Island's Global Waiver is modeled in many ways on Vermont's, there are some key differences (Guyer April 2006; Anonymous July 2006; Crowley and O'Malley 2008; Peoples October 5, 2008). One is that Vermont does not have a single waiver, but operates under two separate Medicaid 1115 waivers—one for acute care services and one for long-term care services, each with separate funding pools. Vermont's Choices for Care long-term care Waiver was approved June 2005 and since extended through September 2015; its Global Commitment to Health acute care Waiver was approved in October 2005 and since extended through December 2013. The basic principle underlying these waivers is similar to Rhode Island's: in exchange for a cap on federal contributions, Vermont received more flexibility to change its Medicaid program. But while both Rhode Island and Vermont continue to operate under Medicaid's traditional matching structure, the federal Government granted Vermont an especially generous funding cap because it was the first state to adopt this type of waiver. Furthermore, Vermont's original coverage levels were considerably more generous, and its population substantially smaller than Rhode Island's. Unlike Rhode Island, Vermont also had a well-developed home- and community-based services system in place and high rates of spending in this area prior to the Waiver, demonstrating commitment to rebalancing and ensuring the capacity of the system to meet resulting increases in demand. It is noteworthy, however, that Vermont pioneered the three-tier level of care system: in this case, "highest," "high," and "moderate," with the only difference from Rhode Island being that those in the middle tier in Vermont may receive either institutional or home- and community-based services, while those in the middle tier in Rhode Island may receive home- and community-based services only, subject to funding availability in both states. It is also noteworthy that very early iterations of Rhode Island's proposal, like Vermont's, consisted of two 1115 waivers.

3 The Politics of Approval

Once the final Global Waiver application was developed, it was sent to the Centers for Medicare and Medicaid Services for review and approval during the waning days of the George W. Bush administration. Unless approved before President Bush left office, state officials faced the prospect of gaining approval from the less sympathetic and less ideologically compatible administration of President-elect Barack Obama. State officials also had to seek approval from the Rhode Island General Assembly, which although skeptical of the Governor's intentions, could prove amenable to any proposal that helped close the state's ever widening budget deficit. This chapter examines how the federal approval process unfolded, including resulting changes in the way Rhode Island's Global Waiver was designed. It also examines the role of Rhode Island's General Assembly, both with respect to approving the Global Waiver and with respect to mechanisms through which the state legislature has overseen implementation and addressed stakeholder concerns about the level of community input.

THE FEDERAL APPROVAL PROCESS

Lack of Transparency in Federal Approval

Together, the lack of detail and transparency during the Waiver development process contributed to distrust on the part of key stakeholders who feared programmatic cutbacks that would, for example, adversely impact successful programs such as RIte Care while creating waitlists for long-term care. This distrust was further exacerbated by the opaqueness of the state's negotiations with the federal government (Baucus et al. June 19, 2008; Alker August 15, 2008; Dingell et al. August 21, 2008; Katz November 4, 2008). Thus, consistent with concerns routinely expressed about the federal approval process (Alker March 2012; U.S. General Accountability Office 2007, 2012), most community stakeholders in Rhode Island reported challenges acquiring information on the status of the state's negotiations with CMS. "I don't believe the advocates felt that they had access to the federal reviewers," recalled one consumer representative. "My recollection is that it was not a transparent process."

Letters written to CMS were one avenue through which key stakeholders expressed their concerns, though the extent to which such communications influenced the agency's deliberations is unclear. Stakeholders reported being particularly troubled by state claims of stakeholder input and consensus (Katz November 4, 2008). "One of the things that got the advocates really upset," reported one consumer representative, "was in the application they said . . . that there was full scale-agreement amongst all parties and they also made a list of all these public meetings that they had had and groups that they met with and so the way we say it here was there was no public hearings or other opportunities for formal organized input into the Waiver itself." Another thing that got advocates really upset was the lack of transparency in CMS' review of the Global Waiver. This is reflected in a letter that expressed frustration because outside stakeholders "have not been able to obtain information about the negotiations between CMS and the state" and urged CMS "to make public the status of the Waiver as well as any major changes that were being considered" and to afford the public "the opportunity to weigh in . . . on these changes, either through written comment or public hearing once it's been provided with advance written information about the revised Waiver submission."[1]

Congressional Delegation as a Conduit for Information

The state's Congressional delegation, including two Democratic Senators and two Democratic Congressmen, came out strongly against the Waiver and served as a potential conduit for stakeholder influence, though to no avail. Through monthly phone calls and other contacts, the state's two Senators and two Congressmen learned about stakeholder concerns. This communication, in turn, spurred letters to the Governor, CMS Director, and U.S. Department of Health and Human Services Secretary whereby members of the delegation and Chairmen of the pertinent House and Senate committees articulated the reservations of consumer advocates and other stakeholders with whom they consulted, including regarding the lack of transparency, opportunity for public comment, and block grant structure of the proposal (Baucus et al. June 19, 2008; Dingell et al. August 21, 2008; Reed and Whitehouse September 23, 2008). It also led the delegation to serve as kind of a clearinghouse for the limited amount of information available on the state's negotiations with the federal government.

"Clearly, there were people [in our congressional delegation]," recalled one state legislative staffer, "who were tracking it and getting information for us and letting us know what they were seeing, what they were hearing. That was one of the few ways that we could really get information." It was recognized that while the Congressional delegation was supportive of community of stakeholders, and took some positive actions in this regard, they could, in actuality, exert very little influence over the process. Thus, one provider representative reported that "we would tell [the Congressional delegation] what we understood were the risks associated with the Waiver. . . . I know [that they] tried to influence CMS and tried to exert some pressure on the process. And in the end it didn't really make a difference because they approved it."

Changes to the State's Waiver Application

Major changes to the state's Global Waiver application were negotiated during the course of the federal approval process. These included the imposition of a dramatically different financial arrangement than the state initially requested—a capped federal-match rather than block grant structure—and imposition of the Waiver's "Special Terms and Conditions" and three-tier system of federal oversight (Weens January 16, 2009). In short, the state agreed to a cap on combined federal and state spending of $12.075 billion over five years (Office of the Governor December 19, 2008). It was estimated that the state would save $358 million during this time period, including $22 million per year from federal dollars provided under the Waiver's Costs Not Otherwise Matchable, or CNOM, provision.

Several reasons were identified for why the state's block grant request was not approved. First, there were doubts about whether CMS had the authority to waive the federal matching structure. Many argued that statutory changes to the Medicaid program statute would need to take place first before the agency could grant requests such as this (Alker August 5, 2008; The Poverty Institute August 15, 2008; Dingell et al. August 21, 2008; Katz November 4, 2008). Thus, reported one state official, "the rationale [for not allowing the block grant] was that it . . . would have taken [federal] legislation to roll back the law. . . . And we [would] have fundamentally changed the nature of what's an entitlement program. . . . CMS said, 'That's not our issue to decide.'" At a minimum, there would have been legal challenges delaying approval of the Waiver until the onset of the Obama administration, which would not have been as positively disposed toward the state's intentions.

Second, CMS would not permit the state to acquire the rights to the federal portion of any savings that might accumulate during the period in which the Waiver would be in effect. "We went into that block grant discussion saying, 'We save money, we want to keep this federal money," reported a state official privy to the negotiations. "In other words, put it back in, and they're saying, 'What is this? You're going to save money and keep the federal share? No, that's our money.'" Essentially, CMS did not want the federal government to spend more under the Waiver than it would have spent without the Waiver, at least as reflected in the spending targets agreed upon based on assumptions about caseload and cost increases applied to five years of baseline funding history. Indeed, CMS ultimately set yearly spending targets to better ensure that the state remained within the overall funding cap eventually negotiated.

In general, outside stakeholders felt better about the capped federal match than about the proposed block grant because the state could only receive federal funding if it spent money itself, thereby better assuring state officials' commitment to the program while limiting the extent to which it could be reorganized. "The most important thing is the state still controls the spending," explained The Poverty Institute's Linda Katz at a March 22, 2010, legislative hearing. "This is still a matched program. So in order . . . to get a federal dollar, the state has to spend a dollar first. So, really the Medicaid program is largely as it was before the Global Waiver was enacted. The question remains how much is the state willing to spend for Medicaid funded services [and] how can the state achieve savings . . . without harming beneficiaries or making unreasonable demands on providers."

But while state officials felt comfortable with the $12.075 billion total funding ceiling negotiated—CMS basically accepted what Department of Human Services/EOHHS staff believed to be fairly inflated estimates (Anonymous February 18, 2009; Alexander January 28, 2011)—outside stakeholders doubted the adequacy of the state's projections, believing that the total cap on expenditures might not be sufficient to fund the program with adverse but as yet unknown implications for RIte Care recipients, elderly long-term care recipients, and other beneficiaries due to the lack of details provided (Peoples December 20, 2008; Needham and Gregg December 23, 2008; Coffey January 2009; Solomon January 2009; Anonymous February 18, 2009; Needham and Gregg January 10, 2009; National Association of Social Workers January 2009; Needham January 13, 2009). "There is not enough information," observed, Dawn Wardyga, Program Director of Rhode Island Parent Information Network, at a January 12, 2009, House Finance Committee Hearing. "There's not enough detail. They have not involved the community from the get-go. If they had, some of the questions we are asking, we might not have to" (Needham January 13, 2009). State officials again pointed to the Global Waiver as a general framework within which specific decisions about the program would be made in time. Thus, at the same hearing, Ann Martino, Policy Administrator at the Department of Human Services, argued that "[the Waiver] really is a blueprint for moving forward. I think that's one of the confusions when people say there is no detail. Essentially, what the federal government did is provide us with authority to do certain things. How we use that authority is part of the implementation process and will be directed in part by the General Assembly and also input from the community" (Needham January 13, 2009).

There was particular concern about the state accepting a cap on federal funding without knowing what the future might hold. According to a consumer advocate, "the state was putting itself at risk because you just don't know what circumstances are going to be over the course of the five years" and, according to a provider representative, "they were going to woefully underestimate what we needed to fund this system." Given perceived limitations associated with the funding cap, there was also concern that state officials would use whatever additional flexibility that had been provided to draw back on its commitment to the program in order to help reduce the state's budget deficit. This outcome had already been seen in Vermont, where funds from the state's Choices for Care long-term care waiver were diverted by the state legislature to close a budget gap, even while wait-lists for home- and community-based services persisted. That Rhode Island's $12.075 billion funding ceiling was decided on before the economic downturn reached its nadir was especially worrisome for some because it did not fully account for higher than expected unemployment and accompanying increases in Medicaid enrollment (Solomon January 2009; Anonymous February 18, 2009; Goodnough January 22, 2009). The Waiver was based on an assumption of a maximum unemployment rate of 4.9%, but during the recent economic downturn, Rhode Island's unemployment topped 10% (Reed et al. January 13, 2009).

In addition, the $12.075 billion cap agreed upon was substantially less than what the state had requested. In its August 2008 Waiver application, the state had asked for $12.386 billion in total program funding over five years. This was subsequently revised to $12.9 billion in October 2008 during the state's negotiations with CMS (Solomon January 2009). The final cap agreed upon was based on historical spending, adjusted with an annual growth rate of 7.8%, which is lower than Vermont's rate of 9.0%, Rhode Island's original August 2008 projection of 9.2%, and its revised October 2008 projection of 10.2% (Solomon January 2009). The 7.8% rate includes a 1.2% anticipated enrollment increase, in contrast to Rhode Island's August and October 2008 estimates of 2.3% and 3.3%, respectively.[2] This discrepancy between what the state requested and what was ultimately agreed upon raised concerns that the total funding level might not be adequate to meet applicants' needs. The uncertain implications of federal fiscal support, an increasing likelihood given the outcome of the November 2008 election and the rapidly deteriorating state of the economy, raised concern a well (Solomon January 2009; Needham and Gregg January 10, 2009; National Association of Social Workers January 2009). Indeed, the federal stimulus package that would soon pass would temporarily increase the state's FMAP from 52% to 64% and require the state to maintain eligibility at July 1, 2008, levels or else risk losing whatever additional federal money might be provided. The latter provision also meant that state officials would have little control over whatever enrollment increases might occur as a result of the recession.

State officials highlighted negotiation of a clause permitting the state to opt out of the Global Waiver should the funding situation become untenable due to unforeseen and emergent conditions (Carcieri January 5, 2009; Anonymous February 18, 2009; Peoples February 4, 2009). Should that happen, however, outside stakeholders were concerned that the program would revert back to the state plan only and, as such, the state would lose initiatives originally authorized under the state's 11 prior waivers but folded into the Global Waiver, including RIte Care and the various home- and community-based services programs serving the elderly, severely mentally ill, developmentally disabled, and other populations (Reed et al. January 13, 2009). "One of the things that was a concern for people," explained one provider representative, "was that if we got into this and accepted it and went forward and then a year into it, or 18 months in it, or two years into it, people were like, 'Man, this is not a great idea for us,' if we walk away, we go back to bringing the Medicaid program under a state plan, which is not what anybody here would want. You don't get to walk back to the RIte Care waiver."

In exchange for the total cap on program expenditures negotiated, the state wished to obtain as much flexibility as it could to make changes (Alexander January 28, 2011). To the surprise of at least one state official, CMS originally countered with a proposal that made few alterations in the existing federal-state partnership. "It was amazing," this individual recalled, "because their first attempt at it was really they wanted to have almost the same authority they have right now." Ultimately, the state negotiated the Global Waiver's "Special Terms and Conditions," which required state officials to be somewhat more explicit about the actual changes they intended to make, say, with respect to operating the state's nursing home diversion and transition programs, enrolling all but those with third-party insurance coverage into managed care, and imposing a new three-tier system for identifying the level of care required by applicants for long-term services and supports (Weens January 16, 2009). Essentially, the state was granted the flexibility to make the changes documented in the Waiver's "Special Terms and Condition" without having to request permission for making those changes from the federal government (Weens January 16, 2009). If, however, the state wished to make changes that were not so specified, then the degree of federal oversight would depend on a three-category system of federal oversight that was also adopted.

Here, explained one state official, "the state can go forward and do, like, Category I changes pretty easily with CMS' approval. . . . Category II needs a little bit more of a public engagement process and is a little bit harder to do. . . . And then [Category] III changes kind of like would really be hard to do." Negotiations between federal and state officials focused on "picking and choosing what went into those categories" and how long CMS had to review changes associated with each. The goal, explained Elena Nicolella, currently the state's Medicaid Director but a consultant while the Global Waiver was being negotiated, at a March 15, 2010, legislative hearing, was "to ensure that the level of review by CMS was commensurate with the scope of that change. Prior to the Global Waiver any change regardless of how involved the change required the same amount of time and process from CMS." While "we didn't get as much as we wanted to," according to another state official, "we got more than we thought we were going to end up getting, ultimately because they moved."

It is likely that the state has faced more scrutiny under the Obama administration than it would have had under a Republican administration. As one knowledgeable observer pointed out, it is a "very different CMS than it was a year ago. [Rather than viewing Medicaid as a] runaway cost that needs to be constrained [it is viewed as] as an effective tool to expand access to health insurance in national health reform." "It's kind of an interesting twist of fate," seconded a consumer advocate, "that the Governor's Office has pursued this waiver thinking that the federal government would give them all sorts of carte blanche to do things, where now I think the administration will be looking very closely at what the state is saying it wants to do."

CMS also agreed to permit the state to draw in federal money for certain state-only programs, although limited to people with incomes up to 200% of the FPL at the insistence of the Federal Office of Management and Budget. State officials believed that CMS was amenable to the state's Costs Not Otherwise Matchable (CNOM) request because they persuasively argued about the potential benefits of doing so for the bottom line. "One of the things that the central office said to us," recalled one state official, "is that of the state's that came in asking for CNOMs, we were the only ones who had come in with a very thought out, legitimate argument that could show that if we CNOM'd this program, and preserved it, and expanded it, it would ultimately, over time, reduce utilization in that case, or utilization of more higher cost services."

THE STATE LEGISLATIVE ROLE

A Tight Time Frame Colored by Promised Savings

The Democratic party-dominated state legislature did not formally approve the Global Waiver but passively provided its consent by not formally rejecting it within 30 days as stipulated previously in state law. Consumer advocates believed that the General Assembly made it too "easy on themselves" by setting up a process whereby approval was assumed unless they voted to reject it. Instead, advocates would have preferred a process whereby the General Assembly had to "affirmatively decide yes or no" before the Waiver could go ahead. Because of the 30-day time frame adopted, the state legislature had limited time to review the agreement—initial federal approval was granted on December 19, 2008, and the General Assembly did not convene again until after the Christmas and New Year's holidays. Thus, "we had to act quickly," reported one legislative staffer. "I think we gave ourselves some date like January 11[,2009] and the legislature convenes January 5. So, we had very little time to make a decision." It was during this brief interval that caucuses were held and legislative staff walked members through the policy and fiscal implications of the proposed agreement. It was also during this brief interval—on January 9 and 12—that two public hearings were held where the Governor and administration officials defended the Waiver while others expressed reservations or outright opposition over 11 contentious hours (Needham and Gregg January 10, 2009; Needham January 13, 2009), a position expressed by the state's congressional delegation in a letter to the Governor (Reed et al. January 13, 2009).

Although characterized as "reluctant participants" and generally distrustful of the state's Republican governor, state legislators recognized that, at a minimum, new federal money would be coming into the state in the form of the Costs Not Otherwise Matchable, or CNOM, programs, a factor highlighted during hearings held at this time (Needham and Gregg January 10, 2009). They also appreciated the safeguards imposed by CMS—that state officials would not have unlimited flexibility to restructure the program but were bound by the Global Waiver's "Special Terms and Conditions" and federal review of Category II and III changes (Weens January 16, 2009). But the decisive factor underlying then House Speaker William Murphy's January 15 announcement that the General Assembly would not vote to block the Global Waiver, despite whatever concerns were expressed, was $67 million in promised first-year Waiver-derived savings built into the state's FY '09 budget the previous June, though it had long been recognized that actual first-year savings resulting from the Waiver would be substantially less due to delays in submission of the Waiver application by the state and subsequent review by the federal government (Anonymous July 29, 2008; Donnelly January 1, 2009; Needham and Gregg December 23, 2009; Peoples January 14, 2009; Peoples and Needham January 15, 2009). At the time, the state was facing a current year deficit of $357 million (Gregg January 7, 2009). If the state legislature did not approve the Waiver, it would have needed to find those savings someplace else, a daunting task given the state's increasingly desperate fiscal outlook. "When you have savings of X [built into the state's budget] document," explained one legislative staffer, "you either have to go along with it, or you have to find a way to add money to cover the savings if you're not going to use those savings. And I think that [was] a huge . . . factor . . . that, 'Okay, if we don't do this, where are we going to get the money?' "

To the consternation of state legislators, the state would ultimately save substantially less than promised (Peoples January 14, 2010). In FY 2009, for example, the state ended up saving $16 million rather than the $67 million promised by the Governor (Hall January 20, 2011). Outside observers felt that the level of proposed "savings anticipated was highly unrealistic" and, as such, "the promise . . . has proved to be totally false." State staff largely attributed the disappointing level of first-year savings to delays in the federal approval process, which took longer than they had anticipated. They attributed the disappointing level of projected second-year savings to the fact that they did not receive as much flexibility as they would have liked to accomplish all that they intended to due to restrictions imposed by CMS, the General Assembly, and the federal stimulus law (described below) (Peoples January 14, 2010).

An Increased Oversight Role for the State Legislature

The General Assembly has used both existing and specially enacted Global Waiver-specific strategies to oversee implementation. The state budget process has represented one traditional strategy. Since "everything budgetary obviously goes through the legislature," explained one legislative staffer, "the easiest way to give oversight is to fund it or not to fund it." There have also been periodic hearings, both on the House and Senate sides, typically divided among state officials and consumer advocates but also provider representatives. Thus, another legislative staffer explained, "the Senate House Committee . . . joint with the Finance Committee . . . almost instantly began having hearings where [they'd] bring [the administration in] to present. . . . What's your infrastructure? Who's there? Who's going to be making these decisions? What's your plan? What's your approach? What's coming first? What's coming next?' And the Senators would have input through that way or at least would make public what the plans were."

The administration has also communicated informally with the General Assembly on Global Waiver-related matters. "Certainly through our normal budgetary processes and other informal hearings," reported one state official, "there is communication and interaction between all the EOHHS departments and the General Assembly's fiscal offices about the Wavier programs. We definitely on an ongoing basis do report on the programs, so I think there is oversight and interaction." Furthermore, state officials believed that fears the administration would significantly alter Medicaid without going through a public process were overblown as most major changes would still need to be approved by the state legislature (Peoples January 14, 2009). "In Rhode island state law . . . the program that established Medicaid," explained one state official, "you want to change that eligibility group—you can't do it unilaterally. You have to go through the General Assembly. . . . At the end of the day, it was a public process that was much broader than anything you can get [going to a public forum]. . . . When these guys up the Hill told us something, we had no choice."

Existing oversight procedures did not satisfy opponents' concerns about "implementing the waiver at the same time you're cutting the budget" and "trusting state government to make more intricate decisions about people's health care." Thus, in response to continued trepidation on the part of providers and advocates, the General Assembly eventually passed legislation putting into place additional safeguards and providing itself with a more formal oversight role in implementing the Global Waiver, although small differences between the House and Senate versions of the bill delayed adoption several months. This legislation, strongly supported by advocates and largely drafted by the Coalition for Responsible Medicaid Reform, an organization that grew out of advocates and providers' concerns about the state's waiver application, was first introduced when the Global Waiver was formally approved by the federal government (Katz January 20–21, 2009). "It was just all the sound and fury about the Waiver," recalled one provider representative. "So when the legislation came out it was perceived as a way to lessen the threats of the Waiver and sort of reduce people's fears about the administration's intentions. . . . The fears were about if the governor was getting all this flexibility, were they just running rough shod over what providers and advocates want."

Although passed by both the House and Senate in February 2009, by the end of May 2009, the state's oversight legislation had still not been enacted due to disagreement about whether it should include protections for RIte Care recipients (Peoples May 29, 2009). Ultimately, the legislation was signed into law on July 1, 2009, nearly six months after federal approval had been received and the same day state implementation of the Global Waiver began. This legislation served several purposes: (1) to create a Global Waiver Implementation Task Force, (2) to establish a legislative oversight committee, (3) to require prior legislative approval for all Category II and III changes, and (4) to offer some protections to people who began receiving nursing home care prior to implementation of the Global Waiver.

In its application to the federal government, the Department of Human Services/EOHHS listed 38 public forums that occurred between February and June of 2008, the period during which the Global Waiver was drafted (EOHHS August 7, 2008). Newspaper articles from this period, as well as the interviews undertaken for this study, highlight stakeholder concerns over the lack of transparency and community input that actually took place. The oversight legislation, therefore, included a Global Waiver Implementation Task Force through which the Department of Human Services/EOHHS was directed to seek out and incorporate input from the broader stakeholder community. However, because passage of the oversight legislation was delayed, it was unclear how many people should serve on the community taskforce, what their specific duties would be, and whether they had any legal authority (Peoples May 29, 2009). Knowing that the legislation was pending and that community support was lacking, the Department of Human Services/EOHHS nonetheless recruited members and established the Task Force several months before the legislation passed, with the first session taking place May 12, 2009 (Rhode Island Government March 9, 2009; EOHHS May 12, 2009). The Task Force originally included 60 members (of more than 200 who asked to participate) and was slated to meet quarterly. The oversight legislation, however, required a smaller 45-member Task Force with more frequent monthly meetings. Rather than explicitly remove members who had already been recruited, the Department of Human

Services/EOHHS decided to rely on attrition to reduce the size of the Task Force to meet statutory specifications; monthly meetings began July 2009 and have continued to the present day.

The oversight legislation also set up a 12-member Joint Legislative Committee specifically charged with overseeing Medicaid and the Global Waiver. This Committee never seems to have met, although members were appointed, at least on the Senate side. The legislation also put into place CMS' three-category system of federal review at the state level. Consequently, all but simple administrative changes must be reviewed by the state legislature before the Department of Human Services/EOHHS can seek approval from the federal government (Peoples February 4, 2009). The implication was that the state legislature would now participate in Category II changes, an area it had previously left up to the administration. The state legislature would also play a more formalized role vis-à-vis Category III changes, an area in which it had already exercised some oversight authority under state statute. Together, the three categories of change requiring varying levels of CMS and legislative review has probably resulted in greater transparency than existed previously because, as one consumer advocate explained, "even if it's not a statutory change that has to happen, they still have to come to the General Assembly and say, 'This is what we're planning to do.'" Concern remained, however, about the absence of a formal process for obtaining community input when such changes were being made. "There has not been consistency in providing the public opportunity to comment on these changes before they are submitted to CMS," observed Linda Katz (March 1, 2013), Policy Director at The Economic Progress Institute (formerly The Poverty Institute). "We request that . . . EOHHS agrees to establish a consistent process for prior notice of Category II (and III) changes with an opportunity for public comment. Often the persons and entities that will be affected by the proposed changes can provide valuable information to OHHS about the impact and viability of the proposed change. Having a standardized and open process also helps to increase the community's trust in the administration of the Medicaid program." In response, EOHHS promised to work with the Global Waiver Implementation Task Force "to improve the process so that there is ample opportunity for public comment" (EOHHS March 18, 2013).

The requirement for prior legislative approval has clearly limited state administrative flexibility. Thus, according to Elena Nicolella (October 22, 2012), the state Medicaid Director, the "Global Waiver has not been as successful in addressing administrative barriers due to the historic structure and culture of CMS and unanticipated state restrictions." Indeed, like community stakeholders, a particular challenge for state officials has been the absence of clear mechanisms through which legislative review and approval for specific changes might be made, particularly since the legislature's Global Waiver oversight committee was never formally established. The result is that state officials now need to plan well in advance to make sure that there is either legislation or a budget article in place before they can go forward with either a Category II or III change. Because the state legislature now involves itself in decisions it previously was not involved in, the result has been a somewhat more burdensome process—certainly more extensive than originally envisioned and, in some ways, greater than if the Global Waiver had not been pursued. "The biggest thing was that imposition that every change that was a Category II or III had to be approved by the legislature," reported one state official. "Certainly the feds did not contemplate that. They gave us the flexibility to avoid doing that. . . . So what we gained in the flexibility from the federal side, we completely lost on the state side. The majority of the Medicaid program is operated under the Waiver authority. It really has expanded the ability of the General Assembly to get involved in decisions." That the oversight process would, in fact, create additional burdens for program administrators was admitted by Democratic House Majority Leader Gordon Fox, who indicated that "we are going to err on the side of having everything come through us. We'll just have to work hard to get through it" (Peoples January 16, 2009).

That the requirement to seek approval from the General Assembly combined with the lack of clear mechanisms for doing so has increased the legislative role in Medicaid is also reflected in the perception of other observers. "I would contend," reported one provider representative, "[that] they ended up with more restrictions than if they had just made some of these programmatic changes [without the Global Waiver]. . . . It seemed like the state had these hoops they had to go through at the federal level and now they have these hoops they have to go through at the state level." "The General Assembly sort of added a whole other layer of approval and everything that [the Department of Human Services] was not anticipating," confirmed a consumer advocate. "They were trying to make this supposedly more flexible and to change the time that it takes to make decisions, and they did . . . shorten the timeframe that CMS has to respond [but] now with the oversight legislation. . . . I don't think that there have been a whole lot of efficiencies in terms of decision making that have really been realized."

A major provider and advocate concern was whether the state would have the power to remove people from nursing homes who moved in under the old level of care criteria, or to not allow them to move back into the nursing home if they had transferred out, if they were classified as "high" rather than "highest" under the new criteria established under the Global Waiver (Coffey January 2009; Needham January 13, 2009; Peoples May 29, 2009). In light of this concern, the oversight legislation "grandfathered" current nursing home residents from the new level of care provisions. First, the legislation included a provision protecting current nursing home residents who did not want to be transferred back to the community by requiring that the state's old institutional level of care criteria be applied to those residents residing in nursing homes on or before June 30, 2009. As such, "if a person was in a nursing home," according to one state official, "we weren't going to be able to touch them . . . unless they explicitly said they wanted to move out. We'd have to use our old level of care every time we assessed them." This provision was deemed both practical and fair because, as one provider representative explained it, "if someone's 'highest' in a nursing home . . . and now they level that person as 'high,' the person's out of the nursing home. . . . Well, they've sold their home. . . . Where are they going to go? They have to reestablish an apartment? Get pots and pans? Learn to cook again? Think about it."

Second, the legislation originally included a provision ensuring that someone who had voluntarily moved out of a nursing home could move back in under the old level of care criteria if they decided that they could not make it in the community. This provision, however, proved incompatible with the federal Waiver agreement, which stated that the new level of care criteria would be applied once someone transferred out of a nursing home, so if they are classified as "high," they could not go back in even if they wanted to. Still, the General Assembly was able to include a provision within the oversight bill confirming that those scoring "highest" could be readmitted, in addition to those facing special circumstances that may adversely impact health or safety, including failed placement. "So, there is some protection," confirmed once consumer advocate, "but it's not the broad protection of who's in a nursing home on this date, 'I agree to go out, I'm always entitled to go back in.'" Moreover, there was concern about what would in fact constitute a "failed placement" (Peoples July 9, 2009). Although watered down, some nonetheless viewed this provision as important for encouraging participation in the state's nursing home transition efforts. Thus, at a March 22, 2010, hearing, Democratic State Senator Charles Levesque reported believing that "there are a lot more people, who in fact, opted into the program because they had that assurance . . . that if it was unsuccessful they could come back into the nursing home."

SUMMARY

Fears about state officials' intentions in pursuing the Global Waiver were exacerbated by the lack of transparency in its negotiations with the federal government. While the state's congressional delegation served, in part, as a conduit for stakeholder concerns, ultimately, it did not influence the outcome of the negotiations. Several major changes were made to the state's Waiver application during the negotiation process. Rather than block grant Medicaid, the state accepted a capped federal match whereby a limit was placed on combined federal and state spending over five years and the state was still required to expend its own resources before it received money from the federal government. Furthermore, rather than gaining nearly unlimited flexibility to shape the program, as initially requested, state discretion was limited to specific proposals outlined in the Waiver's "Special Terms and Conditions," with additional changes being subject to the Waiver's three-tier system of federal oversight. Although more acceptable than a block grant, outside stakeholders were concerned about the adequacy of the expenditure cap, believing it might prove inadequate in light of the state's rapidly deteriorating fiscal environment. Other especially salient components of the final Waiver agreement included provisions permitting the state to draw in additional federal matching dollars for programs that would otherwise have been funded entirely by the state (i.e., the Global Waiver's Costs Not Otherwise Matchable, or CNOM, authority) and a clause permitting the state to opt out of the Global Waiver, basically at any time. The implications of withdrawal for populations previously served by separate Waiver programs remained a concern for some. There was fear that if the state ended the Global Waiver, populations previously served by the state's prior waiver programs would no longer be eligible for needed services.

After federal approval, the state legislature had an opportunity to prevent implementation of the Global Waiver. However, it chose to permit the Waiver to go into effect, largely because of millions of dollars in promised savings and the ability to draw in new federal money under the Waiver's CNOM authority. Both possibilities were deemed critical to helping fill the state's growing budget deficit. Once approved, the General Assembly used both existing and newly established mechanisms to oversee implementation. Existing mechanisms have included the state budget process, periodic hearings, and routine communication between the legislative and executive branches of government. Waiver-specific mechanisms, which derived from specially enacted oversight legislation, include a Global Waiver Implementation Task Force and Joint House-Senate oversight committee, though the latter never seems to have been put into effect. They also include a requirement that all but simple administrative changes be approved by the state legislature before being submitted for federal approval. Current nursing home residents were grandfathered from the new level of care provisions as well. Overall, the larger role reserved by the state legislature in Medicaid program decision making has limited state administrative flexibility to adopt desired changes, at least according to some observers.

NOTES

1. The content of this letter was read aloud by one of the consumer representatives interviewed.
2. It was assumed that per member per month annual costs would increase by 6.8%.

4 A Primer on the Global Waiver

The politics of federal and state approval resulted in the final Global Consumer Choice Compact Medicaid Waiver implemented by the Department of Human Services in concert with other departments within the Executive Office of Health and Human Services. This chapter reviews the major components and activities conducted under the final Waiver agreement. Most provisions pertain to rebalancing long-term care away from institutions toward home- and community-based services. Although the language of the Global Waiver largely focuses on elders in need of long-term services and supports, the state has sought to apply the philosophy of providing care in the least restrictive settings possible, not only to older adults but to people with developmental disabilities, adults with physical disabilities, the mentally ill, and children with special health care needs. Other major provisions of the Global Waiver include requiring most Medicaid beneficiaries to enroll in managed care as well as reforming the way in which the state contracts and pays for services. New authority to draw in federal matching dollars for previously state-only funded programs is examined as well, in addition to changes in the level and timing of federal and state oversight.

LONG-TERM CARE REBALANCING

Like Rhode Island's Perry-Sullivan legislation and Real Choices Systems Change grants, the Global Waiver seeks to attain a 50–50 spending split between nursing home and home- and community-based services by 2013. Indeed, it has been noted that prior efforts such as Real Choices "paved the way for the Global Waiver's efforts to rebalance the system of long-term services and supports" and that "many Global Waiver objectives and strategies are closely related to those of the Real Choices grant" (Anonymous May 23, 2011). A number of ongoing efforts fed into the Global Waiver's strategy for rebalancing long-term care. These include evaluating the needs and experiences of both institutionalized and community-based long-term care recipients and developing educational materials—brochures, videos, booklets—to inform client decision making. These also include training discharge planners and community groups about available long-term care options and identifying quality indicators to be tracked across systems over time. Still other efforts include: assessing the capacity of program administrators and providers to expand community-based options; centralizing and standardizing the clinical and financial long-term care eligibility process; applying savings deriving from reduced institutional placements to further expansion of home- and community-based options; and initiating and documenting stakeholder meetings about state efforts to reduce reliance on institutional placements through increased use of alternative settings in the community.

Perhaps the most prominent Global Waiver-related rebalancing task has been the adoption of a three-tier level of care determination process for eligibility for Medicaid long-term care: "highest," "high," and "preventive." Previously, there had been only one basic level of eligibility, with all those meeting the state's clinical eligibility requirements being eligible to receive nursing home care or to participate in one of the state's home- and community-based waiver programs if a slot was available. Now only those deemed "highest" need have an entitlement to nursing home care, though they may also choose a home- and community-based placement. Those deemed "high" are eligible for home- and community-based services only and those deemed "preventive" are restricted to a package of home care benefits—limited certified nurse aide (CNA)/homemaker services and minor home modifications, given available funding. The CNA/homemaker services benefit includes a maximum of six hours per week for a single individual and 10 hours per week for two or more eligible individuals living within the same household. The provision of respite, physical therapy, and occupational therapy services have also been considered as part of the package of benefits made available to those deemed preventive.

Rhode Island's criteria for the preventive level of care include: has a chronic illness or disability and requires supervision with two or more activities of daily living (i.e., toileting, bathing, eating, dressing, transferring) or extensive assistance with at least three instrumental activities of daily living (e.g., meal preparation, laundry, shopping, cleaning). Rhode Island's criterion for the "high" needs cohort is the same as what was formerly used to determine eligibility for long-term care prior to the Global Waiver. This means that a group that was previously defined as needing an institutional level of care and guaranteed access to nursing home services now does not have that option, even if funding is available.

The state has reported the distribution of level of care determinations each quarter since implementation of the Global Waiver began (Department of Human Services January 2010–February 2013; EOHHS January 2011–April 2013). In each instance, the vast majority of individuals were reported to be assessed at the "highest" level of care, followed by "high," and "preventive." Thus, of 23,425 level of care determinations made between July 1, 2009, and December 31, 2012, 66.6% were assigned a "highest" designation,

26.2% a "high" designation, 5.7% a "preventive" designation, and 0.5% to no designation at all. Because the new level of care provisions do not apply to the developmentally disabled population or to those receiving behavioral health services, it does not impact residential care placement in either of these settings.

The state also developed and implemented what it refers to as an Assessment and Coordination Organization (ACO) to better promote uniformity in the administration of Medicaid-funded long-term care services, including with respect to information and referral, eligibility and referral and care planning and care management. Here, the goal has been to create a central interagency mechanism for making level of care determinations, supporting community-based placements, implementing consistent case management practices, and conducting high-cost case reviews and other functions across the state's health and human services agencies. Under this system, all long-term care referrals are directed to the Department of Human Services' Office of Medical Review at which level of care determinations are made centrally by six Office of Medical Review nurses. Referrals for long-term care derive from the state's long-term care field offices, hospital discharge planners, and nursing homes, which communicate the information necessary for Office of Medical Review nurses who determine eligibility based on the use of a common level of care assessment tool. Determinations are subsequently communicated back to the referral source. Complex, high costs cases are also referred to a new Office of Community Programs in which four registered nurses and two social workers are charged with undertaking case management and oversight. The Office of Community Programs also supports community-based placements more generally, including managing services received by "preventive" level of care recipients who are not eligible for Supplemental Security Income. Clients who are eligible for Supplemental Security Income receive case management from social case workers at Department of Human Services' long-term care field offices. Those who are not medically complex may also receive case management from the Department of Elderly Affairs from one of six case management agencies located throughout the state.

Concomitant with this centralization, the state removed delegated authority from discharge planners to make level of care determinations, though a role for discharge planners in making discharges on weekends and holidays was retained when state staff is unavailable. Several efforts have been made to better educate discharge planners and other long-term care referral sources about services and housing options available in the community. This includes an April 28, 2011, discharge planning conference attended by about 200 individuals. It also includes development and implementation of Community Options Training for hospital and nursing home discharge planners in the way of webcasts and printed materials. The state developed and launched its Rite Resources website, an electronic database whereby discharge planners, patients, and their families are provided up-to-date information on the availability of services provided by nursing homes, assisted living facilities, home health agencies, adult day agencies, and other home- and community-based providers contingent on client demographic, clinical, and service need characteristics (EOHHS November 28, 2011b). The state has also established a Long-Term Care Options Counseling Program within the state's Aging and Disability Resource Center, The Point, to better provide individuals and their families with the information necessary to make more appropriate decisions about themselves and their loved ones.

Major Waiver-related rebalancing tasks have also included designing and implementing nursing home transition and diversion projects beginning July 1, 2009, and January 1, 2010, respectively. The state's nursing home transition program was initially operated by an outside vendor, the Alliance for Better Long-Term Care, which also runs the state's long-term care ombudsmen program. The Alliance would go into nursing homes and work with the facility, Departments of Health Services and Elderly Affairs staff, residents, and their families to identify persons who were both willing and able to be move safely back into the community. Individuals and families also self-referred to the program based on brochures, posters, and other marketing materials that had been distributed in nursing homes throughout the state. Once the decision to transfer had been made, the Alliance would work with Departments of Human Services and Elderly Affairs before, during, and after the transition to ensure the provision of the necessary community support. Subsequently, the state made the decision not to renew the Alliance's 18-month contract. As such, beginning July 1, 2010, the Department of Human Services' Office of Community Programs has been charged with the transition program in collaboration with the Department of Human Services' Office of Medical Review and Department of Elderly Affairs' Office of Community Programs, which also has experience transitioning. Beginning the last quarter of 2011, the transition program has been supplemented by receipt of a $24.6 million five-year federal Money Follows the Person Demonstration Grant, which is set to expire March 31, 2016. Planning activities under both programs have been aligned, and the state has examined the possibility of expanding respite and transition care services under Money Follows the Person, known as the Rhode to Home Program in Rhode Island.

During the 18 months in which the Alliance for Better Long-Term Care ran the state's transition program (January 2009–June 2010), 133 nursing home residents were transitioned back into the community (Department of Human Services January 2010–February 2013). In the 30 months since the state took over (July 2010–December 2012), 316 individuals were transitioned, approximately one-quarter (26.0%) of the 1,213 individuals initially referred to the Office of Community Programs for this purpose during that time period. Of those transferred since the state took over, 78.7% have been transferred home with core home- and community-based services and 14.0% to assisted living.

The diversion project includes several elements, which, in addition to better educating discharge planners and others about available options within the community, involved tasking an onsite registered nurse at Rhode Island Hospital in collaboration with hospital social workers, to identify Medicaid beneficiaries who might be discharged safely back into the community. This nurse was subsequently reassigned to the state's primary care case management program, Connect Care Choice. It has been estimated that Rhode Island diverted 546 persons from nursing home placement between July 2010 and May 2011, including 84 persons identified through Connect Care Choice and 480 assigned a "high" level of care, i.e., those believed to be eligible for nursing home care under the old leveling system but not under the new three-tier process adopted as part of the Global Waiver (The Lewin Group December 6, 2011). For each beneficiary transferred or diverted from a nursing home to home with services, the state assumes average savings of $3,060 per month (The Lewin Group December 6, 2011). For each beneficiary transferred from a nursing home to assisted living, the state assumes average savings of $3,510 monthly. For each beneficiary transferred from a nursing home to home without services, the state assumes average savings of $4,560.

Efforts have also been made to expand access to and the availability of certain home- and community-based supports, including shared living, home health, assisted living, adult day, and preventive services. Prior the Global Waiver, shared living was only available to people with developmental disabilities. Since implementation of the Waiver, it has been extended to elderly and adult disabled Medicaid eligibles who cannot live independently and meet the state's "highest" or "high" level of care designations. Shared living permits financially and clinically eligible individuals to receive care in a host home that is supervised by a shared living agency (Department of Human Services April 2010). The host caregiver can be a friend, relative, neighbor, acquaintance, or someone else; he or she cannot be a spouse or legal guardian. Host caregivers are responsible for being on call 24/7, providing socialization, a homelike environment, personal care, homemaker services, chore services, meals, and transportation. Through a competitive contracting process, two agencies—The Homestead Group and Caregiver Homes—were awarded contracts by the state to manage the shared living program, including recruiting, training, and monitoring host homes and caregivers (who receive stipends ranging from $13,000 to $18,000 per year), providing registered nurse services and caregiver respite, and implementing shared living service and safety plans. Medicaid pays the caregiver stipend only which, depending on income, might include a cost share from the care recipient; it does not pay for room and board. This, instead, is paid for out of the beneficiaries' Social Security or Supplemental Security Income checks. The shared living program grew from six to 75 clients between September 2010 and December 2012. As of September 30, 2012, Rhode Island's Medicaid Shared Living Program is known as RIte @ Home.

Other Waiver-related initiatives include a negotiated rate increase for assisted living facilities, from $36.32 to $42.16 per day, effective July 1, 2010; provision of a $206 monthly payment to Supplemental Security Income recipients in assisted living facilities that do not take Medicaid, and development and implementation of new criteria for Medicaid-participating home health agencies, including participating in the state's "Enhanced Reimbursement Program" whereby agencies can earn additional reimbursement by meeting standards beyond minimal licensing requirements. Prior to the Global Waiver, the state had implemented a 10% increase in homemaker, personal care, home health aide, and adult day care reimbursement effective July 1, 2008. Additional efforts include identifying assisted living facilities that meet "qualifying residence" requirements under Money Follows the Person, exploring the possibility of acuity-based reimbursement in adult day care and pursuing rebalancing options under the Patient Protection and Affordable Care Act.

CARE MANAGEMENT

A major Waiver-related task has been to implement mandatory enrollment in Medicaid managed care for all those without third-party medical coverage. Previously, children and families on Medicaid were enrolled in managed care through the state's RIte Care program, and those with low incomes but too high to qualify for Medicaid in the state's premium sharing program, RIte Share. By contrast, enrollment in the state's managed care program for adults, Rhody Health Partners, was optional. This was also true of children with special health care needs but with respect to RIte Care. Beginning in July 1, 2009, Medicaid eligible adults with no health insurance coverage other than Medicaid were required to enroll in either Rhody Health Partners or primary care case management via Connect Care Choice, while children with special health care needs were required to enroll in RIte Care.

Connect Care Choice includes 17 participating practices where physicians partner with an onsite nurse care manager to create a medical home for patients to better ensure all necessary services are effectively managed and coordinated. Participating practices must also coordinate with behavioral health providers if necessary and adopt e-prescribing, e-billing, and computerized decision guidelines. Rhody Health Partners consists of two participating health plans, Neighborhood Health Plan of Rhode Island and United Healthcare Community Plan of Rhode Island, where care management is provided by interdisciplinary teams of providers. Mandatory enrollment was phased in, with clients being permitted to switch between Connect Care Choice and Rhody Health Partners up to December 31, 2009, after which they were locked into their plans for one year until the next open-enrollment period began. If clinically eligible, aged or disabled enrollees may choose to enroll in the state's integrated delivery system for individuals dually eligible for Medicaid and Medicare, the Program for All-Inclusive Care for the Elderly (PACE).

To improve outcomes, the state imposed Communities of Care on high utilizers with complex needs enrolled in the state's managed care plans (RIte Care, Rhody Health Partners) and on high emergency department utilizers enrolled in the state's primary care case management system (Connect Care Choice). The state also developed targeted interventions on behalf of high utilizers of pharmacy benefit services, both in Medicaid fee-for-service and managed care. The state implemented Screening, Brief Intervention, and Referral to Treatment (SBIRT) services for beneficiaries enrolled in Connect Care Choice (effective February 2011) and managed care (effective summer 2011) who either had or were at risk for substance abuse.

By mandatorily enrolling Medicaid beneficiaries in care management, state officials wish to promote personal responsibility, prevention, and wellness, and to assist beneficiaries with accessing care coordination and community-based services. This is also true of related efforts to develop, implement, and monitor medical home standards and to expand the use of managed long-term care. The state further intended to adopt incentives for enrollees to take greater responsibility for the self-management of care, in addition to revising the state's Medicaid buy-in program for adults with physical disabilities who seek to gain or maintain employment (i.e., the Sherlock Plan). The former include Health Opportunity Accounts, which would establish personal health care accounts for higher-income populations, and Healthy Choice Accounts, which would create itemized spending and rewards for lower-income populations to spur healthy behaviors and choices. Both these initiatives have yet to be implemented.

The state engaged in a comprehensive planning and design process under its Integrated Care Initiative to pursue state and federal opportunities to integrate care for populations and services previously excluded from Medicaid managed care, including Medicaid beneficiaries who are also eligible for Medicare and Medicaid-only beneficiaries in need of long-term services and supports. The aim of this initiative is to "achieve improved health and well-being, better healthcare, and lower costs" by "[transforming] the delivery system through purchasing person-centered, comprehensive, coordinated, quality health care and supports services that promote and enhance the ability . . . to maintain a high quality of life and live independently in the community" (Mauro July 23, 2012). This includes improving the coordination of primary, specialty, hospital, behavioral, and long-term care services, addressing fragmentation in coverage between Medicare and Medicaid, and aligning financial incentives across payers and providers.

Key to this effort will be participation in CMS' Financial Alignment Demonstration to support state efforts to integrate care (CMS May 10, 2013). The Affordable Care Act created a Federal Coordinated Health Care Office within CMS to identify ways in which Medicare and Medicaid might work jointly to improve care for individuals dually eligible for Medicare and Medicaid. It also created the Center for Medicare and Medicaid Innovation to test innovative payment and service delivery models designed to reduce program expenditures while maintaining or improving quality of care. Together, the two centers have committed over $1 billion to assess various care coordination strategies and incentives. This includes CMS' Financial Alignment Demonstration through which 26 states have developed proposals to assess models for integrating primary, acute, behavioral health, and long-term care services for dual eligibles. Under the demonstration, participating states will be permitted to test strategies for integrating care over three years. These include a capitated model whereby a health plan enters into a three-way contract with the state and CMS to provide comprehensive and coordinated care in return for a prospective blended payment. These also include a managed fee-for-service model whereby the state enters into an agreement with CMS permitting the state to benefit from savings to both Medicare and Medicaid stemming from initiatives that lower costs and enhance quality. The state submitted its proposal to CMS on May 31, 2012, after which the federal agency held a one-month public comment period (June 1–July 1, 2012) (CMS July 1, 2012).

Under its proposal, the state intends to enroll dually eligible and Medicaid-only recipients in need of long-term services and supports into enhanced versions of its managed care and primary care case management programs for people with disabilities, Rhody Health Options and Connect Care Choice *Community Partners*, as well as PACE if level of care and other criteria are met. The state is currently in the process of procuring these services. Letters of intent for both programs were solicited February 18, 2013. Proposals were subsequently received and reviewed. The intention is to stagger enrollment over four months, from July 1 to October 1, 2013. Qualifying beneficiaries will receive a letter after which they will have four weeks to choose a health plan, either a Rhody Health Options plan, Connect Care Choice *Community Partners*, or PACE. Enrollment will take place eight weeks after the original letter is dated.

SMART PURCHASING

Major Global Waiver-related initiatives include several activities meant to promote the "smart," efficient contracting of Medicaid services whereby the state has sought to use its leverage and purchasing power to ensure payment for high-quality, cost-effective services. The purpose in employing selective contracting is to incentivize quality and cost improvements and to enhance the value of Medicaid dollars spent. It is also intended to promote a more uniform payment structure as compared to the prevailing system whereby the state often pays varying rates for the same services offered by different providers. Selective contracting has been pursued in three areas: durable medical equipment, prosthetics, orthotics, and supplies (DMEPOS); shared living; and managed care.

Through a competitive bidding process, the state successfully identified and contracted with two vendors to provide shared-living services to the elderly and disabled. Although the state had received bids in an effort to re-procure DMEPOS, no bid proved sufficiently attractive and, as such, no contract was ultimately awarded as part of this initiative. However, competitive bidding was used to re-procure health plans serving the state's RIte Care and Rhody Health Partners managed care programs. Bids were received from Neighborhood Health Plan of Rhode Island and United Healthcare Community Plan of Rhode Island, with one provider, Blue Cross Blue Shield of Rhode Island, opting not to continue its association with the RIte Care program after having done so for 16 years. Currently, two-thirds of managed care enrollment in Rhode Island is in Neighborhood Health plan (91,405 members), and the remaining one third is in the United Healthcare Community Plan (44,299 members) (IPRO October 2012). Of 135,704 total managed care enrollees, 84% (114,069) represent the core RIte Care population, 5% (6,727) children with special health care needs enrolled in RIte Care, 2% (2,591) children in substitute care enrolled in RIte Care, and 9% (12,617) in Rhody Health Partners. Neighborhood Health Plan's entire product line is Medicaid. In contrast, Medicaid constitutes 57% of United Healthcare Community Plan's product line, with the remaindering consisting of Medicare (22%) and commercial (21%) products.

The state continues to develop and pursue selective contracting strategies in capitated Medicaid managed care, managed long-term care, and primary care case management. The state used re-procurement as an opportunity both to reduce costs and to institute other changes. The latter, for example, includes enhancing mandatory CMS requirements by requiring each plan to conduct four quality improvement projects annually, including ones focused on children with special health care needs, disabled adults enrolled in Rhody Health Partners, and members enrolled in the state's Communities of Care initiative. The latter also includes reinforcing the importance of National Committee on Quality Assurance accreditation whereby any denial of accreditation results in termination of the plan's contract with the state.

In addition to choosing Medicaid contractors competitively, the state's "smart" purchasing strategy has involved nursing facility and hospital reimbursement reform. In both cases, the state's intention has been to replace the prevailing cost-based system with a price-based system grounded in average nursing costs in the case of nursing homes, adjusted for resident acuity, and diagnostic related groups (DRGs) in the case of inpatient hospital care. Implementation of hospital DRGs took place in 2010. Starting October 1, 2012, the state began a four-year transition to a new nursing home reimbursement system whereby the direct-care component of each nursing home's payment rate is adjusted for the acuity of individual residents. To minimize the impact of the new methodology, the state will ensure that no nursing home experiences a loss in direct care during the transition, and that gains or losses on all other rate components will be limited to $5.00 per resident per day during the first transition year and progressively smaller amounts during the remaining transition years. Beginning in year 2, the state intends to incorporate pay-for-performance incentives, rewarding facilities that achieve certain quality outcomes including in relation to staffing stability and, potentially, other measures. The state may also adjust payment for behavioral health or dementia care. The state had intended to increase cost-sharing to enhance personal responsibility, encourage cost-effective service use, deter crowd-out, and reward healthy choices. These efforts, however, were eventually blocked by CMS due to maintenance of effort requirements included in the federal health reform law. Planned increases to home health payments are still in process.

COSTS NOT OTHERWISE MATCHABLE

As noted, CMS granted Rhode Island the authority to obtain federal matching funds for populations and services previously covered only by the state. The purpose in granting the state this authority was to determine if such a strategy was cost-effective over the long run by slowing down or preventing the trajectory towards full Medicaid eligibility. These are known as CNOMs, or Costs Not Otherwise Matchable. Each EOHHS Department has benefited from CNOM dollars. The Department of Behavioral Healthcare, Developmental Disabilities, and Hospitals is the largest recipient, as CNOM money covers all of the Department's outpatient substance abuse, partial hospitalization, and intensive outpatient programs. During the Waiver's first four years—January 2009–December 2012—Behavioral Healthcare, Developmental Disabilities, and Hospitals received $41,882,254 in federal CNOM money (Department of Human Services January 2010–February 2013). Another particularly noteworthy CNOM initiative is the Department of Elderly Affairs' Co-Pay Program, which previously relied entirely on state dollars and beneficiary cost-sharing to fund home health, adult day, and case management services for low income people aged 65 years or older with incomes too high to qualify for Medicaid but in need of supportive services. During the Waiver's first four years, Elderly Affairs received $18,037,038 from the federal government for this program (Department of Human Services January 2010–February 2013). In all, Rhode Island received $6,434,905, $16,834,550, $19,502,121, and $17,624,952, respectively, in federal matching dollars during state FY 2009, FY 2010, FY 2011, and FY 2012 for state expenditures of $5,801,081, $15,414,550, $17,335,506, and $16,657,935 on programs that had been "CNOMed" (Department of Human Services January 2010–February 2013; EOHHS January 2011–April 2013).

OVERSIGHT

As reported earlier, the Rhode Island General Assembly passed a July 1, 2009, oversight bill which requires that certain categories of Medicaid program changes be approved by the legislature first before the Department of

Table 4.1 State and Federal Oversight Requirements

	Description	State Requirement	Federal Requirements
Category I	A change that is administrative in nature that the state has authority to change under the State Plan or demonstrations Special Terms and Conditions. Does NOT affect beneficiary eligibility, benefits, overall healthcare delivery systems, payment methodologies, or cost sharing.	Changes must be presented to the permanent joint legislative committee on the Global Waiver for approval prior to implementation.	State must notify CMS of change (informal). CMS approval not required for implementation.
Category II	A change that could be made as a State Plan amendment or through 1915 waiver authority without a change in the waivers Special Terms and Conditions (STC) or the section 1115 waiver and expenditures authorities. May affect benefit packages, health delivery systems, cost-sharing levels, and post-eligibility contributions to cost of care. Does NOT affect beneficiary eligibility.	Changes must be approved by the General Assembly prior to implementation. DHS/EOHHS must also comply with existing public notification and hearing process prior to implementation.	State must comply with State Plan public notice process. State must notify CMS in writing prior to implementation, and must provide justification and assurances that such changes are consistent with program goals, improve program operation, would be permissible under a State Plan or section 1915 waiver, and are cost-effective. CMS approval not required before implementation, but federal matching funds will not be provided for changes that are implemented but not approved.

(*Continued*)

Table 4.1 (continued)

	Description	State Requirement	Federal Requirements
Category III	A change requiring modifications to the current waiver or expenditure authorities or Special Terms and Conditions and any change not clearly defined as Category I or II[1]	Changes must be approved by the General Assembly prior to implementation. DHS must also comply with the existing public notification and hearing process prior to implementation.	State must comply with the State Plan public notice process. State must notify CMS in writing and submit a demonstration amendment. CMS approval necessary prior to implementation.

1. Examples: all eligibility changes; changes in mandatory benefits; spend-down level changes; cost-sharing in excess of 5% of family income; benefit changes not in accordance with existing federal statute; post-eligibility treatment of income; and amendments requesting change to budget neutrality cap.

Human Services/EOHHS could seek permission from CMS to implement those changes. These categories, termed I, II, and III and defined by CMS when it authorized the Waiver, were designed for purposes of establishing federal oversight protocols and to make federal review more commensurate with the scope of changes proposed. Category I, II, and III changes and associated federal and state oversight requirements are described in Table 4.1. Between July 2009 and December 2012, the state made eight Category I requests, eight Category II requests, one Category III request,[1] and 12 amendments to the state plan (Department of Human Services January 2010–February 2013; EOHHS January 2011–April 2013). Most were approved by CMS; however, some such as proposed limits on the number of emergency department visits (a Category II request) and proposed increases in RIte Care Premium Cost Sharing (also a Category II request) were denied.

SUMMARY

Under the Global Waiver, Rhode Island sought greater administrative flexibility in pursuit of three major programmatic goals: (1) Rebalance the publicly funded long-term care system to increase access to home- and community-based services and supports and to decrease reliance on institutional stays; (2) Ensure all Medicaid beneficiaries have access to care management whereby primary and acute care is managed and coordinated with other services and supports; and (3) Procure Medicaid-funded services through cost-effective payment and purchasing strategies that align with programmatic goals. The state also obtained the ability to receive federal matching funds for populations and services previously covered by state-only funded programs. The level of federal and state legislative oversight and scrutiny was made more commensurate with the scope of future program changes as well.

NOTE

1. Elsewhere, the state reports no Category III requests (Nicolella October 2012).

5 External Factors and Implementation

Despite the heightened role for the state legislature, some Global Waiver opponents have not been satisfied, believing that the General Assembly had not engaged in effective oversight, both of EOHHS in general and of its constituent departments. That the joint oversight committee has not met and that Global Waiver oversight has occurred "catch-as-catch-can from budget meetings" has proven problematic for some observers, particularly given the absence of assurances of how the legislature's oversight role would be fulfilled when the General Assembly was not in session. That the Department of Human Services/EOHHS has submitted budget articles listing all the Category II and III changes it would like to put in place but not providing any additional details about how such changes would look has tried the patience of some outside observers as well. "They've come in with the budget article that says these are the changes we're planning to make under the waiver," reported one consumer advocate, "and they're asking the General Assembly to give them approval to go to CMS to get approval to do that, and a big problem now is that the details of that are not spelled out. I mean, they're proposing to save $40 million but not specifying how that $40 million would be saved." More broadly, there was concern whether a part-time state legislature such as Rhode Island's would have the time or level of expertise to execute detailed oversight (Peoples February 4, 2009).

This chapter looks beyond the state legislature to consider other factors external to the Department of Human Services/EOHHS that may have had a strong influence on implementation of the Global Waiver. It starts with the Global Waiver Implementation Task Force authorized by the General Assembly. Next, it examines the implications of the Global Waiver for increasing cooperation among key stakeholder groups representing different populations and service modalities. It concludes by examining fiscal and budgetary pressures that have influenced the way in which the Global Waiver has been implemented.

GLOBAL WAIVER IMPLEMENTATION TASK FORCE

Task Force Has Been Heavily State-Directed

Although established to provide a conduit for the public input that was lacking during the development of the Global Waiver, there was general dissatisfaction with the way the Global Waiver Implementation Task Force operated, at least early on. Indeed, most interviewees felt that the Task Force has not had much influence on state implementation efforts despite state lawmakers' intentions in this respect. One frequently cited criticism is the lack of productive dialogue. Communication has tended to be one-way. The agenda has been set by the Department of Human Services/EOHHS with meetings consisting largely of state officials informing Task Force members about progress and activities administering the Waiver. "It was mainly just show-and-tell by Department of Human Services," reported one consumer advocate, "but not much chance for input and discussion." "They're not really asking them to give any input," confirmed another advocate for consumers. "They're really just sitting them in a room and reporting off that this is what we've accomplished, sort of, this month. It's just too bad, because they could use those resources."

Part of the challenge has been varying interpretations of the Task Force's mission. In particular, there was disagreement as to whether the Task Force should simply be advising the Department of Human Services/EOHHS on Global Waiver implementation or actively participating in the implementation process itself. This disagreement arose, in part, due to the language included in the state's oversight legislation, which directed the Task Force to "work collaboratively with the Executive Office of Health and Human Services and the Department of Human Services to plan, design, and implement changes to the Medicaid program under the demonstration and to evaluate the impact of such changes and of the demonstration."[1] Some felt that Task Force members should get involved in the "nitty-gritty of implementing the program" since, well, "it's called an Implementation Task Force." Others felt that too much stakeholder involvement would result in an unwieldy and cumbersome process that could slow down and inhibit progress.

Interestingly, the size of the Task Force has been criticized by both state officials and Task Force members. The inclusion of 60 people representing such a diverse array of interests has served both to limit the amount of influence that could be exerted by any one Task Force member and to complicate the incorporation of whatever input might be provided into the state's implementation efforts. This view is reflected in the observations of one provider representative who reported that the size of the panel has "almost led to an inertia and to make it harder to change things because there are so many interests involved all the time, it's very confusing." This view is also reflected in the observations of one state official who reported that "the thing that [the government] has to have is a vision of the entire program, rather than looking at it piecemeal. Everybody [on the Task Force] has their own piece they're looking at. . . . That's part of the challenge."

Another part of the challenge has been the absence of community leadership. The oversight bill required the appointment of both administrative and community co-chairs of the Global Waiver Implementation Task Force. While Ann Martino, now Deputy Secretary for Policy at EOHHS, was appointed administrative co-chair when the Task Force was first established, a community co-chair was not appointed until October 2011, nearly two and a half years after the Task Force began meeting. Indeed, it was not until newly elected Independent Governor Lincoln Chafee appointed former Democratic House Finance Committee Chair Steven Costantino as EOHHS Secretary in 2011, that a committee co-chair was identified. "A good portion of that frustration," reported one provider representative, "is directly related to the fact that there was no community chair who is involved in setting agendas, and setting the goals and vision for the Task Force." This was not entirely the fault of Department of Human Services/EOHHS, however. On the one hand, the administration imposed strict criteria on the selection process, that it could not be someone who received money from the state or would have a potential conflict of interest. On the other hand, attempts were made to recruit someone to fill this role but, as one local Medicaid expert put it, "no one wants to [do it] because they feel if they take a leadership role it shows that they're supportive of it." In the interim, state officials established a Community Executive Council consisting initially of the chairs and co-chairs of the Task Force's work groups, to review and to prioritize recommendations based, in part, on the level of proposed budget savings achieved. Eventually, only three applications for the community co-chair position were received after a renewed effort to recruit someone for the position was announced June 2011. In October 2011, former State Senator Thomas Izzo, a Democrat from Cranston, was chosen and introduced as the community co-chair.

In addition to delays appointing a community co-chair, some interviewees were frustrated that the state had released the names of individuals recruited to serve on the Task Force but not their organizational affiliations. Their concern stemmed from resulting difficulties determining whether the Department of Human Services/EOHHS had recruited representatives from all the various stakeholder groups required under the Task Force's authorizing statute.[2] Still others were surprised by the omission of medical providers from the Task Force's membership. In response, the state revived its Medical Care Advisory Committee, which had lain dormant for several years, although one knowledgeable observer could not reconcile the content of these quarterly meetings, which focused mostly on medical issues, with implementation of the Global Waiver. There was also concern about the manner in which the state acquired input from actual consumers. "The Global Waiver Task Force has few members who qualify as consumers," observed Anne Mulready (February 28, 2013), a Supervisory Attorney at the

Rhode Island Disability Law Center, "and it is not clear that the state has any formalized means of obtaining feedback directly from consumers. Focus groups and other kinds of targeted meetings with consumers are more likely to result in feedback from consumers than formal public comment opportunities. We urge the state to incorporate these other methods of obtaining consumer feedback on the quality and adequacy of services."

Lack of Responsiveness to Task Force Recommendations

The lack of effective dialogue between the Department of Human Services/ EOHHS and the stakeholder community was widely noted. The most frequently cited example was the lack of state responsiveness to recommendations developed by the Task Force's work groups. Initially, state staff established six work groups: Housing, Employment, Long-Term Care Insurance Partnership, Katie Beckett, Dual Eligibles, and Medicaid Benefit Redesign. At the insistence of Task Force members, however, the Medicaid Benefit Redesign was divided into two separate work groups, Acute/ Primary Care and Long-Term Care, with the latter being further divided into two subgroups, Adults/Elders and Individuals with Developmental Disabilities. At the insistence of participants, the scope of the Katie Beckett Work Group was broadened to include all children with special health care needs, while the Long-Term Care Partnership Program work group extended its purview to include private long-term care financing issues more generally.

State officials directed the Task Force's work groups to develop specific recommendations that could be pursued as budget articles, waiver changes, legislative proposals, or rule changes. Beyond this general instruction, however, there was very little charge. "Basically, the Department said, 'well, if you could do whatever you wanted do, what would you do in this area?' " according to one provider representative. "This didn't make a lot of sense, because it's not like it was a blank slate. That was frustrating to people, although I think people tried really hard; they gave their best effort." There was also tension between what members viewed as the state's imperative and, perhaps, even charge that the Task Force and its work groups focus on achieving reductions in costs, and members' desire to enact longer-term changes that might improve care quality and program efficiency. Indeed, at the very first Task Force meeting, it was announced that "all policy recommendations must be developed with financial constraints and affordability in mind" and that all should include fiscal analysis of how they would save money or achieve long-term savings if investment was required (EOHHS May 12, 2009). But although "we all know that Medicaid can be improved in different ways," explained one consumer representative, "very few things can happen quickly and save a lot of money and help people. So . . . we have ideas like over the next two, three, four years if we change the system from one way to another it would save money; people would get better care, but it's not going to save you $17 million . . . or whatever you need to save in the next two months, that's just not the way good planning happens."

Most work groups met several times before turning in reports outlining their recommendations. These reports, which were delivered in November 2009, were subsequently reviewed by state staff who did not comment on the recommendations until the end of January 2010, at which point Task Force members were provided a 31-page matrix indicating which recommendations the state might go forward with and which they had chosen not to pursue. Task Force members expressed frustration with the lack of discussion, both with regard to the work group concept itself and with regard to the recommendations that were ultimately produced. In relation to the work group concept, one consumer advocate recalled that "[the Department of Human services] actually proposed the idea of these work groups, and it was a very odd situation, because they came to a meeting and said, 'Here's what the work groups are going to be.' There was no discussion of what do we think ought to be done. It was like, 'Here's the work groups; everybody needs to sign up for a work group.' " In relation to the work group recommendations, one provider representative described it as "all very one-way. It's all very, 'Give us the information, we'll make a decision.' There's not that sort of reciprocal process." Task Force members were especially frustrated that their work group efforts seem to have been for naught. "We have no evidence, no proof that any of the work we did, any of the writing, any of the recommendations" informed implementation of the Global Waiver, according to one provider representative; a consumer advocate added that once they handed out the matrix, "it's sort of like they've moved on, like that was something they gave out last time. There was never any real discussion about what are we going to do and what are we not going to do. And in the meantime the Governor comes out with his budget, which contains cuts, and which everybody goes crazy about because they're not using the recommendations that people had made."

It was felt that community input would have been more productively translated into policy if the Task Force's work groups had been better supported by state personnel. While state staff helped set up the meetings, organizing the rooms and sending out notices, some were more helpful than others, for example, providing data and reporting about the policy areas studied. It was also felt that the Task Force's work groups would have worked better if they were tasked with giving feedback about particular Waiver-related tasks or initiatives rather than brain storming generally about specific populations. "What we really want is some work groups that are task oriented," explained one consumer advocate. "That would include state agency people and community people to really tackle some of the issues going forward, and not just sort of these broad groups." It was also felt that the Task Force's work groups would have worked better if there had been greater interaction with the state's own internal work groups. Without such interaction, "there's a danger of what I'll term 'parallel play,'" explained one executive branch official, "wherein . . . there's tremendous actual stakeholder involvement . . . but [not] in the area where the actual decisions are . . . being made."

Eleven internal work groups were formed by the Department of Human Services/EOHHS, each organized around a major task proposed in the Global Waiver agreement. Thus, for example, the state had a work group called the "Assessment and Coordination Organization" team, which was charged with implementing a smoother, easier to understand long-term care eligibility process and consisted of staff from the Departments of Human Services and Elderly Affairs and other pertinent agencies. Most Task Force members felt that "there hasn't been enough cross communication between the internal groups and the external groups." Some simply wished to be kept informed of the state's internal activities—they felt it was part of their charge. Others felt that that greater collaboration with community stakeholders was the key to successful implementation of the Global Waiver's provisions, particularly since the state did not have enough of its own staff to accomplish what needed to be done. "There are some really hard things that have to happen, and tough decisions, especially in bad budget times," explained one consumer advocate, "but when you do it together, when you do it collaboratively, you make a lot more progress. Not everybody is going to be 100 percent happy, but you can at least support each other going forward. . . . The state has what they refer to as . . . the external task force, that's us, and the internal work groups. Why aren't we working together? I don't get it."

Recognizing frustration among Task Force members, state staff issued a survey at the January 25, 2010, meeting with the goal of "being more responsive to membership concerns, issues, and topics that would make the Task Force more productive and meaningful going forward" (EOHHS January 25, 2010). However, it was not until a year and a half later, after the changeover in gubernatorial administration that newly appointed Secretary Costantino thanked Task Force members for their service and identified several changes, including appointing a community co-chair and plans to reorganize the Task Force to better integrate its work with other EOHHS initiatives, advisory bodies, work groups, and councils focusing on Medicaid issues, including the state's Health Reform Commission and subgroups (EOHHS May 23, 2011; Costantino June 23, 2011). This too was the objective of the new community co-chair, Tom Rizzo, who hoped to increase the amount of productive interaction between the Task Force and EOHHS (EOHHS November 28, 2011a). Specific proposals included making Task Force Agendas and summaries available ahead of time, more actively engaging departmental directors, inventorying all initiatives undertaken as part of the Global Waiver, and providing Task Force members opportunities to support and offer input into policy and budget initiatives in this area (EOHHS December 19, 2011).

The Task Force and Other Bodies Have Been a Useful Conduit for Stakeholder Input

Despite widespread criticism, some interviewees believed that the Task Force had worked well as a means of canvassing input from such a diverse group of stakeholder interests. Thus, one consumer advocate reported being "impressed with the degree to which the officials in the state of Rhode Island go to be inclusive with the advocacy community and providers," while a legislative staffer saw it as a "positive thing" that "they did make an effort to get a lot of different voices heard on that Task Force."

Others believed that the Department of Human Services/EOHHS has been fairly open in its communication with the stakeholder community, both at Taskforce meetings and at other venues. "I think people [have been] given an opportunity to say what their idea are," observed one state official, "I haven't seen anything that's secretive; it's been very open to that extent." "Although it's been bumpy at times," observed Maureen Maigret, Policy Director at the Senior Agenda Coalition at a March 22, 2010, legislative hearing, "there certainly has been a greater opportunity for people in the community to have a dialogue with their respective departments. . . . [This] is very much appreciated and something that needs to continue to happen if we want to have the kind of transparency that the Global Waiver talks about." It was pointed out that the Department of Human Services/EOHHS has also been very open and visible with the state legislature, "meeting with the legislature whenever those meetings were called, providing as much information as possible, trying to get clarification to them as expeditiously as necessary." In addition, state officials have met with various groups on a one-on-one basis, in addition to providing regular updates and answering questions at the Lieutenant Governor's Long-Term Care Coordinating Council.

Still others highlight payoffs deriving from the amount of work the Department of Human Services/EOHHS has devoted to gathering stakeholder input. "I would say that [EOHHS] and [the Department of Human Services] puts a lot of energy into meeting with consumer advocacy groups," observed one state official, "hearing their concerns, working with them, getting input from them to inform the process. And I think . . . our programs have benefited from it, and our clients have certainly benefited from it." For their part, state officials pointed to a few examples where they acted on recommendations made by the Task Force's work groups. These included proposed legislative changes to the state's Sherlock Plan, or Medicaid buy-in program for working adults with disabilities, that grew out of the Task Force's Employment Work Group. These also include submitting legislation to increase insurers' payment for children with special health care needs based on recommendations from the Task Force's Katie Beckett work group.

In addition to identifying a community co-chair, the role of the Task Force was reconsidered and independent evaluation results were obtained after newly elected Independent Governor Lincoln Chafee appointed

Democratic Steven Costantino as EOHHS Secretary in 2011. These decisions served, in part, to reduce stakeholder distrust and facilitate greater levels of cooperation between the broader community and program administrators. So too have concerted efforts to acquire and incorporate stakeholder input into recent program initiatives, including the state's Integrated Care Initiative, a Category II change first submitted to CMS January 2013 as part of the federal government's Financial Alignment Demonstration, and the state's request to renew the Global Waiver, which is set to expire December 31, 2013, for another five years submitted to CMS March 2013. Both proposals seemed to benefit from substantial community involvement and support. Indeed, in its Financial Alignment proposal to CMS, EOHHS reported that "[Rhode Island] Medicaid is committed to an open, transparent and accountable process with the diverse constituencies of Rhode Island stakeholders from planning through implementation of the demonstration program" (EOHHS May 31, 2013). The state held 17 meetings between September 16 and December 14, 2011, with community stakeholders to inform its draft proposal. The state then conducted two public forums and a 30-day public notice process, as per Rhode Island law, during which 178 questions and comments were received, mainly from consumer and provider constituencies (EOHHS September 22, 2012), before the final proposal was submitted to CMS on May 31, 2013. Subsequently, state decisions about procurement have been informed by three work groups—Services and Supports; Oversight, Evaluation and Continuous Improvement; and Outreach and Information—each of which met three times with substantial stakeholder involvement during the summer of 2012. During each stage, EOHHS consulted with the Global Waiver Task Force.

Community stakeholders appear to favor the changes being instituted with the Integrated Care Initiative although disagreement about certain program details remain (Flynn and Maigret June 30, 2012; Hayward February 26, 2013; Katz, Flynn, and Mulready July 1, 2012; Neighborhood Health Plan of Rhode Island February 22, 2013; Sharma and Regan June 29, 2012). There also seems to be general appreciation for state efforts to involve consumer stakeholders although concerns remain regarding the extent of beneficiary/family member engagement and the need for concrete mechanisms to ensure continuing stakeholder input over time. "We do not doubt EOHHS' commitment to stakeholder engagement and 'meaningful beneficiary input' in the planning and implementation of the Demonstration,'" wrote representatives from three major consumer advocacies—The Economic Progress Institute, Senior Agenda Coalition, and Rhode Island Disability Law Center—in a joint letter to CMS, reflecting a remarkably different tone from the Global Waiver's early days (Katz, Flynn, and Mulready July 1, 2012). "But," the letter continues, "we think it is important for CMS to ask EOHHS to spell out specifically how it will work with stakeholders and especially with beneficiaries (consumers) and their family members. . . . CMS should require EOHHS to specify what happens after [the July/June 2012 meetings], to inform CMS about the membership of work groups to ensure that consumers/family members are engaged and to plan for additional consumer input. . . . We also think it is important that EOHHS establish a stakeholder advisory group that will work with the state on an on-going basis . . ."

In seeking to renew the Global Waiver, Rhode Island has explicitly followed the new rules and time frame promulgated by CMS under provisions contained within the Affordable Care Act meant to increase transparency and community participation in the waiver design and approval process. From January 18 to March 1, 2013, three public meetings were held and opportunities for public comment provided after which responses to nearly 125 questions and comments from 25 groups, mainly consumer and provider advocacies, were submitted and the Waiver renewal application revised in light of the comments received before submittal to CMS (EOHHS January 18, 2013, March 18, 2013, March 2013). Furthermore, according to EOHHS, the work of the Global Waiver Task Force, Medical Care Advisory Committee, Integrated Care Initiative work groups, and Consumer Advisory Committee[3] informed the state's draft renewal proposal and eventual submission to CMS (EOHHS March 18, 2013). Public comments on the state's draft proposal demonstrate agreement with the general provisions of the renewal (EOHHS March 18, 2013). Thus, for example, Linda Katz (March 1, 2013), a former critic of the Global Waiver Task in its original incarnation, key member of the Global Waive Task Force, and Policy Director of The Economic Progress Institute (formerly The Poverty Institute) reported that "we believe that the Extension request includes many proposals that will improve access to appropriate health care for Medicaid participants by addressing the complex needs of low-income populations and promoting quality-based services for people who require long-term services and supports. The proposal will ensure that federal and state investments are used efficiently to promote the purposes of the Medicaid program."

Public comments on the state's draft renewal proposal further demonstrate agreement with the role community stakeholders played in developing specific provisions (EOHHS March 18, 2013). Thus, "[w]hile [the Rhode Island Health Center Association] was initially concerned about the implementation of the Global Waiver here in Rhode Island," reported its President and CEO and former EOHHS Secretary Jane Hayward (February 26, 2013), "many of those concerns were formed due to the lack of information and public process around the development of the Global Waiver. The state has instituted a much improved process. In this application, community input and suggestions are already reflected in several of the proposed initiatives. It is our hope and expectation that this current round of hearings and written comments will lead to further strengthening and improvements of a waiver renewal application that starts off in a very good place." Some, however, expressed concern that the state did not include a provision in the extension request committing itself to continuing the Global Waiver Implementation Task Force or some other form of obtaining systematic community input during the five-year waiver extension period. One suggestion was to reimage the Global Waiver Implementation Task Force as the state's Medical Care Advisory Committee, organized into three subcommittees focused on children and families (including children with special health care needs), adults (including seniors and childless adults), and adults with disabilities (Katz March 1, 2013).

INTERSECTOR COOPERATION

Traditional Relations Across Population Sectors: Still Siloed

Several different populations can qualify for public assistance, including children, the elderly, physically disabled adults, the developmentally disabled, and the mentally ill. These populations have typically been cared for by separate systems and, as such, have developed very different traditions about how they have been funded and served. Not surprisingly, therefore, advocates and providers networks representing different populations have focused on their own particular interests as they compete for scarce resources. Some observers believe that these silos have largely remained intact since implementation on the Global Waiver began. "Out in the community the provider network is still siloed," explained one executive branch official, "and there's still divisions. . . . I don't think we've broken those walls down as we've tried to put reform in place." "[Different populations are] still [pitted against one another]," added another state official. "Advocates and providers know what they know and they generally do not know what's going on outside of the little area in which they operate. Even when they were talking to each other, they were talking past each other."

Waiver Promotes a Broader Perspective and Cooperation

Despite remaining divisions, a number of interviewees perceived greater cooperation among provider and advocacy groups representing different populations and service modalities. This has been driven, in part, by the perceived need to unite provider and advocacy interests in light of the changing needs of the populations served. A prime example is the developmentally disabled population which, because they are starting to live longer, is increasingly requiring aging-related services. "Things are sort of converging in terms of where these people fall," explained one provider representative. "Some of these [Behavioral Healthcare, Developmental Disabilities, and Hospitals] providers, they're almost like assisted living now, since the populations are that old. . . . The Homestead Group, which is a big provider up in Woonsocket that does the groups homes and . . . cares for the real developmentally disabled population, [is] opening an adult day center in their facility, initially to care for their own clients as they age but also . . . other populations. . . . So I think there's going to be more convergence."

Increased cooperation has also been driven by the program-wide scope of the Global Waiver. Through participation on the Global Waiver Implementation Task Force, individuals representing different groups have joined together and, in so doing, acquired a broader perspective than if the conversation focused exclusively on their own populations. "For the first time, you have a very diverse, extremely large group," reported one state official. "You have a real combination of providers as well as other advocates really at the table trying to deal with the whole Waiver implementation . . . in the same room listening to the same language, and the same reporting mechanism. It really helps in the broader perspective of any conversation that takes place related to services for any population." Thus, it was felt that participation at both Task Force and work group meetings had promoted dialogue and increased understanding and awareness among different types of providers and advocates.

A broader perspective has also arisen due to participation in the Coalition for Responsible Medicaid Reform. In short, the Coalition is a largely informal group that has served as a clearinghouse for information and grievances and convener where providers and advocates impacted by the Global Waiver can come together to analyze information coming out of the departments and develop strategies with which to influence the direction of state policy in this area. As such, it has "[served in] something of a watchdog capacity," according to one Coalition member, "to kind of make sure that individual consumers and families are considered at each step of the process, because, as a collective, we felt that wasn't happening." It was reported that traditionally, provider and advocacy groups representing different populations rarely spoke with one another. The Global Waiver, however, provided an impetus to bring people together across the spectrum that serve and advocate for children, seniors, and adults with disabilities. The melding together of the stakeholder community in the Coalition was, perhaps, one of the unintended consequences of the Global Waiver. "It was good for the advocates and the providers," reported one provider representative, "[that] they created this kind of loosely assembled group that made them acknowledge that they are all a piece of this Medicaid pie. Instead of having the [developmentally disabled] people against the kids or against the old people in the nursing homes, there was some semblance of putting us all together at the same table."

FISCAL AND BUDGETARY CONSTRAINTS

Waiver Implementation Driven by Fiscal and Budgetary Environment

It was widely recognized that implementation, like development of the Global Waiver, has been driven primarily by the fiscal and budget environment prevailing within the state. Indeed, a dominant and recurring theme was the effect of the fiscal crisis on Medicaid, which has enhanced the focus on cost control, limited the amount of state dollars available for the program, and made it difficult to distinguish Waiver-driven changes from budget-driven changes. The latter, in particular, is reflected in proposals to substantially reduce reimbursement for certain hospitals and to lower overall funding for the nursing home sector while adopting a new methodology for paying providers. "I'm not sure if those are results of the Global Waiver," explained one consumer advocate, "or just the fiscal situation we're in." And "the General Assembly . . . in their desire to have a balanced budget," explained another consumer advocate, "[doesn't] have any other solution [but to] say, 'Okay.' "

Regardless of their proximate causes, changes such as these led most of the provider representatives and consumer advocates interviewed to conclude that decisions made under the Global Waiver have been weighted more heavily toward cutting costs rather than on achieving savings and improving care through programmatic improvements such as rebalancing. One interviewee pointed out, for example, that 42% of the savings documented by [the Department of Human Services] in its 2010 budget derived from rebalancing long-term care as compared to 58% that derived from cuts in provider rates and administrative costs. Said one provider representative, "I'm not quite sure how we're going to achieve the goals that are stated from the outset. . . . The deficit we're facing in Rhode Island definitely impacts on opportunities that we as a state might be able to recognize under the Waiver if circumstances were better." Said a consumer representative, "it's all about the money. . . . What the state is doing is squeezing money out of Medicaid."

In addition to lowering hospital and nursing home reimbursements, specific proposals and initiatives cited both in the interviews and other sources include: generating savings through re-procurement of all managed care contracts at lower rates; precluding those deemed "high" need on the state's new level of care assessment instrument from accessing nursing home care although they may have done so previously; reducing dental coverage; adopting a generics-first pharmaceutical benefit policy; reducing spending on behavioral health services; redesigning the state's developmental disability system; restricting the number of emergency room visits; increasing beneficiary cost-sharing; and rolling back parent eligibility under RIte Care (EOHHS 2013; Holahan and Rifkin February 2012; Peoples March 20, 2009; EOHHS December 21, 2009; Department of Human Services January 2010; Liberman June 2010; EOHHS June 28, 2010; Gregg and Marcelo June 7, 2011; Marcelo August 26, 2011). Examples also include delaying planned reimbursement increases for community-based providers and forgoing a planned $400 increase in the amount of monthly income beneficiaries could keep to help pay for housing, transportation, and other costs necessary to remain in the community. The latter, in particular, was a prime example of what many perceived to be a small short-term investment that could have considerable long-term consequences in terms of reductions in nursing home placement. But it was not implemented because, as one consumer advocate explained, "the state is in such dire need of money."

Consumer advocates also highlighted what they perceived to be subtle "backdoor" efforts to restrain spending, including slower application processing speeds and reductions in the number of service hours authorized (Liberman June 2010). "What's happening," one consumer advocate asserted, "is that because of the state budget crisis people are slower to get services and sort of, again, the state is just trying to save money, so it's not acting on applications as quickly as previously, and we lack information about the scope of services that people are getting." Several reported that it was taking longer for people with developmental disabilities to receive community services while children previously eligible for Katie Beckett services were being disqualified upon recertification. Advocates recognized, however, that these perceptions were anecdotal and that state officials would deny that any formal changes in state policy had taken place to encourage such behavior on the part of program administrators.

While state officials admit that "the budget gap . . . has] taken precedent over everything else at this point in time," they also assert that efforts were made to maintain quality, eligibility, and service levels to the extent possible given the state's very challenging budgetary situation. This has also been the observation of some outside observers who reports that "yes, the department could have just charged ahead and said we don't care, but they haven't been that callous. . . . They've at least sat down and discussed the issues. . . . They haven't rushed forward just to save dollars." One example cited by Craig Stenning, Director of the State's Behavioral Healthcare, Developmental Disabilities, and Hospitals Department, at a March 15, 2010, legislative hearing, is the continuation of work begun under the state's developmental disability waiver. "I firmly believe that some of the changes that we're making will result in a better system," Stenning reported, "a more transparent system, and a better level of care for individuals. If we were doing that without attempting to achieve savings, this would be a piece of excellent work. Unfortunately, we are doing it under the umbrella of attempting also to provide a savings target that, yes, has presented a lot of stress both to the community and for our own staff, as well." The intersection of fiscal with programmatic considerations will continue to be at the forefront of state decision making for the foreseeable future. "One of the explicit reasons the State pursued the original waiver was to rein in spending on the Medicaid program," EOHHS explains in its application to renew the Global Waiver for another five years. "In the four years of implementation of the current 1115 waiver, there has not been significant change in Rhode Island's economic outlook. . . . The need to reform the Medicaid program so that it is a cost-effective and sustainable investment still exists."

Federal Stimulus and Health Reform Legislation

The federal stimulus package adopted under the American Recovery and Reinvestment Act (ARRA) of 2009 provided states with significantly enhanced federal fiscal support which, in the case of Rhode Island, reduced the state's Medicaid contributions from 47.43% to 36.11% of program costs from October 1, 2008, through December 31, 2010, subsequently extended through June 30, 2011, though at somewhat lower levels, thereby increasing federal contributions by a total of $523 million during this time period (Cross-Call and Solomon March 16, 2012). Interestingly, there was some concern that Rhode Island might not be eligible for the enhanced federal fiscal support provided under the ARRA despite Governor Carcieri's initial claims that the Global Waiver would not preclude state participation in a federal stimulus (Anonymous February 18, 2009; Peoples January 29, 2009, February 4, 2009, February 12, 2009). In order to be eligible for additional federal matching dollars, states could not adopt more stringent eligibility requirements than those existing as of July 1, 2008.[4] However, the state had delayed implementation of a previously negotiated and federally approved change in program eligibility until September 29 of that year, thereby making it potentially ineligible for federal stimulus money. Rhode Island nonetheless remained eligible because the state's senior Senator, Jack Reed, inserted language into the ARRA stating that a state implementing a change in eligibility after July 1 could still receive the enhanced match as long as the change in question was in process before that date.

The ARRA helped reduce advocates' fears about the Global Waiver (Prah May 11, 2010). They particularly appreciated the stimulus' eligibility provisions which, according to state Medicaid Director, Elena Nicolella (October 22, 2012), "have negatively impacted the flexibility anticipated." "Well, the main thing that the ARRA funding has done is to protect the state from rolling back eligibility for parents," reported one consumer representative, "and implementing the premiums in the RIte Care program, because I'm 100 percent certain that if the ARRA hadn't been in effect the state this year would have [done so] since they've done it in less severe fiscal times." "All I can say is thank goodness for the federal stimulus package," added another consumer advocate, "because if we didn't have these federal requirements, what's called the MOE, the Maintenance of Effort requirements, I think RIte Care would be sliced and diced in a million ways to Sunday by now, and luckily health care reform also put in MOEs beyond what the stimulus MOEs are." Indeed, the number of Medicaid eligibles has increased considerably during the course of Global Waiver implementation, from 181,288 in July 2009 to 199,139 in December 2012, due largely to increases in the state's unemployment rate (Department of Human Services January 2010–February 2013). Most growth in Medicaid enrollment derived from increases in the number of parents and children in the program, from 119,448 to 133,037 during this time period.

The emphasis on restraining spending continued after the January 4, 2011 changeover in gubernatorial administration from Republican Carcieri to Independent Chafee. Once federal stimulus funding expired, for example, the Department of Human Services/EOHHS sought to increase cost-sharing to a full 5% of income for RIte Care parents with incomes over 150% of the FPL and to adopt premiums of 3% of income for RIte Care parents between 133% and 150% of the FPL, with the aim of achieving $670,000 in general revenue savings (Marcelo August 26, 2011). Although these changes were included in the Global Waiver's Special Terms and Conditions and previously authorized by the Rhode Island General Assembly (Weens January 16, 2009), they were put on hold due to the federal stimulus. Subsequently, in order to make these changes, state officials needed to first obtain permission from the General Assembly—increasing premiums and cost sharing are considered to be Category II changes, and then, from CMS. Ultimately, CMS rejected the state's plans as violations of the Maintenance of Effort provisions contained within the Affordable Care Act.[5] The state, however, was able to reduce spending on this population through its managed care re-procurement process where RIte Care was combined into a single contract with Rhody Health Partners, with the goal of reducing spending 6% or $42 million over the previous contract (EOHHS February 22, 2010). Through re-procurement, the state also sought to impose Communities of Care for beneficiaries with complex care needs.

Overall, additional federal financing provided under the ARRA helped to support caseload increases resulting from the recession while, perhaps, ameliorating the state's emphasis on restraining program spending and giving it time to prepare administratively for changes planned under the Global Waiver. Indeed, the ARRA saved the state $148 million and $207 million, respectively, in state FY 2009 and FY 2010 (EOHHS June 2011). "In general, the enhanced FMAP delayed or prevented the need to make some really, really tough decisions," explained one state official. "It allowed us to go forward and do some things with implementation, because there was an influx of money coming in where we may have [otherwise have] been in a position where we were reacting to the deficit. A lot of best made plans get tumbled when we get, 'come up with $90 million,' you know?" Explained another state official, "I don't think the Waiver would have worked without the federal Medicaid enhancement and stimulus . . . because in order to do the rebalancing that needed to happen, that's like 18 months to two years' worth of just internal work about redesigning programs, retraining-recruiting staff." There was significant concern about what would happen once the additional federal support provided by the stimulus expired (Marcelo December 15, 2010). "The state is now in a place where it used to contributing very little money to programs," argued a provider representative, "so we're concerned about what that's going to mean . . ."

Like Medicaid, Governor Chafee and members of his administration have expressed strong commitment to health care reform and the Affordable Care Act. This is reflected in creation of the Rhode Island Healthcare Reform Commission led by the Lieutenant Governor (chair), who, as a Democratic and strong proponent of reform, was left out of most decision making in the prior Republican administration, in addition to the health insurance commissioner, EOHHS secretary, governor's policy director, and director of the Department of Administration. It is also reflected in establishment of the state's health insurance exchange through executive order. Rhode Island has made substantial progress toward getting its exchange up and running. The state successfully competed for a federal planning grant ($1.00 million) and level-one establishment award ($5.24 million). It was also the first state to qualify for a three-year $58.51 million level-two establishment award (Holahan and Rifkin February 2012). Not only is the Governor committed to taking advantage of favorable federal matching incentives to expand Medicaid coverage for all Rhode Islanders up to 138% of the FPL, including childless adults, the main population currently not covered by the state's Medicaid program, but EOHHS has sought to take advantage of favorable federal financial incentives within the federal health care reform law to, for example, facilitate state rebalancing efforts, improve the state's data and information processing infrastructure, and integrate care for Medicaid beneficiaries who are also eligible for Medicare.

Federal Cap Has Been a Non-Issue

Rhode Island was not in danger of losing its federal Medicaid match despite initial fears that it might exceed the targeted amount agreed upon with the federal government. At $1.76 billion during the Waiver's first demonstration year (calendar year 2009), the state had spent $842.66 million less than its $2.60 billion expenditure target (Department of Human Services January 2010–February 2013). The same is true for 2010, 2011, and 2012. At $1.86 billion in 2010, the state spent $537.88 million less than the $2.40 billion federal cap. At $1.84 and $1.78 billion in 2011 and 2012, respectively, the state spent $459.48 and $618.99 million less than the $2.30 and $2.40 billion targets imposed. So far, Medicaid spending in Rhode Island has come in $2.46 billion under the cap during the Waiver's first four years (Total Cap: $9.70 billion; Total Expenditures: $7.24 billion). Especially in the current fiscal climate, the limiting factor has been the level of state appropriations and spending; there is just no way the state can come up with enough of its own funding to exceed the federal cap. "You have to remember under the cap our Medicaid expenditures are driven by state spending," explained one state official, "and we just knew the state didn't have the money. . . . The way general revenue was moving, even if things had improved substantially, we knew we weren't going to hit the cap, and we knew we had a fiscal and an administrative cushion because of the incoming CNOM."

This cushion also derived from overly generous assumptions regarding the rate of program growth. The state's expenditure target was based on a five-year average, trended forward on the basis of expected enrollment and utilization increases. One reason that actual spending levels have been so much lower than projected levels is that the trend factor used did not take into account the actual levels of spending the state would experience due to the prevailing fiscal crisis. Another reason is that the state purposefully built in a substantial amount of leeway into its projections. "Rhode Island is well within its budget protection," one state official explained. "We built in a caseload growth factor in the vicinity of 6.5%. . . . We thought we'd be within 4 points on a real basis, but we wanted to put on some cushioning there, because of the unemployment. . . . [So we] thought we had enough money and it's shown itself out now. . . . The number [in the revised waiver application was $12.9 billion] over a five year period—we're trending right now to spend $10 billion. . . . We didn't want to sign a deal if we thought we were going to lose money."

Both provider representatives and consumer advocates recognized that fear about the spending cap had been somewhat over blown (Pugh June 12, 2011; Cross-Call and Solomon March 22, 2011). This is reflected in statements such as "the cap is really not a cap . . . the cap is like star wars. . . . I mean they couldn't spend $12 billion if they tried in five years"; "in hindsight, some of the good news is it looks like the cap that the state was able to negotiate with CMS will be sufficiently high"; and "the federal cap is so high that it's almost a red herring. It provided an opportunity for everybody to stand up and say there's a cap on the federal dollars, but the likelihood of getting there was slim and none. There are not enough state dollars to ever reach that cap." Indeed, the state has asked CMS to remove the cap in its March 2013 request to extend the Global Waiver through December 31, 2018 because state officials believe that the "federal funding cap's specific value and impact to Rhode Island's Medicaid spending . . . has been minimal" (EOHHS March 2013). Removing the cap provision is strongly favored by community stakeholders (Beckwith March 1, 2013; Haward February 26, 2013; Katz March 1, 2013; Maigret March January 28, 2013; Mulready February 28, 2013; Spears February 15, 2013).

SUMMARY

Because the oversight committee has never been formed, state administrators have lacked clear mechanisms for obtaining state legislative approval for making desired changes. Moreover, most stakeholders have not been satisfied with the way the Global Waiver Implementation Task Force has been administered, at least early on. Because the Task Force has not served as a useful conduit for public input, it has not had much influence on the way in which the Department of Human Services/EOHHS has implemented the Global Waiver's provisions. The Task Force is too large and cumbersome. The dialogue tends to be one-way, with state officials dominating the proceedings. Community-leadership has nearly been absent; indeed, a community co-chair was not appointed until two and a half years after implementation of the Global Waiver began. There has also been a lack of perceived responsiveness to the Task Force's recommendations. Greater support by state administrative personnel and greater integration with ongoing implementation efforts within the Department of Human Services/EOHHS were deemed critical for increasing the effectiveness of the Task Force's role. Despite criticisms such as these, some believe that Department of Human Services/EOHHS had done a good job canvassing stakeholder input, both at Task Force meetings and other venues. It seems that state officials did a much better job at incorporating stakeholder input once new leadership took over the reins of state government.

Several patient populations cared for by different service delivery systems rely on Medicaid. This has resulted in competition for scarce program resources among the provider and advocacy groups that represent them. Whereas some believe that silos across population sectors have remained largely intact, most observe increased cross-sector cooperation since the Global Waiver was designed and implemented. This has been driven, in part, by the changing needs of the populations served (e.g., the aging of people with developmental disabilities). It has also been driven by the program-wide scope of the Global Waiver. This is reflected in participation in both formal and informal entities through which a variety of different perspectives could be heard and common interests identified and acted upon.

There is general agreement that decisions made under the Global Waiver have been driven largely by the adverse fiscal and budgetary environment facing the state. As a consequence, the emphasis has largely been weighted toward controlling costs rather than achieving savings and improving care through programmatic changes. The provision of hundreds of millions of dollars in federal stimulus money, however, helped the state support caseload increases resulting from rising unemployment levels while softening the state's emphasis on reducing spending and providing it with some breathing room vis-à-vis implementation of the Global Waiver's provisions. That the state had to maintain eligibility levels at July 1, 2008, levels to qualify for federal stimulus support, a provision since extended by the federal health reform law, has also helped to ameliorate stakeholder concern regarding the Waiver's impact on the populations served. So, too, has been recognition that the state would not come close to losing its federal match as a result of exceeding the funding cap agreed upon with the federal government. This was both because of the generosity of the funding cap itself and because the level of state appropriations and spending were simply not high enough to exceed the cap due to the current fiscal climate.

NOTES

1. RI 2009-H 5112 Substitute C.
2. This pertinent provision of the oversight statute is as follows: "There are distinct populations that receive services funded through the Medicaid program including: children and youth with special health care needs, adults and children with developmental disabilities, adults with serious and persistent mental illness and/or addiction disorders and children with severe emotional disturbance, adults with disabilities, adults age sixty-five (65) and older and low-income children and families. It is the intent of the general assembly that the taskforce includes members who are knowledgeable about the needs of these populations and the services currently provided to them. Members of the taskforce shall be appointed by director of the department of human services. The membership shall include: for each distinct population two consumers or family members of consumers, one member of an advocacy organization and one member of a policy organization; a representative from organizations that either provide or represent entities that provide services to Medicaid beneficiaries including, but not limited to, health plans, hospitals, community health centers, community mental health organizations, licensed substance abuse treatment providers, licensed health care practitioners, nursing facilities, and home and community-based service providers."
3. The state's Consumer Advisory Committee meets six times per year. It focuses mainly on Medicaid managed care programs for children and families, children with special health care needs, and children in foster care.
4. This was also true of the Medicaid provisions included within the Patient Protection and Affordable Care Act of 2010.
5. The Affordable Care Act requires that states maintain current income eligibility levels through 2014 for adults and 2019 for children.

6 Internal Factors and Implementation

The need to manage the Global Waiver Implementation Task Force has posed challenges for state officials. These challenges have arisen, in part, because distrust generated during the design of the Global Waiver has continued through the implementation process even though those state officials working directly with Task Force members were not necessarily the same as those who designed the Global Waiver. As one provider representative pointed out, "some of the people who are currently involved in trying to operate the Task Force and do some other things, they were not involved in this process of doing the waiver, so a lot of them are suffering the disappointment, and unhappiness, and resentment of people when they had nothing to do with the original process to begin with. They're living with this pain of the past, and the sins of the past." State administrative personnel are also, in some ways, living with the sins of the present to the extent that they are blamed for decisions over which they have no control. "One of the things that we've really struggled with," reported one state official, "is their recommendations come through, we may have put together a piece of legislation or a budget article, but we don't have the final say. . . . It goes to the Governor's Office and to the Budget Office, and ultimately, we lose control, and we can't even tell you what we were pursuing."

Challenges managing the Global Waiver Implementation Task Force have also arisen, in part, because state agencies can only do so much given the amount of time, energy, skills, and staff available to get things done. "We're not using the Task Force as well as we could," admitted one state official. "It's a huge drag to meet these people every month; I mean, it's hard, because you have to stop your work. . . . We also have to have staff supporting each one of [the work] groups in addition to doing their own jobs, and trying to carry on, on a day-to-day basis." Minutes from a June 28, 2010, Task Force meeting reported that the state Medicaid Director, Elena Nicolella, expressed concern about the numerous projects state staff members were involved in and, as such, there would need to be some restraints on their Task Force-related activities given internal matters that also required their attention (EOHHS June 28, 2010). It did not help that the state's human service agencies had recently lost hundreds of key personnel. In light of challenges deriving from prevailing resource limitations, this chapter examines internal factors that have influenced implementation of the Global Waiver. This includes the state's capacity to successfully administer the Waiver, both due to the number of experienced administrative personnel and due to the presence of the requisite data and informational architecture. It is also with respect to the amount of coordination that has taken place across the state's administrative agencies.

ADMINISTRATIVE PERSONNEL

Inadequate Numbers of Experienced State Personnel

Concerns that Rhode Island lacked the administrative experience and staff to properly execute the Global Waiver were considerable (Trapp November 17, 2008; The Lewin Group December 2008; Needham and Gregg December 23, 2008; Anonymous February 18, 2009; Reed et al. January 13, 2009; Peoples February 2, 2009, February 4, 2009, March 3, 2009; McKay and Nyberg February 9, 2009; Woodcock February 28, 2010). In particular, the state's capacity was questioned due to the loss of significant numbers of experienced state administrative personnel. Thus, interviewees reported that "they don't have a lot of resources to actually get things done, so it's tough for them" (consultant); "if you look at the numbers of people that were available a couple of years ago to what's available now, it's pretty frightening" (consumer advocate); "because of all the staff cuts that we've had in all the different agencies, I don't know if there's enough people that have the expertise to implement the Global Waiver the way it was meant to be" (consumer advocate); and "we had very serious concerns with the ability of the administration to implement any of it, they had absolutely no staff" (legislative staff). Between July 1 and December 31, 2008, the Department of Human Services lost 101 workers, or 11% of its employees; the Department of Behavioral Healthcare, Developmental Disabilities, and Hospitals, 209 workers (14.4%); the Department of Elderly Affairs, 10 workers (30%); the Department of Children, Youth, and Family Services, 63 workers (8.8%); and the Department of Health, 43 workers (10.5%) (Peoples February 2, 2009).

This reduction in state personnel was due, in part, to changes in the state's retirement system adopted with the expressed aim of reducing the size of the state's workforce (Gregg October 1, 2008). This was driven both by Governor's Carcieri's ideological belief in smaller state government and by the exigencies of the state's budget crisis. Essentially, it was mandated that anyone who did not retire by a certain date would have to pay 20% of their retiree health insurance premiums. Those who did retire, however, could still retain the benefit entirely at the state's expense. Thus, explained one provider representative, "we've had dramatic reductions in the state employee workforce. There have been huge retirement changes that have seen people leave in droves. I think that depleted manpower has certainly affected the state's ability to implement some provisions of the Waiver." This was true not only with respect to central administrative personnel but also frontline staff who interface with individual beneficiaries and providers, including trained nurses and social workers capable of handling eligibility assessment, case management, and other functions.

The prevailing lack of state administrative personnel has been reinforced by EOHHS' heavy reliance on consultants. It was reported that state officials had brought in consulting firms such as ACS, EDS, and Maximus to provide expertise that did not exist within the state's administrative apparatus and to help manage programs such as RIte Care. This public-private partnership "continued to grow and grow until the point where," according to one state official, "[these firms were] involved with program management, policy development, payment method supports" and grant writing. Some felt that both EOHHS and its constituent departments had become so reliant on consultants that it lacked the staff and expertise necessary to perform some functions on its own. "The Medicaid agency is incredibly heavily reliant on consultants," explained another state official. "Without the consultants the staff is dead in the water. Over time they've become infantilized with just giving stuff to the consultants."

The extant shortage in state staff has been exacerbated by prevailing fiscal and budgetary conditions with rising caseloads stretching existing resources and revenue reductions slowing down the rate of new hires, which have not kept up with projections (Peoples February 2, 2009). While increased demand for Medicaid has placed greater burdens on existing resources, disincentives to spend limited state dollars on additional administrative personnel have impeded implementation of the Global Waiver. "With the state of the economy being what it is," explained one state official, "and the state a little reluctant to put additional admin money out there, I think [the Departments of Human Services, Elderly Affairs, and Mental Health, Retardation, and Hospitals] have been [unable to bring] additional staffing on," even though "maybe a dozen people in key positions at certain points . . . could help move the agenda" forward. The state has had trouble filling both old and new positions necessary to implement the Global Waiver (Peoples February 2, 2009). Thus, at the time of the interviews, neither the Department of Human Services' new Office of Community Programs, which is responsible for care coordination for medically complex high-costs cases, nor its new Office of Medical Review, which reviews and processes clinical levels of eligibility, had been fully staffed up. Eventually, however, the state made some progress, eventually completing the necessary hiring in priority areas such as these.

The widely reported shortage in administrative personnel has increased stress among remaining staff, hampering their ability to complete day-to-day functions, let alone the added burdens associated with the Waiver, including presenting, taking, and incorporating feedback from community partners. "People are overwhelmed," explained one provider representative. "I think that anybody that's been there for any length of time is being asked to do a wide range of activity, some of which they have no expertise in, and they're kind of dancing as fast as they can to catch up, but that's very hard." The necessity of having to manage a normal workload in addition to the increased demands associated with the Global Waiver largely explains why (a) state staff do not feel that members of the Global Waiver Implementation Task Force appreciate all of the work that they have devoted to implementing the Global Waiver, at the same time that (b) Task Force members feel that state staff have either neglected their input or failed to set up a process whereby it could be usefully integrated with the state's own efforts. The loss of institutional knowledge was a particular concern for some interviewees. One department, for example, was tasked with introducing an entirely new financing methodology for certain groups of providers, but there was no one on staff with experience adopting new payment systems. The result, one provider representative reported, was "people being to the wall with their work at the state level, and it's made everybody testy, it really has. The level of stress out there is huge."

It is largely due to concerns about staff shortages and inexperience that there was controversy about whether the Department of Human Services should take over the state's nursing home transition program, which had been operated by the Alliance for Better Long-Term Care. At a March 15, 2010, legislative hearing, the state's Medicaid Director, Elena Nicolella, admitted that the Alliance had done a fine job transitioning around 100 persons from nursing homes to the community about a year into their 18-month contract with the state. However, the state made the decision that beginning July 1, 2010, the Department of Human Services' Office of Community Programs would be charged with this task. Two reasons were specified for this change in policy. First, the Department of Human Services believed that they could administer the program at half the cost of the Alliance's $550,000 contract. Second, the Department of Human Services believed that administering the program entirely within the state bureaucracy would result in a more streamlined process capable of more effective care coordination than under the system where cases must be handed from Alliance to state control 30 days after someone had transitioned back into the community.

The state's ombudsman, Kathleen Heren, Executive Director at the Alliance, took issue with the state's claims. At the same March 15, 2010, hearing, she argued that the Alliance's contract included the start-up fees necessary to get the program up and running and, as such, it could now run the program at about $264,000 per year, close to the same price that the state was claiming. She pointed out how effectively the Alliance ran the program, with only two failed transitions to date; one because the patient could not afford the state's co-payment, the other because the patient had died due to congestive heart failure. She also pointed out that Alliance personnel were always available to assist transferees, conduct follow-up, and help move transferees back into the nursing home if necessary, even after the 30-day transition period expired. She further expressed concern that while the state had indeed hired long-term care nurses to perform this function, none of these individuals had experience discharging nursing home residents, including helping them make the right choices given their circumstances and available resources. Other stakeholders were also concerned about whether the state would have the requisite resources to implement the nursing home transition program successfully. It was pointed out, for example, that the Office of Community Programs was only recently established and had new personnel with other significant responsibilities on their plates. This, indeed, was a primary concern of two Rhode Island State Senators. At the March 15 hearing, Democratic Senator Juan Pirchardo reported being "concerned about . . . not putting a lot of additional burden on staff that's already stretched out," whereas Democratic Senator Charles Levesque reported that the state's intention to take over the transition program "creates confusion in me because I still know people over at [the Department of Human Services] and I know that they are high level of stress. I know that they don't have the personnel necessary to do day-to-day functioning."

It was also recognized that there were limits to the number of individuals that could be transferred out of nursing homes no matter who ran the program. First, you cannot transfer someone who does not want to transfer. Second, you cannot transfer people who have had one or more failed placements. Third, you cannot transfer somebody who may be at risk within the community, either because they might be provided insufficient services and supports, including unpaid family care, or have alcohol, substance abuse, or other problems that auger against successful placement. Fourth, it was inevitable that the number of potential transferees would decline over time after what Senator Levesque referred to as the "low hanging fruit, people who actually perhaps should not be there," have been transitioned out.

Insufficiently Experienced Leadership Within the State

Some interviewees expressed concern that while prior state agency leadership had significant experience with Medicaid and a long history of working with provider and advocacy organizations, some—though not all—of the new leadership had little experience with Medicaid populations or working in partnership with the community. It was reported that large numbers of long-time senior employees had left because of the retirement changes implemented. The result, according to one provider representative, was that "the brain trust, the historical knowledge within Medicaid, the people who knew how Medicaid ran in Rhode Island were all gone." Thus, a major concern was how could significant changes reconfiguring the way in which the Medicaid program operated be proposed without the leadership necessary to implement those changes. Rhode Island's Acting Medicaid director, Frank Spinelli retired in 2008 in the midst of the Waiver application process. It was a year before the position was permanently filled again in August of 2009. Consider the comments of another provider representative: "There were big changes where [former acting Medicaid Director] Frank Spinelli had sort of started it and then he retired, because they had that whole state retirement sort of fiasco in the middle of it, where all their senior people all retired. Certainly the Department of Human Services has said that they've had some difficulties with staffing, and Elena Nicolella is the new Medicaid Director, it's just she's so bright and energetic, but you just wonder how much one person can do, you know?"

In the meantime, leadership at EOHHS and the Department of Human Services was shifting. Temporary deputy directors were appointed whose experience and qualifications with Medicaid populations was questioned. Rhode Island advocates also noted that the new head of EOHHS, Gary Alexander, did not have a background in Medicaid, which was also concerning. In particular, it was felt that some of the senior staff put in charge of the process, including then EOHHS Secretary Alexander, "didn't know that there was a deep history of working together with advocates in the state in these different [health and human services] areas," nor knew "how to work with the people that were doing it, and become partners with them, rather than just go ahead and do what you want and not ask until it's all over." Indeed, it seemed that adoption of the top-down strategy taken on the part of agency leadership to designing and implementing the Global Waiver did more than anything else to alienate potential allies and to engender opposition among the stakeholder community.

INTERAGENCY COORDINATION

Divided Responsibility for Medicaid Across Departments Still Poses Challenges

As noted earlier, development and implementation of a uniform, coherent policy affecting Medicaid has been inhibited by administration of the program across five separate EOHHS departments. This dynamic has been compounded by the uncertain role of the Health and Human Services Secretariat, which lacks formal administrative and budgetary authority over the five constituent departments ostensibly under its auspices. Although some believe that relationships among the various departments have improved somewhat under the Waiver, most, including The Lewin Group (December 2008) in its *Administrative and Staffing Recommendations for Implementing the Global Compact* report, and the Hilltop Institute in its *Resource Mapping* report (Woodcock et al. February 28, 2010), identify continued challenges associated with these arrangements. "[The waiver] certainly does provide a framework for a truly integrated coordinated system of care," reported one state official, "but the institutional structures don't allow for that, and unless that changes, we will not be in a position where we can ultimately [get as far as we would like to go]." Thus, while the directors of the various departments were certainly interested in receiving additional federal funding through the state's Costs Not Otherwise Matchable (CNOM) authority, they continue to resist having their policies and budgets changed under the Waiver's provisions. "You have separate directors who do have their separate authority," explained another state official, "and [the state's] ability to hold other entities accountable for how they spend those Medicaid dollars is always going to be an issue, because the money and the policy from the perspective of the Directors is in their own domain."

A continuing lack of clarity regarding the role of EOHHS remains the primary obstacle to greater interdepartmental coordination. This is especially true of the Medicaid program which, while formally sitting in the Department of Human Services at the time the interviews were conducted, funds programs in other departments. As reported, EOHHS was created, in part, to address fragmentation resulting from this arrangement. But there has been a great deal of pushback. "Functionally, the Secretary has authority over all of them," reported one state official, "but in reality . . . the scope of the Secretary is largely a function of how much support you have in the Governor's Office, or from the legislature, and that's variable; it depends on the issue, almost." It was pointed out that even in situations where a director wanted to move their department in a direction contrary to the goals of the Global Waiver, there would be little, if any recourse for the Secretary's Office to move them in a different direction. Thus, although the goals of the Global Waiver tended to align with the goals of most directors, particularly with regard to maintaining beneficiaries in the least restrictive settings possible, such alignment need not have been case. "Quite frankly," added another state official, "all of these directors didn't want to let their stuff go. . . . Politically, this was a very difficult consolidation to do and we never really pulled it off."

Beginning July 1, 2011, EOHHS became the Single State Medicaid Agency within which the Medicaid program is officially housed. This entailed relocating key administrative and policymaking staff of Rhode Island's Medicaid program from the Department of Human Services to EOHHS, in addition to most Medicaid funds previously allocated to that Department (Chafee 2011). Although this change should provide EOHHS with greater authority to coordinate Medicaid policy across the various human services agencies under its purview, further progress may require centralizing all Medicaid funding. Thus, while "[w]e strongly support any efforts to improve the coordination of financing across all EOHHS agencies," explained Jane Hayward, former EOHHS Secretary and current President and CEO of the Rhode Island Health Center Association, "[w]e recommend that EOHHS consider pooling the funds for the Medicaid delivery system at EOHHS, and move funding from the agencies to EOHHS where the former [Department of Human Services] Medicaid funding has already been situated. We believe that this will foster the goal of a more cohesive approach to policy development and implementation." EOHHS recognizes that continued efforts must be made to strengthen coordination across the state agencies responsible for Medicaid (Nicolella January 28, 2013).

Waiver Promotes Collaboration and Understanding Across Departments

There is some evidence to suggest that the Global Waiver has helped promote greater communication, collaboration, and understanding across departments despite persistent challenges posed by prevailing bureaucratic divisions (Nicolella October 22, 2012). It was reported, for example, that the state's internal work groups have provided health and human services personnel with opportunities to get to know one another and the respective missions of their departments of origin. "Part of the reason this was a rewarding experience," reported one state official, "was it did give us an opportunity to really collaborate closely with our partners [in the other departments]. . . . Even though this is a tiny state . . . people don't know what each other does. We're now learning what is available through other departments. . . . That's a good thing, because sometimes we serve similar populations, or even the same population."

Placing all money in one pool under a single waiver has helped break down the prevailing silo mentality. Instead of protecting one's own budget, there has been increased emphasis on meeting beneficiaries' cross-departmental needs. Several examples were provided. One is a move to develop a better coordinated, consolidated transportation system for all clients rather than separate systems for, say, populations served by the Department of Human Services versus the Department of Behavioral Healthcare, Developmental Disabilities, and Hospitals. Another is collaboration between the Departments of Human Services and Children, Youth, and Families to interpret the language of the Waiver's Special Terms and Conditions for children and families because it is largely oriented toward the adult disabled and elderly populations. Still another is increased collaboration between the Departments of Human Services and Elderly Affairs, now a Division within Human Services, in administering home- and community-based service for elderly and disabled people. Yet another is collaboration across EOHHS departments vis-à-vis interagency planning for long-term care, including a Long-Term Care Consolidation Summit and subsequent follow-up activities. It has been reported that state agencies have worked closely in the administration of the program's CNOM authorities as well (EOHHS March 2013).

A particularly salient example is collaboration between the Departments of Human Services and Behavioral Healthcare, Developmental Disabilities, and Hospitals in developing the Behavioral Health Acute Stabilization Unit, a service designed to divert people from emergency rooms and subsequent inpatient behavioral health stays to more appropriate and effective community-based settings. It is likely that this initiative would have been dead in the water without the Global Waiver. This is because while the Department of Human Services, as the payer of the state's share of inpatient psychiatric stays, would have accrued the savings resulting from implementation, the Department of Behavioral Healthcare, Developmental Disabilities, and Hospitals, as the primary funder of the state's community-based behavioral health service system, would have been subject to the costs. With the Global Waiver, however, the two departments were able to come together to design and implement this new Medicaid benefit. "So, we came to an agreement," reported Behavioral Healthcare, Developmental Disabilities, and Hospitals Director Craig Stenning at a March 15, 2010, hearing, "that in fact because the savings come to [the Department of Human Services] that [the Human Services] would fund the service, but [Behavioral Healthcare, Developmental Disabilities, and Hospitals] wrote the regulations and program plan while both departments administer and manage the benefit together. That was a very positive development, and it's been a beneficial service that's now available."

Among the priorities for state FY 2013–2014 established by Secretary Steven Costantino and the heads of EOHHS' constituent department is to "share data—eliminate silos preventing transparency and EOHHS-wide collaboration" (EOHHS 2013). Indeed, the extent of collaboration across EOHHS, its constituent departments, and other state entities seems to have grown since the Chafee administration took over the reins of state government (Holahan and Rifkin February 2012). Under the Affordable Care act, for example, Rhode Island is known as a leader in pursuing integration between its health insurance exchange and other programs. This is largely due to high levels of interdepartmental cooperation. According to Holahan and Rifkin (February 2012), "[e]xchange efforts in Rhode Island . . . have benefited from strong leadership and interagency collaboration among dedicated individuals. The interagency workgroup—co-chaired by the health insurance commissioner, the Medicaid director and the lieutenant governor's chief of staff—has taken an active role in much of the exchange planning and implementation to date." The ultimate goal is to develop processes and tools that meet the eligibility determination and other needs, not only of the exchange but the state's Medicaid and other human service programs.

DATA AND INFORMATION SYSTEMS

The Lack of Requisite Data and Information Resources

The state tracks various data elements through a variety of existing systems. It was reported, for example, that Hewlett Packard administers claims processing for all state programs. Each EOHHS department receives a Medicaid report which presents monthly and year-to-date spending, and estimates total spending for the remainder of year. This latter figure is then compared to what was budgeted by the General Assembly in order to project whether or not the department is likely to go over what was appropriated. Each department is also provided a utilization report which presents the number of units of service and clients served. Departments have their own databases as well; for example, Elderly Affairs has all case management agencies' input data on clients into a central system. Based on this information, it can identify the number of units of case management utilized while determining total costs at a given rate of reimbursement.

Despite a multiplicity of systems, a number of interviewees suggested that the state lacked the requisite electronic data and information systems to effectively administer and evaluate the Global Waiver. "There's a lack of technology," admitted one state official, "it's been a huge problem for many years. We're trying to tackle that." "Anything we do," admitted another, "any change, no matter what the direction is, costs money, because we have archaic systems that need to be programmed." Especially problematic areas include program eligibility and quality assurance. As part of the Global Waiver, for example, the state was required to submit a quality plan to CMS that identified the kind of data elements that would be gathered in order to evaluate progress. Developing this plan proved somewhat challenging because some of the data needed for this purpose were not readily available. While the state had good access to claims data, it faced challenges analyzing its assessment information because its case records had yet to be automated.

It was pointed out that government has gotten increasingly complicated over the last 25 years but that the state's information, human resource, and other systems had not kept up with this complexity. Thus, the state continues to rely on antiquated information technology, which requires substantial time, energy, and money to maintain, impedes the sharing of information easily across other state and federal systems, and precludes timely access to the key data points necessary to track and evaluate progress, either because the various data elements needed are not integrated or readily accessible. This has proven frustrating not only for state officials but for outside stakeholders. "I've gone to . . . [the heads] of the [Department of Human Services] offices and everything," explained one provider representative, "and this antiquated system, like this computer system, just doesn't even allow them to spit it out. I said, 'You mean your system can't tell me on a weekly basis this, this, this, and this? 'No.' It's like you're kidding." Said a consumer representative, "there are no metrics, because they don't have a lot of staff and they don't have a really good data system. . . . It's really hard to judge or to measure what success they've had. Is it financial success? Is it the number of clients being serviced in home care versus nursing homes? They don't have good data, so you could argue that this is a failure very easily. . . . Or you could argue that it's a total success. I wouldn't know what was true."

Concomitant with implementation of the Global Waiver, EOHHS began a series of modernization efforts in light of widely recognized problems with the state's information architecture. This is reflected in the convening of a Modernization Steering Committee by EOHHS with "the goal of modernizing access to human service agency programs in a consistent manner" and "encouraging the EOHHS Departments to utilize consumer centered approaches to service design and delivery that expand their capacity to respond efficiently and responsibly" to the people served (EOHHS October 7, 2009, December 2, 2009). General needs identified included updating network, hardware, and software resources; instituting data sharing across agencies; implementing centralized monitoring and reducing redundancy; and adopting a centralized portal for all EOHHS programs (Alexander March 20, 2010). Specific projects included modification of the state's Medicaid management information and claims processing system (MMIS) and Medicaid eligibility determination/redetermination system (InRhodes), and initiatives to promote more widespread adoption of electronic health records, including Medicaid beneficiary enrollment in current*care*, the state's electronic medical record for Medicaid.

Specific projects also include an initiative funded by a $3.6 million Information Technology planning grant provided by CMS in conjunction with the Global Waiver. Known as the CHOICES Project, the goal of this initiative is to develop a Data Warehouse for comprehensive real-time data reporting, and to develop a Community Systems Management system for managing long-term care application processing and care management functions. The latter has included development of new databases with which to store beneficiaries' clinical information in a HIPPA-compliant manner. It has also included a web-based software program—OMAR—whereby data collected by Office of Medical Review nurses conducting level of care reviews in the field due to the provision of insufficient clinical information from referral sources will automatically be uploaded from laptops to the CHOICES Data Warehouse where it will be integrated with claims and billing data. This information, in turn, could be used to generate detailed reports on either an ad hoc or standardized basis. The goal is to improve the state's program management and evaluation capabilities, and to improve coordination across departments. The CHOICES Data Warehouse is being phased-in over time.

Current leadership at EOHHS has expressed even clearer commitment to promoting an analytical orientation throughout the secretariat, including "[using] measurement and analysis to innovate, promote excellence, foment change" (EOHHS 2013). Indeed, since Governor Chafee took office, Rhode Island has been a leader in preparing the data and information processing groundwork for health care reform, not only with respect to the health insurance exchange and Medicaid but the interaction between these two major components of the Affordable Care Act and other state programs. Rhode Island, for example, has partnered with the New England Collaborative Insurance Exchange Systems project, a $35.5 million federally funded initiative charged with developing information technology components for the exchanges (Holahan and Rifkin February 2012). Especially important for Medicaid is Affordable Care Act requirements that states adopt electronic rather than paper-based eligibility determination processes that work in real-time, permit enrollment or renewal online or over the telephone, operate in conjunction with the exchanges, and share information with other state and federal databases (Courtot and Coughlin November 2012). The state must also put into a place a "no wrong door" approach to applying and enrolling in Medicaid, the Children's Health Insurance program, and subsidized coverage in the health insurance exchanges. Especially important for meeting this requirement in Rhode Island is the Unified Health Infrastructure Project, a joint initiative between EOHHS, the Rhode Island Health Benefit Exchange, and the Office of the Health Insurance Commissioner, for purposes of designing and implementing an integrated web-portal for determining eligibility for health insurance, Medicaid, and other non-health human services programs. State efforts in this area have not gone unrecognized. "The state has been steadily moving towards a more integrated experience for Rhode Islanders accessing services," observed Jane Hayward, former EOHHs Secretary and current President and CEO of the Rhode Island Health Center Association. "This integration is helpful and necessary within the Medicaid program itself across various departments, as well as across agencies and programs more broadly. The [Unified Health Infrastructure Project] to integrate eligibility systems for Medicaid and the Exchange, as well as other programs . . . is a giant step in the right direction."

The Need to Incorporate Additional Information into State Processes

It was felt that the provision of certain additional information would improve state decision making, but especially when determining whether and to what extent individuals would be eligible for long-term services and supports. In particular, both provider representatives and consumer advocates expressed concern about the data used to inform decisions under the state's new system for leveling long-term care applicants. As noted, the Department of Human Services' Office of Medical Review was granted sole responsibility for reviewing and processing clinical levels of eligibility using the new level of care instrument developed by the state. One provider representative felt that the new instrument did not adequately account for the needs of individuals with Alzheimer's disease and other dementias. The result, it was feared, was potential limitation or denial of services to those who otherwise should get them. "The level of care form is unfair to those that have dementia and related diseases," this individual explained. "It doesn't really correlate with the fact that many folks with dementia actually are very capable with their [activities of daily living] and yet can't make good decisions and would wander into the streets."

A more general criticism pertained to the Department of Human Services making leveling decisions via desk review of information collected and delivered to them by providers. Prior to the Global Waiver, Department of Human Services nurses determined whether or not someone met nursing home-level criteria based on information providers submitted directly to the state on a commonly used form. Under the new system, providers perform an assessment, send that information to the Office of Medical Review which, in turn, transfers the results onto a second form on the basis of which level of care determination—"highest," "high," or "preventive"—is made. That the state now requires providers to submit information on a separate form than that used by the Office of Medical Review does not make sense to some observers. That the Office of Medical Review makes their determinations typically without seeing the applicants or taking into account applicants' preferences did not make sense to others. "There's no allowance for client participation," argued one provider representative. "This assessment is done blind, by a nurse in an office, who gathers medical information about this person. Never once is the customer or client asked what they want or what they think they need.

A Need to Capture Additional Data Elements in Order to Analyze Progress

A recurring theme among most types of interviewees but especially provider and consumer representatives was the need to collect and report certain additional data elements over time. "Here's my gripe about the whole process," reported one provider representative, "what we don't get is data! We don't get it . . . I want to see raw numbers." Particularly important for stakeholders was having the ability to follow pertinent data elements both across departments and over time to better assess whether the waiver was, in fact, successful, and whether the state was investing enough resources to achieve its goals. Several felt that while the state may have been tracking the necessary data internally, it had yet to be shared with the Global Waiver Implementation Task Force and other interested parties. Thus, "the other thing that we wanted," explained one consumer advocate, "was greater transparency in reporting data on what was happening, so we could keep score on rebalancing and also costs, of how this was going."

There was also concern about the state's proposed evaluation plan, which was submitted to the federal government in July 2009, within the 120 day post-approval deadline period imposed by CMS (EOHHS July 17, 2009). Here, it was felt that state's emphasis on documenting general trends in spending and utilization, say, across nursing homes and various home- and community-based settings, only told part of the story. What was missing were data on beneficiaries' experiences, both in terms of service scope and quality. The most frequently cited examples where additional data elements needed to be captured were in relation to the state's attempt to rebalance long-term care. It was recognized that the Department of Human Services/EOHHS had indeed released some basic data, including the proportion of long-term care applicants assessed at the "highest," "high," and "preventive" levels of care and number of nursing home transitions and diversions that had taken place. A number of interviewees, however, expressed concern with the assumptions underlying some of the data that had been released. In determining the number of diversions that had taken place, for example, the state includes all those identified for diversion by its primary care case management program, Connect Care Choice. It also includes 30% of those assigned a "high" level of care under the assumption that they would have chosen a nursing home rather than a community-based placement if the option had been made available to them. A number of interviewees took issue with this decision. "It's a lot of really loose assumptions that are the basis for what they report out as their success," explained one provider representative. "If they put somebody in a high category and that person's living at home, they take some percentage of that and say well that person would have gone into a nursing home if we hadn't done this. Well, who knows if they would have gone into a nursing home or not. . . . It's never really been understood how they came up with that and how much they're actually doing."

Most interviewees wished the state would release more detailed data at more frequent intervals. This included data whereby cost savings attributable to rebalancing could be readily tracked and identified, as a provision in the state's Perry-Sullivan statute requires that a portion of any savings resulting from reduced use of Medicaid nursing home care be invested in initiatives expanding the use of home- and community-based services. This also included weekly or monthly data on long-term care applicants and referrals and types and amount of services received across each of the major population groups served (e.g., the elderly, developmentally disabled). "We don't know how this is working," explained one consumer advocate, "because we need to know how many applications for Medicaid funded services are filed each month. . . . How many are approved? How many are denied? . . . If people are found eligible, what's the scope of services?" Thus, in addition to the number of applicants, interviewees wished to see data on the number of nursing home referrals and number and types of home- and community-based service referrals, including hours served. They also wished to see data on application processing times; that is, the number of days it took from when an application was submitted to when it was approved and services provided. The number of appeals and their outcomes and presence and size of program waitlists were identified as well; so too was the need for quality measures so that the consumer experience in long-term care settings could be documented and assessed, including with respect to quality of care and quality of life and satisfaction with the services rendered. "If we're making changes, no matter how small they might seem," explained one consumer advocate, "we should be evaluating that, and that doesn't mean just counting numbers. The state should be looking at the impact on human beings in this state. . . . I so far have really not seen anything concrete in terms of like how do we know that those they diverted from nursing homes are satisfied, feel supported, that kind of thing? . . . Now, I'm not saying it's not happening; I'm just saying I haven't seen it. . . . That's the transparency issue."

Quarterly progress reports to CMS and the Rhode Island General Assembly have subsequently provided some of the additional data requested (Department of Human Services January 2010–February 2013; EOHHS January 2011–April 2013). The Department of Human Services/EOHHS began submitting *Section 1115 Quarterly Progress Reports* in January 2010 to CMS. These reports initially presented a quarter-by-quarter update of Global Waiver activities and basic data. The latter, in particular, reported counts of Medicaid eligibles; number of level of care assessments and assignments; number of nursing home transfers and discharges; shared living enrollment; managed care enrollment; CNOM enrollment; and actual and projected spending levels across different populations and service categories, including the total amount under the cap. As of the January–March 2011 report, additional analytical information has been provided. This reflects the incorporation of information previously only included in the state's quarterly *Designated Medicaid Information* reports, which EOHHS began submitting to the Rhode Island General Assembly's Senate Committee on Health and Human Services October 2010. EOHHS makes these submissions in compliance with a June 8, 2010, Senate Resolution enacted in response to continuing stakeholder concerns regarding the implementation of the Global Waiver evident during Senate Committee on Health and Human Services' oversight hearings. In addition to data on RIte Care and other programs, data on long-term care includes: number of application approvals and denials; number and units of care received and total and average costs by service, age, and Department; percent distribution of spending for institutional and home- and community-based services by population; number on waitlists; application processing times; clinical eligibility processing times and appeals; average length of nursing home stay for transferees and post-transfer arrangements; and causes of unsuccessful diversions/transitions. Early in 2012, the state began releasing nursing home transition data monthly on the EOHHS website.

SUMMARY

The Global Waiver Implementation Task Force has been burdensome for state officials, not only because of distrust that arose during the Waiver development and approval process but also because of prevailing resource limitations. Due to changes to Rhode Island's retirement system, there was widespread concern that the state did not have sufficient numbers of administrative personnel to properly implement the Global Waiver. This concern was exacerbated both by heavy reliance on outside consultants and by prevailing fiscal and budgetary conditions that increased demands on the Medicaid program while slowing down the rate of new hires. The result was increased stress among program administrators when performing day-to-day functions, let alone the added burdens associated with administering the Global Waiver. A particular worry was the dearth of experienced leadership within the state with a history of working collaboratively with providers and advocates. It was pointed out that the top-down strategy taken on the part of agency leadership in designing and implementing the Global Waiver contributed greatly to alienating potential allies among the stakeholder community.

Medicaid-funded programs are administered by several departments ostensibly operating under EOHHS. Most believe that this arrangement has posed challenges as the directors of the various departments continue to resist having their policies and budgets directed from a central authority, though all appreciate the additional federal money acquired under the Global Waiver's Costs Not Otherwise Matchable or CNOM provisions. It seems that the major obstacle precluding greater interdepartmental coordination has been a continued lack of clarity regarding EOHHS' role, though it has since been made the single state Medicaid agency, which may help matters in this regard. Moreover, some believe that greater communication, collaboration, and understanding have taken place since implementation of the Global Waiver began. This is reflected in cross-departmental cooperation deriving from participation in the state's internal working groups. It is also reflected in growing emphasis on meeting beneficiaries' cross-departmental needs regardless of budget source. Preparation for implementing health care reform has promoted interdepartmental cooperation as well.

Although the state tracks a variety of key data elements across a number of different information systems, most felt it lacked the requisite data and information processing capacity to effectively administer the Global Waiver. Instead, the state relies heavily on antiquated technology that requires considerable resources to maintain and prevents timely access to the data needed to track and evaluate progress. The state has thus sought to modernize its information technology architecture as part of its Global Waiver implementation strategy. This includes modifications, both to the state's Medicaid management information and claims processing systems. It also includes development of a data warehouse for comprehensive real-time data reporting; a new system for managing long-term care application and care management functions; and a central portal for determining eligibility for private insurance, Medicaid, and other programs. Despite initiatives such as these, continued need for improvements in the information used to inform level of care determinations was noted. Moreover, several additional data elements were identified that should be collected and reported, both routinely and as part of the state's evaluation plan for the federal government. Quarterly progress reports to CMS and the Rhode Island General Assembly has subsequently provided some of the additional data requested.

7 Service Delivery and Implementation

There is substantial variation in long-term care policy and market characteristics, both within and across states. This variation is reflected in differences in the policies that state and local governments adopt, say, with respect to Older Americans Act programs, state-only funded initiatives, and, of course, Medicaid, whether in relation to provider regulation, payment, eligibility, benefits, or overall spending (Feinberg et al. 2004; Ng et al. December 2012; Howard, Ng, and Harrington December 2011; Kitchener et al. February 2007; Miller 2002; Synder et al. November 2012; Reinhard et al. September 2011; Woodcock et al. June 14, 2011). This cross-state variation is also reflected in differences in the demand and need for care, for example, the number and proportion of chronically ill and frail elders, adults with physical and developmental disabilities, and children with special health care needs, as well as differences in the need for government assistance, perhaps as best indicated by the unemployment rate and proportion of individuals at or near the poverty level (Synder et al. November 2012; Reinhard et al. September 2011). This cross-state variation is further reflected in differences in the supply of service providers, whether family caregivers (Arno 2006), nursing home operators (Harrington et al. June 2008; Harrington et al. October 2011), assisted living/residential care facilities (Mollica September 2009; Stevenson and Grabowski 2010), home care agencies (CMS April 2011), adult day care centers (Rosato, Lucas, and Howell-White May 2005), home health and personal care aides (Seavey and Marquand 2011), and options for transportation and housing (Farber et al. December 2011). The costs of care vary substantially as well (Metlife Mature Market Institute November 2012; Reinhard et al. September 2011).

This chapter examines the impact of the Global Waiver on the state's capacity to provide necessary care within Rhode Island. This includes the role that provider capacity has played in the implementation process, both in relation to adult day care, assisted living, homemaker, and other home- and community-based services, as well as the nursing home sector. It also includes the role that the state's ability to obtain federal matching dollars for previously state-only funded programs, i.e., its Costs Not Otherwise Matchable (CNOM) authority, has played during the course of implementation.

PROVIDER CAPACITY

Uncertainty about the Availability of Necessary Community-Based Resources

There was widespread doubt about the capacity of the provider community to serve greater numbers of clients under the Global Waiver (Needham and Gregg December 23, 2008; Goodnough January 22, 2009; McKay and Nyberg February 9, 2009; Spears February 15, 2013). In particular, interviewees expressed concern that there would be insufficient provider capacity to meet the increased demand for services resulting from nursing home diversions and transitions. The general perception was that while some progress toward rebalancing had indeed taken place, the state had not accomplished what it had hoped to up to that time. This was largely attributed to the level of community-based resources available. "You can't move people out of a high level of care into the community without a sufficient safety net to assist them," explained one provider representative, "and I think some of it may be that those community based resources were not all in place, or at least not to the extent that would be needed to support the influx that was anticipated."

Specific areas of concern included assisted living, subsidized housing, adult day services, home health care, transportation, and the paraprofessional long-term care workforce (Allen, Gozalo, and Steinman June 30, 2011; McKay and Nyberg February 9, 2009; Neighborhood Health Plan of Rhode Island February 22, 2013; McKeon February 28, 2013; Mulready February 28, 2013; Nyberg February 12, 2013; Rhode Island Association of Facilities and Services March 22, 2010; Spears February 15, 2013; Woodcock et al. February 28, 2010). It was reported that the state lacked sufficient assisted living and other housing stock to care for those diverted or transitioned out of nursing homes, and that there were limited slots (and therefore long waitlists) available for the state's subsidized housing programs. It was reported that the transportation needs of seniors and disabled people had yet to be addressed although problems in this area had long since been acknowledged. It was reported that many home-care agencies might not be able to meet the weekend, overnight, and evening needs of an increasingly frail and debilitated service clientele; that while "there are lots of good players out there and there are some interesting models," there was a need for additional standards and coordination, particularly given the influx of new providers into the state. It was reported that additional attention needed to be paid to workforce development, training, and compensation; otherwise, there might not be enough caregivers to go around even if the number of agencies proved sufficient.

Several interviewees pointed to a lack of planning on the part of the Department of Human Services/EOHHS to ensure the availability of appropriate levels of community-based resources. State officials "anticipated that provider capacity [was] going to be a problem" and that while they "[could] try to drive it to make sure there are some institutional alternatives . . . [they could not] control it." Others, however, felt that the state could have been much more proactive in this area. "If I'm a car company," explained one state official, "and my designers design a car, at some point those designers have to talk to the production people, because they can't design something with materials that don't exist. . . . And then they've got to test that design with the consumers that are going to use it. This is just business school 101. None of that went on with this. These guys just made stuff up with no regard for what the system could actually do."

To their credit, the Department of Human Services/EOHHS had contracted with The Hilltop Institute at the University of Maryland-Baltimore County to conduct resource mapping (Woodcock et al. February 28, 2010). Unfortunately, The Hilltop report was not delivered until February 28, 2010, nearly nine months after implementation of the Global Wavier began. As such, the state began its nursing home transition and diversion programs well before it had a clear idea of what the capacity of the community was to meet the expected increase in the demand for services. Moreover, the results of The Hilltop study were not particularly useful, not least of which was because just 84 of the 268 providers of long-term services and supports surveyed responded, for an overall response rate of just 31%.

Community Providers Have Responded with Increased Capacity Under the Global Waiver

Some believed home- and community-based and assisted living providers would rise to meet expected demand, particularly if accompanied by increases in reimbursement. Thus, one state official reported telling the General Assembly that they "believed that home care providers would put people on their payrolls and train them if there was opportunity to pay them for it and I haven't heard of too many instances that that hasn't been happening. Adult day providers were a limited source and they need some brick and mortar, but again, if we were able to find slots for those individuals and maybe give them additional funding . . . they would open their doors." Still others pointed to a "profusion of new home care agencies starting up, new assisted living, new adult day care."

Indeed, it was reported that once the Global Waiver was approved, businesses that had an interest in serving these populations began to take advantage of available opportunities. This is reflected in reported growth in (1) the number of home care agencies applying for licensure; (2) the number of nursing home operators converting nursing home beds to assisted living beds; and (3) the number of assisted living facilities willing to take Medicaid beneficiaries because, while the rate of Medicaid reimbursement may be lower than the private pay rate, the additional clientele was attractive, particularly for those facilities having trouble filling private-pay beds. Increased utilization of the Department of Elderly Affairs' assisted living program was also reported, which state officials attributed, in part, to the nursing home transition and diversion efforts conducted under the Waiver's auspices. In addition, the Global Waiver enabled the state both to expand its shared living program for the developmentally disabled and to establish shared living as an option for seniors and other disabled adults.

Community Providers Have Not Responded with Increased Capacity Under the Global Waiver

Most interviewees were less sanguine about the responsiveness of the market to the Global Waiver. It was reported that most community-based providers had experienced little to no increase in their censuses since the Waiver began. Thus, while some adult day care centers may have had experienced growth in the number of Medicaid recipients served, most censuses remained flat, having not seen an increase in referrals (Rhode Island Association of Facilities and Services March 22, 2010). It was argued that if most new home- and community-based referrals derive from nursing home transfers and diversions, reimbursement rates would need to increase to better reflect the growing acuity and complex service needs of the population served (Maigret January 28, 2013; McKeon February 28, 2013; Nyberg February 12, 2013). "Rebalancing long-term care cannot happen without strong, adequately paid community supports," argued Kathleen McKeon, a Supervisor at the Office of Community Programs and Catholic Charities at the Diocese of Providence. "Agencies that could play a much greater role in community support, such as Adult Day Centers, are funded at a rate significantly below the actual cost of the service. State funds to support respite care for family caregivers, and state support for RI Meals on Wheels have decreased during the 4 years of the global waiver. These are only a few such examples" (McKeon February 28, 2013). Furthermore, rather than paying adult day centers and other community service providers a single rate, multiple rates might be developed to better account for the varying resource needs of the clients cared for. "Adult day services [currently receives] one straight rate," explained Maureen Maigret, Policy Director of the Senior Agenda Coalition at a March 22, 2010, legislative hearing. "One thing that could be done that would be helpful is to provide for an enhanced rate for those adult day programs that are serving persons with dementia . . . [or] . . . who need skilled care"; for example, wound care, heavy medication management, and glucose monitoring."

The general perception was that it would be difficult to bolster provider payments to those levels necessary to spur investment due to the current fiscal climate (McKay and Nyberg February 9, 2009; McKeon February 28, 2013). "One of the ways you build capacity in the community," explained one provider representative, "is look at the rates that you're currently paying community providers. . . . If you're actually trying to attract more people into that line of business then maybe . . . put together a series of incentives that would help them to make a decision to come into that marketplace. There's no resources for doing that." Planned rate increases for home care have been delayed. While adult day providers received a funding increase under the Perry-Sullivan legislation, it was felt that this increase was inadequate. This is reflected in the views of one provider representative who reported that "adult day health in Rhode Island has had one of the lowest funding rates [in the nation] . . . [though] just last year [it] got a pretty significant rate increase . . . from about $40 a day to about $50. . . . But it is still far below other states."

Progress increasing access to assisted living has also been stymied by low reimbursement (Maigret January 28, 2013; McKay and Nyberg February 9, 2009; New England State Consortium Systems Organization December 22, 2009; Nyberg February 12, 2013; Rhode Island Association of Facilities and Services March 22, 2010). Indeed, it was reported that only about one-third of the state's assisted living facilities accept Medicaid. Assisted living facilities receive two payments from Medicaid beneficiaries—one for board and care, which comes from the beneficiary, and the other for the services rendered, which comes from Medicaid. Combined, these two payments cannot compete with what an assisted living facility can receive from a privately paying client. "Assisted living is like the linchpin of rebalancing," asserted one provider representative. "[But] it's just not available yet. . . . Medicaid pays assisted living $1,830 a month and most assisted [living facilities] charge their private residents maybe twice that. It's not an inviting thing if you're an assisted living provider."

Limited Ability to Monitor the Quality of Community Providers by State Agencies

Concern was expressed regarding the ability of the state's Department of Health to monitor the quality of care provided by an influx of new home- and community-based service providers, particularly given recent staff reductions. "In the last 15 months [there have been] 14 new applications [from home care agencies looking to enter the state]," reported a provider representative. "We could be up to 76. Give me a break! The Health Department's staff is probably down a third, the ones that are supposed to be overseeing these people." Said a consumer representative, "it's fine to do all these things, but Health has one inspector doing home care and they're swamped. . . . If you start putting all these people in home care agencies, how is anybody going to monitor it? . . . If you got 50,000 agencies opening up, there's no way you can keep track of them and there's no way to know what they're all doing. . .You want to do all this stuff and then you cut the legs out from the state agencies. I mean, you need people to be able to do these things." Supported by advocates, the leading home care association in the state lobbied the General Assembly to adopt a two-year moratorium on new licensed home care agencies (Peoples May 23, 2010). This proposal was likely motivated, in part, by the economic self-interest of existing agencies who wished to prevent entry of additional competition into the Rhode Island market, thereby maintaining their own censuses and revenue streams. However, it was also motivated, in part, by a genuine concern both for the quality of care provided by new entrants into the market and the ability of the state's Department of Health to monitor it.

Nursing Homes and the Global Waiver

Clearly, a major goal of the Global Waiver was to reduce the number of Medicaid long-term care recipients using nursing home care. This is reflected in the promotion and development of additional home- and community-based services options. It is also reflected in the state's nursing home transition and diversion programs. Not surprisingly, there was some concern among nursing home operators "that rebalancing was pretty clearly intended to contract our industry." Still, industry leaders acknowledged that "there's no putting your head in the sand" as rebalancing was going to happen with or without the Global Waiver. It was widely recognized that Rhode Island ranked near the bottom of states vis-à-vis the proportion of Medicaid spending directed toward non-institutional long-term care options. It was also recognized that the state had undertaken a number of initiatives over the years to reverse this trend, not least of which included its nine prior 1915(c) home- and community-based waivers, the Perry-Sullivan legislation, and Real Choices Grants. Some corners of the industry further recognized that there was a limit to how much the nursing home sector could be downsized given the aging of the state's population and recognition that the state's nursing home transition and diversion programs had not had much of an impact so far. Whatever concerns the nursing home industry had about these provisions were overshadowed by plans to implement a new acuity-based reimbursement system concomitant with reductions in overall expenditures within the sector.

Both the state and industry recognized that if comparatively lower care residents were transferred or diverted, nursing homes would be left with a frailer, sicker, higher acuity population. Thus, there is general agreement that the base nursing home payment rate should be adjusted for resident acuity to better account for the amount of resources nursing homes devoted to caring for their residents (McKay and Nyberg February 9, 2009; New England Consortium Systems Organization 22, 2009; Rhode Island Association of Facilities and Services March 22, 2010; Rhode Island Health Care Association March 29, 2010). The nursing home industry was concerned, however, with a proposed $2.6 million reduction in nursing home funding (Nyberg February 12, 2013; Rhode Island Health Care Association January 5, 2010). This trepidation was shared by other observers, including members of the Senate's Health and Human Services Committee who, at a

March 15, 2010, hearing voiced concern about the implications of reducing nursing home funding for staffing and, in turn, quality at the same time facilities were being asked to serve an increasingly fragile clientele. At the same hearing, the state's Medicaid Director, Elena Nicolella, admitted that "if we were simply changing the payment methodology in a truly budget neutral environment then it would be much easier to implement" but indicated that the proposed reduction was actually quite small as the state's share of Medicaid "expenditures on nursing homes, all funds, is approximately $300 million" and "we are seeking to decrease that expenditure by $1.3 million" (i.e., the state's share of Medicaid nursing home spending). The nursing home industry is further troubled by the state's desire to pay a fixed price for the direct nursing component of their base rate, regardless of actual costs, based on the median cost in this area across all facilities during the previous year (Rhode Island Health Care Association January 5, 2010, March 29, 2010). "In moving from a cost to price based reimbursement system," argued one provider representative, "they're just sort of taking it from one and giving it to another; redistributing the same dollars in a fashion that really has very little to do with resident acuity."

COSTS NOT OTHERWISE MATCHABLE

Successful in Bringing in Additional Federal Dollars via CNOM Programs

The state has been successful in using its CNOM authority to obtain additional federal dollars for services and populations that do not typically qualify for the federal Medicaid match—that is, programs previously funded entirely through general revenue funds, including for people who do not meet state Medicaid eligibility criteria and services for people who are eligible for Medicaid but do not typically receive a particular type of benefit. The state's CNOM authority appears to be one of most popular aspects of the Global Waiver (Beckwith March 1, 2013; EOHHS March 2013; Freyer April 11, 2011; Hayward February 26, 2013; Maigret January 28, 2013; McKeon February 28, 2013; Mulready February 28, 2013; Nyberg February 12, 2013). Indeed, the only value deriving from the state's current budget neutrality arrangement with CMS (i.e., the federal funding cap), according to EOHHS (March 2013), is the ability to fund populations and services that would otherwise be excluded as Medicaid expenditures, a provision the state does not want to jeopardize should the Waiver be renewed without a cap, as requested. Thus, "the greatest thing that came out of it for the state," enthused one provider representative "was the CNOM areas where they were able to grab Medicaid dollars that they hadn't been able to get before." This is because the ability to CNOM state programs has saved the state money, in some cases supporting expansions, in others helping to prevent service cuts. Indeed, there is general agreement that CNOMs, which have provided the state with much needed fiscal relief, have been used to maintain service levels and benefits that otherwise would have been reduced or eliminated due to prevailing budgetary difficulties. "A good part of the waiver in these economic times," explained one consumer advocate, "is that those state funded programs might have been cut were it not for the ability to get the federal matching dollars. . . . [A program] that had been proposed to be cut, for example, last year [because it was state funded], now it wasn't on the chopping block . . . because . . . now it's federal and state funded."

The infusion of federal CNOM dollars has enabled the Department of Behavioral Healthcare, Developmental Disabilities, and Hospitals to provide services to adults with mental health or substance abuse services at risk for hospital care who were previously dependent entirely on state funds and would never have been eligible for Medicaid. "Most of these initiatives predate the Global Waiver," Craig Stenning, Director of Behavioral Healthcare, Developmental Disabilities, and Hospitals reported at March 15, 2010, legislative hearing, "[but] in the area of behavioral health [the CNOMs] have allowed us to continue some programs which otherwise would have faced reductions without the waiver." Although Behavioral Healthcare, Developmental Disabilities, and Hospitals' programs for the developmentally disabled have benefited less from the influx of CNOM money because most state dollars in this area are already federally matched, the proportion of people being served in residential settings has declined as use of community-based supports, including day placements and shared living, has risen.

In the Department of Children, Youth, and Families, the infusion of federal dollars through the state's CNOM authority has enabled the Department to continue its prevention and early intervention work aimed at keeping families intact and children out of residential treatment through the provision of specially targeted community-based services. "Given the economy, given the state crisis that we've seen in the last . . . 18 months," observed one state official, "a lot of our system of care transformation, especially in the first phase . . . had it not been for the CNOMs . . . would have lost probably half of that funding."

By permitting the state to "CNOM" the Department of Elderly Affairs' Co-Pay program, which funds home health, adult day, and case management services for low income people aged 65 years and older with incomes up to 200% of the FPL, the Global Waiver enabled the state to save general revenue funds and prevent cutbacks during a period of fiscal austerity. The federal government approved the use of federal dollars in this manner because it agreed that the Co-Pay Program was a good preventive strategy for keeping people in the community and out of nursing homes, thereby slowing the trajectory toward full Medicaid eligibility. "The Global Waiver allowed us . . . [to fund] the [co-pay] program at a slightly higher level [and accrue] savings [in] general revenue funds, because we had the federal match" reported a state official, "so we were extremely happy that it was accepted and approved by CMS . . . to qualify as a CNOM." The Co-Pay Program, observed Jim Nyberg, Executive Director of LeadingAge Rhode Island, "has greatly benefitted from the Waiver by providing stability in the financing and delivery of these services."

Being able to CNOM this program has also helped eliminate waitlists for home- and community-based services. Indeed, a major concern among consumer advocates had been the potential expansion and imposition of waitlists under the Global Waiver as only those long-term care applicants deemed "highest" on the state's level of care assessment instrument now have an entitlement to either nursing home care or home- and community-based services. This is in contrast to those applicants deemed "high" and "preventive" for whom the receipt of home- and community-based services is dependent on available funding, even though those included in the "high" needs group would have previously qualified as needing an institutional-level of care and would have been entitled to at least nursing home services with no waiting lists[1] prior to the Waiver. The latter, in particular, generated fears that people with "high" care needs may not have access to any services, leaving them with significant unmet care requirements. Despite widespread concern, no one has been placed on a waitlist since implementation of the Global Waiver began, both according to our interviews and Department of Human Services (January 2010–February 2013) and EOHHS (January 2011–April 2013) quarterly reports to CMS and the General Assembly. One state official believed that no one designated as "high" or "preventive" would, in fact, be denied home- and community-based care under the Global Waiver and, as such, the worst-case scenario would be a reduction in the scope of services made available, say, in the number of hours of home-based therapy allocated from 18 to 12 hours per week.

The current absence of waitlists in Rhode Island contrasts with the situation that existed before the Global Waiver was implemented. When the Co-Pay Program was entirely general revenue funded, for example, admissions would often be frozen and waitlists established half way through the fiscal year when program administrators realized that they were going to overspend their budget. Since federal funding has been added to the mix, waitlists have been non-existent for this and other programs. "Every year in the past it's been frozen . . . as the state sort of ran out of money as the fiscal year went on," reported one provider representative, "but as part of the waiver that population became eligible for a federal match . . . and at the end of the day, they've seen a slight budgetary increase and they haven't had problems with the waiting lists for the last two years. [That's] probably one of the main, big successes of the waiver for the home and community based providers."

CNOM Programs Increase Administrative Burdens but Juice Still Worth the Squeeze

Although there was near consensus about the benefits of the Global Waiver's CNOM authority, implementing CNOM programs has imposed additional administrative burdens on state agencies and providers. To CNOM a program, a state agency must promulgate new rules and protocols for services previously not funded under Medicaid if it wishes to receive the federal match. This includes developing new Medicaid eligibility standards, case management protocols, and claims processing requirements. "CNOMing" previously state-only programs, therefore, has not been a negligible undertaking for the state staff involved. "The extent of the changes [the Department of Elderly Affairs had] to make in [the] copay program," reported one state official, "for example . . . writing a policy, changing all the forms, changing all the eligibility . . . took longer than [they] thought, not so much because of any communication delay [in obtaining necessary guidance from CMS], but it was such a detailed process that to do it correctly, it took a great deal of time."

Providers face additional burdens as well. This is because once a program has been "CNOMed," providers must work out new claims processing and documentation procedures while developing processes with which to determine which clients are reimbursable in this manner. This has been perceived as particularly burdensome in the behavioral health sector. "If you ask the providers today," reported one representative, "we're not necessarily in love with [the CNOM authority], because it's been a pain and nightmare. They haven't worked out the billing procedures for CNOMs and sort out the rules of the game of who can get a CNOM funded service. . . . [It's] also proven to be quite an administrative burden, as we are now required to gather and maintain a significant amount of documentation on clients that wasn't previously required."

Despite complexities such as these, most agreed that the juice was worth the squeeze and, as such, both state officials and provider representatives reported looking out for additional CNOM opportunities (Maigret January 28, 2013). State officials, for example, reported looking into the feasibility of "CNOMing" both Department of Elderly Affairs' pharmaceutical assistance and respite programs and the Department of Children, Youth, and Families' burgeoning home- and community-based initiatives. As one state official explained it, "the one thing that I learned from our experience was don't be afraid to be creative, to look for opportunities that might not otherwise be a Medicaid funded service and really understand how those services link to the Medicaid universe in terms of either keeping people off Medicaid or keeping them out of long-term care facilities."

At the time of the interviews, consumer advocates highlighted two populations not eligible for Medicaid that the state has already been authorized to cover under the Global Waiver's CNOM authority but which it has not moved forward with yet. One population is persons living with HIV/AIDS with incomes below 200% of the FPL. Currently, most such individuals are not eligible for Medicaid coverage. The other population is RIte Care parents who had their children temporarily removed by the Department of Children, Youth, and Families due to substance abuse and behavioral health issues. Typically, if a parent had their children taken away, they would lose their RIte Care coverage because they no longer had them in custody. The intention in maintaining coverage for these individuals is to preserve access to the medical and behavioral health services necessary to resolve their behavioral health issues and work toward reunification. The state's five-year extension request keeps this provision intact (EOHHS March 2013). Consumer advocates, however, would like to see it broadened so that parents could maintain coverage no matter why their children were removed from the home (Beckwith March 1, 2013; Katz March 1, 2013).

The state's extant CNOM initiatives, including the Elderly Affairs' Co-Pay Program and Behavioral Healthcare, Developmental Disabilities, and Hospitals' program for at-risk mentally ill adults, basically extended federal financing to programs previously funded exclusively by the state treasury; as such, the addition of federal matching funds reduced the fiscal burden on the state. Indeed, the state's five-year extension request includes a provision increasing income eligibility for the Co-Pay program from 200% to 250% of the FPL while broadening eligibility for the state's at risk program for mentally ill adults (EOHHS March 2013). By contrast, extending coverage to RIte Care parents who lost their children and to those living with HIV/AIDS would represent entirely new investments on the part of the state, thereby explaining, in part, why the state had not moved forward with these initiatives yet in light of prevailing fiscal circumstances. Thus, concluded one consumer advocate, "I would say that the CNOMs have probably protected some of the state funded services that otherwise might have been cut in this environment; on the other hand, it's prevented putting into effect expansion of coverage for those [people with HIV/AIDS and RIte Care parents who had their children removed] because it requires new state dollars."

Still, the state has kept all current CNOM authorities in its extension request, thereby suggesting that CNOM programs that remained unimplemented during the first five years might be implemented in the next if fiscal circumstances improve sufficiently. It should be pointed out that some of the state's CNOM programs will prove unnecessary once Medicaid eligibility in the state is expanded to include all those under age 65 years with incomes below 138% of the FPL. Alternatively, it will be critical that the state maintain others such as the Elderly Affair's Co-Pay program since the 65 and over population is explicitly excluded from the expansion (Nyberg February 12, 2013). In general, there is broad support among community stakeholders to identify additional CNOM opportunities; for example, providing respite to " 'pre-Medicaid eligible populations' makes good economic sense and is a compassionate way to assist those who make great personal sacrifices to care for loved ones" (McKeon February 28, 2013).

SUMMARY

Doubt was expressed about the ability of providers to serve significantly greater numbers of long-term care recipients within the community. This has served, in part, to impede the state's long-term care rebalancing efforts. Specific areas of concern include the availability of subsidized housing, assisted living, adult day, home health, and transportation services, as well as the paraprofessional workforce more generally. Lack of planning on the part of the Department of Human Services/EOHHS to ensure the availability of appropriate levels of community-based resources was highlighted. Whereas some pointed to signs that the home- and community-based and assisted living sectors had begun to take advantage of opportunities deriving from the Global Waiver, most were less optimistic, believing that reimbursement levels, a casualty of the current fiscal climate, were still too low to stimulate sufficient levels of market growth. There was also concern that even if the number of providers increased significantly, the state's Department of Health would lack sufficient capacity to monitor the quality of care provided in light of reductions in staff. Nursing home providers generally recognized the need to increase the use of home- and community-based service options within the state. Moreover, whatever concern the industry had about the Global Waiver has been overshadowed by the development of a new, price-based reimbursement system that, among other things, adjusts the level of payment received for resident acuity. Adjusting for resident acuity is deemed necessary in light of the growing complexity and severity of the nursing home population due to the transition and diversion of lower care beneficiaries to home- and community-based settings.

Perhaps the most popular aspect of the Global Waiver has been the state's ability to use its CNOM authority to draw in additional federal matching funds to help finance programs previously paid for entirely out of the general treasury. This provision was particularly appreciated as the state's budget situation would have otherwise resulted in significant reductions in these efforts. Thus, the infusion of federal CNOM dollars enabled agencies such as Behavioral Healthcare, Developmental Disabilities, and Hospitals; Children, Youth, and Families; and Elderly Affairs to both eliminate waitlists and to continue providing behavioral health/substance abuse, prevention/early intervention, and assisted living/adult day care services, respectively, to populations who did not meet typical requirements for Medicaid eligibility. Although desirable, "CNOMing" previously state-only funded programs is not necessarily easy, with additional administrative burdens being placed on both state agencies and providers. The general consensus, however, was that the benefits of doing so far outweighed the costs and, as such, both state officials and provider representatives reported looking out for additional opportunities in this area. Foremost among these opportunities are populations that the state already has authority to CNOM under its agreement with CMS but which it has not moved ahead with yet because doing so would represent entirely new investments on the part of the state. This is in contrast to the populations that have already been "CNOMed" because doing so enabled the state to reduce rather than increase its own spending.

NOTE

1. Although these individuals could have been placed on waitlists for home- and community-based services under previous waivers, they were entitled to and guaranteed nursing home services prior to the new three-tier level of care system adopted.

8 Waiver Achievements and Lessons

Former Rhode Island Executive Office of Health and Human Services Secretary Gary Alexander reported more than $100 million in savings deriving from Rhode Island's Global Consumer Choice Medicaid Waiver over its first two years (Alexander January 28, 2011). Since that time, conservative commentators and Republican politicians have held up the Global Waiver as a successful example of what could be achieved nationally if the entire Medicaid program was block granted (Anonymous March 28, 2011; Howard September 2012; Lawless and Ferrier June 15, 2011; Pugh June 12, 2011; Roberts May 15, 2011; Senate Finance Committee July 14, 2011; Volsky March 30, 2011). This assessment is not supported by the data. First and foremost, the Global Waiver is not a block grant but a capped federal match whereby the state is still required to expend its own resources before receiving contributions from the federal government. In addition, the state did not receive significantly more discretion to administer Medicaid under its agreement with the federal government but instead acquired permission to make certain program changes under the Waiver's Special Terms and Conditions, with additional changes being subject to the three-tier system of federal oversight adopted. Moreover, no block grant proposal would permit states to opt out at any time due to unseen or untenable fiscal circumstances as is currently the case with the escape clause included in the Waiver agreement between Rhode Island and the federal government. This chapter looks beyond the block grant rhetoric to assess the Global Waiver's impact. It also draws lessons and recommendations from Rhode Island's experience with the Global Waiver, both regarding the design and administration of state health reform generally and long-term care rebalancing specifically.

ACHIEVEMENTS OF THE GLOBAL WAIVER

Block grants aside, did the Global Waiver live up to expectations? This section examines the impact of the Global Waiver, both overall, on savings and expenditures, and with respect to each of the three major programmatic areas targeted: long-term care rebalancing, care coordination, and "smart purchasing." It also examines provisions of the state's Waiver renewal request in light of the lessons learned. General provisions of the state's renewal request include removal of the aggregate global cap of the original Waiver and adoption of a more traditional approach to determining budget neutrality (EOHHS March 2013). General provisions of the renewal request also include continuation of all authorities provided under the original Waiver, say, with respect to RIte Care, home- and community-based services, and Costs Not Otherwise Matchable. Perhaps, most importantly, EOHHS proposes development and implementation of additional eligibility, benefit, and service delivery changes, to both increase access and to ensure that the care provided is responsive and appropriate to beneficiaries' needs, while improving system performance, use of information technology, and coordination with other publicly financed programs and sources of health insurance coverage.

The Impact of the Global Waiver on Overall Spending and Savings

In short, most of the Medicaid program savings achieved by Rhode Island during the period in which the Global Waiver has been in effect derive not from the Global Waiver but from other sources, including increased spending on the part of the federal government. Indeed, analysts at the Center for Budget and Policy Priorities conclude that one reason Rhode Island spent less under the Global Waiver was the provision of millions of dollars in federal stimulus support and the institution of cost-savings measures that could have been implemented independently, either of a federal waiver or the global cap (Cross-Call and Solomon March 22, 2011). Center for Budget and Policy Priorities analysts also conclude that the federal government actually spent more money under the Global Waiver than it would have otherwise spent, not only because of the federal stimulus but because the state was able to draw in additional federal matching dollars for programs previously funded entirely by the state through the Waiver's CNOM authority and because the cap on total spending was set well above what the state expected to spend. In its original waiver application, the state requested a $12.386 billion cap although it anticipated only spending $10.761 billion. That the state has subsequently spent substantially less than it could have spent under the Waiver agreement—$7.24 versus $9.7 billion during the first four years—reflects the overgenerous ceiling put into place, not "savings" or "surpluses" claimed by some block grant advocates.

Consistent with Center for Budget and Policy Priority analyses is an independent evaluation contracted by EOHHS once the Waiver's original advocates, Republican Governor Carcieri and former EOHHS Secretary Alexander, left office. Overall, the results of this evaluation, conducted by The Lewin Group, reveal just $22,944,888 in total Medicaid program savings deriving from the Global Waiver provisions approved by CMS in January 2009 during the first two fiscal years of implementation (2009, 2010), all of which could have been implemented under other authorities without a global cap and a far cry from the $100 million purportedly saved during the first 18 months (The Lewin Group December 6, 2011). Those provisions contained explicitly within the Global Waiver include the state's nursing home transition and diversion programs, nursing home acuity adjuster, mandatory managed care enrollment and re-procurement, selective contracting of shared-living and hospital-outpatient services, and redesign of the state's habilitation and personal choice programs. Combined with $42,771,921 in additional federal matching dollars brought in under the Waiver's CNOM authority, the state reduced its total spending by $65,716,217 as a result of provisions included within the Global Waiver. Of course, this additional $43 million saved by the state does not represent reduced Medicaid program spending but, in fact, increased spending on the part of the federal government.

Other initiatives implemented during this time period also saved the state money but cannot be attributed to the state's Global Waiver agreement with the federal government and certainly do not depend on a global cap. These can be divided among savings deriving from initiatives requiring additional CMS approval—$9,396,325—and program management initiatives requiring state agency and/or legislation action—$22,892,894. Examples of initiatives requiring CMS approval include: hospital reimbursement reform, various rate reductions, a generic first prescription policy, and participation in the Money Follows the Person Demonstration. Examples of initiatives requiring stage agency/legislative action include: nursing home rate reductions, lower administrative payments for managed care, transportation rate reductions and redesign, efforts to improve program integrity, and enhanced estate recoveries.

The Impact of the Global Waiver on Long-Term Care Rebalancing

Some incremental progress toward long-term care rebalancing has been made while the Global Waiver has been in effect. The Lewin Group (December 6, 2011) identified a 3.0% reduction in the average number of monthly nursing home users between state FY's 2008 and 2010 (from 5,565 to 5,398).[1] Although annual nursing home expenditures generally remained steady, increasing by only 0.8% (from $296 to $299 million), total nursing home days declined as the cost per resident per day increased by 4.4% (from $148.03 to $156.80), suggesting growing acuity among the population served. By contrast, the average monthly number of home- and community-based services users grew by 9.5% (from 3,082 to 3,375), concomitant with a 45.1% increase in annual expenditures (from $42.8 to $54.0 million).[2]

Most home- and community-based service utilization in Rhode Island occurred in one of four areas: personal care services, adult day care, home health care, and assisted living, with personal care services accounting for the majority of users and expenditures. Between state FYs 2008 and

2010, monthly personal care spending and participants increased markedly, from about 2,050 to 2,875 and $2.6 to $4.2 million, respectively. Whereas monthly adult day care users and expenditures increased from approximately 300 to 400 and $200,000 to $300,000 during this time period, users and expenditures of assisted living remained somewhat steady, at ~175 and ~$180,000, while home health declined from 350 to 250 and $180,000 to $120,000. In all, the average monthly number of long-term care users—nursing home and home- and community-based—increased by 1.5% (8,646 to 8,772) and total expenditures by 4.1% (from $339 to $353 million) during the time period analyzed.

The Lewin Group's findings are reinforced, in part, by a study conducted by researchers at Brown University (Allen, Gozalo, and Steinman June 30, 2011). This investigation found a 10% reduction in the proportion of new nursing home admissions that remain institutionalized for more than 90 days, from 63% to 53%, between 2008 and 2010. It also found evidence of increased impairment with activities of daily living (ADLs) both among new nursing home entrants and those staying institutionalized for longer than 90 days, particularly among those admitted directly from the community. Furthermore, the proportion of admissions from home defined as "low care"—that is, with no late loss ADLs—declined from 5.2% to 2.5% and 10.9% to 6.1%, respectively, among short- and long-stay nursing home residents. Together these results suggest a modest impact of Rhode Island's rebalancing initiatives, especially with respect to increased acuity among the state's nursing home population and reduction in the proportion staying long term. That approximately one-quarter of residents who stay longer than 90 days reacquire enough functioning to be characterized as "low care" suggests that further refinement to the state's transition program may be necessary.

Overall, despite improvements on the margin, there has been general disappointment with the impact of the Global Waiver on long-term care rebalancing (Caffrey January 28, 2013; EOHHS March 2013; Maigret January 28, 2013; McKaig February 11, 2013; Nicolella January 28, 2013). In its extension request, EOHHS (March 2013) admits that its nursing home transition and diversion strategies have fallen short of expectations. "We, too, are disappointed with the progress on rebalancing," reported Maureen Maigret (January 28, 2013), Policy Consultant at the Senior Agenda Coalition, a consumer advocacy. "The latest report to the state Senate on the Global Waiver shows 15.44% of funds spent on long term care for elders in the 3rd quarter of FY 2012 were for home and community services and 84.56% on institutional care. This is virtually unchanged from the 1st quarter of FY 2010. . . . According to the AARP's State Long-Term Care Profiles Report, Rhode Island ranks 49th among the states in rebalancing perceptive, despite efforts to date." Indeed, according to official state estimates, the relative distribution of Medicaid expenditures between community-based and institutional services has remained steady during the Waiver's first four years, both for elders (~15% community, ~85% institutional) and persons with disabilities (~41% community, ~57% institutional, 2% Tavares Pediatric Center) (excluding the developmentally disabled) (Department of Human Services January 2010–February 2013; EOHHS January 2011–April 2013).

In light of continuing challenges, EOHHS has opted to take a more comprehensive approach to meeting beneficiaries' long-term care needs, both by focusing on people's overall health and taking a broader view of long-term services and supports (EOHHS March 2013; Nicolella January 28, 2013). The state's new strategy is largely reflected in its Integrated Care Initiative in which, as noted previously, disabled Medicaid beneficiaries in need of long-term services and supports and Medicaid beneficiaries who are also enrolled in Medicare will be enrolled into enhanced versions of the state's managed care and primary care case management programs for people with disabilities, Rhody Health Options and Connect Care Choice *Community Partners*. The scope of covered benefits will be expanded to include the long-term services and supports necessary to prevent avoidable emergency room visits and hospitalizations while enabling beneficiaries to remain in the community. Although submitted previously as a Category II change request, EOHHS included the Integrated Care Initiative in its Waiver renewal proposal to ensure the extension of the program throughout the Waiver renewal period and to demonstrate its commitment to delivery system reform.

The state's revised rebalancing strategy also includes expedited eligibility for a limited package of three days of adult day care and 20 hours of personal care/home maker services weekly, and limited skilled nursing services for up to 90 days based on self-attestation of financial eligibility. This is a potentially important provision given that it takes 49 days, on average, for the state to determine financial eligibility, thereby forcing many individuals who might otherwise be able to remain in the community to enter a nursing home in order to receive needed care (Maigret January 28, 2013). While community stakeholders strongly favor this provision, many feel that the package of services made available during the period of presumptive eligibility would, for many individuals, be inadequate to prevent nursing home placement (Katz March 1, 2013; Maigret January 28, 2013; McKaig February 11, 2013; Neighborhood Health Plan of Rhode Island February 22, 2013; Nyberg February 12, 2013). It was suggested that the state authorize additional days of adult day care, more hours of home care, and additional benefits such shared living. EOHHS maintains that additional services beyond the minimum will be made available on a case-by-case basis to those who need them (EOHHS March 18, 2013).

The state's revised rebalancing strategy includes plans to develop and implement a Consumer Assistance Program, which in building on the Access and Coordination Organization put into place under the current Waiver, would "support and help to coordinate all of the information and referral, options counseling, eligibility assistance, and case management that occurs across" state agencies (EOHHS March 2013). EOHHS intends to incorporate the activities of the state's Aging and Disability Resource

Center, The Point, into the Consumer Assistance Program. The state also intends to offer peer supports and mentoring to community-based Medicaid enrollees to, in part, "link members with a multitude of resources in order to assist them in overcoming barriers to appropriate medical and community based service use; assist members to be responsible, accountable, and self-sufficient health care consumers; and serve as their mentor and coach to achieve positive health and wellness outcomes" (EOHHS March 18, 2013). Both peer mentoring and consumer assistance are supported by community stakeholders (McKeon February 28, 2013; Mulready February 28, 2013).

Several provisions within the state's Waiver renewal request seek to maintain at-risk individuals in the least restrictive settings possible for as long as possible through the provision of supportive housing and employment supports. This reflects the view, according to state Medicaid Director Elena Nicolella (January 28, 2013), that there is a need "to explicitly recognize housing and employment as significant determinants of health and self-sufficiency," a perspective shared by both consumer and provider representatives (Maigret January 28, 2013; McKeon February 28, 2013; Mulready February 28, 2013; Nyberg February 12, 2013). The emphasis on housing is reflected in a provision increasing the personal needs allowance for certain beneficiaries eligible for long-term services and supports so that they have sufficient resources to keep and maintain a home. Qualifying individuals include those transitioning back to the community after 90 days in a nursing home whom the state deems financially unable to stay in the community without being able to keep more of their income. The emphasis on housing is also reflected in the provision of housing stabilization services, including substance abuse and financial counseling, life skills training, and medication management to Medicaid eligible and near-Medicaid eligible individuals at risk of losing their homes, residing in a homeless shelter or transitional housing, or requiring long-term restorative interventions to maintain stable housing.

To support employment, the state proposes to implement a Healthy Works Initiative that provides supported employment, prevocational, and habilitative services that wrap around largely rehabilitative-oriented employment services already made available under the program. Qualifying individuals include: (1) non-elderly adults who qualify for Medicaid on the basis of a disability and (2) chronically ill adults between ages 27 and 64 years with incomes up to 200% of the FPL eligible for or at risk of becoming Medicaid eligible. The state also plans to implement a small pilot project to provide employment rewards and supported employment, prevocational, and habilitative services to young adults aged 18 to 30, independent of disability status. Enrollment in this latter initiative will be limited to 200 participants annually.

A number of provisions within the state's Waiver renewal request target certain at risk populations for early intervention. This emphasis on early intervention is reflected in the provision of in-home behavioral health programs (e.g., child, family, and group therapy; parental training; intensive care management) to children in or at risk of being placed in Department of Children, Youth and Families custody due to problematic behaviors. This emphasis on early intervention is also reflected in modification of several CNOM programs. This includes broadened eligibility for the state's Co-Pay program from 200% to 250% of the FPL for elders aged 65 years or older, in addition to adults between ages 19 and 64 diagnosed with Alzheimer's disease or other dementia, also with incomes up to 250% of the poverty line. This also includes language clarifying that eligibility for the state's at-risk program for mentally ill adults with incomes up to 200% of the FPL includes both uninsured *and underinsured* individuals who lack coverage for specialized behavioral health and substance abuse services that may otherwise help prevent hospitalization and the trajectory to full Medicaid eligibility because, say, housing and employment can be maintained (EOHHS March 2013). The emphasis on early intervention is further reflected in the inclusion of new CNOM authorities; for example, permitting pre-Medicaid eligible adults with incomes up to 200% of the FPL to qualify for housing stabilization services.

The Impact of the Global Waiver on Care Coordination and Smart Purchasing

Beyond procurement of managed care, EOHHS (March 2013) has concluded that provisions for selective contracting contained within Rhode Island's original Waiver agreement were ineffective. The state, for example, proved unsuccessful in applying selective contracting to durable medical equipment. It also focused on obtaining the lowest price which, in and of itself, does not necessarily improve performance. Going forward, EOHHS plans to take "a more comprehensive approach in which selective contracting is implemented as part of an overall strategy to ensure care and services are delivered in the most cost-effective manner" (EOHHS March 2013). Importantly, the state's Waiver extension request includes a provision removing co-payments for all services but extended family planning. This change is clearly supported by consumer advocates (Beckwith March 1, 2013; Katz March 1, 2013), though the state rejected advocates' request that RIte Care premiums be removed as well.

In general, Rhode Island's Medicaid-managed care options have performed very well, both overall and with respect to the new, disabled populations incorporated into such programs under the Global Waiver. As per CMS regulations, Rhode Island contracts with an External Quality Review Organization, IPRO, to annually assess the accessibility, timeliness, and quality of services provided by the plans that participate in the state's Medicaid managed care programs: Neighborhood Health Plan of Rhode Island and United Healthcare Community Plan of Rhode Island. The most recent IPRO (October 2012) report indicates that in 2011, both health plans had achieved an Excellent accreditation rating by the National Committee on Quality Assurance (NCQA). Moreover, of 213 health plans nationally, Neighborhood Health Plan and United Healthcare Community Plan ranked 8th and 16th, respectively, based on NCQA criteria (IPRO October 2012). The same was true in 2012, with Neighborhood Health Plan and United Healthcare Community Plan ranking 5th and 18th out of the 227 health plans reviewed (EOHHS October 2012). Indeed, Neighborhood Health Plan has been ranked in the top 10 for eight consecutive years.

Since 1998, Rhode Island has measured and rewarded performance based on health plan performance relative to national benchmarks in administration, access, and clinical quality with the percentage of incentive payment being distributed across six domains: Member Services (12%), Medical Home/Preventive Care (48%), Women's Health (10%), Chronic Care (20%), Behavioral Health (8%), and Cost Management (2%) (EOHHS October 2012). In 2011, both Rhode Island plans exhibited "strong performance on access to care and provision of well care and preventive screening services for children and adolescents, excellent access to ambulatory and preventive care for adults and generally high levels of member satisfaction" (IPRO October 2012). Neighborhood Health Plan also exhibited strong performance on a variety of acute and chronic care measures, though neither plan met goals for conducting timely initial health screenings for special enrollment populations, including disabled adults served by Rhody Health Partners and children with special health care needs served by RIte care. Based on its performance United Healthcare was required to put into effect a corrective action plan to improve performance in several domains, including initial health screens and care management for the special enrollment groups.

For its part, the Lewin Group's (December 6, 2011) evaluation suggests that it was more cost effective to enroll children with special care needs and adults with disabilities in managed care than unmanaged fee-for-service. The Lewin Group report also suggests that populations enrolled in managed care tended to receive care in more appropriate, less costly settings, with lower emergency room and higher physician service utilization being exhibited when compared to their unmanaged fee-for-service counterparts. This latter finding is reinforced by analyses comparing the locus of care before and after specific individuals transitioned from unmanaged fee-for-service to managed care. Here, both children with special needs and adults with disabilities experienced a decrease in emergency room visits and increase in physician visits after the transition took place.

If approved by the state legislature, EOHHS plans to submit a state plan amendment expanding Medicaid eligibility to all adults without dependent children with incomes up to 138% of the FPL. Through the Waiver extension, the state seeks authority to enroll this population into managed care. Also, as noted, EOHHS intends to build on its success in managed care by enrolling Medicaid-Medicaid dual eligibles and disabled Medicaid-only eligibles in need of long-term care into Rhody Health Options and Connect

Care Choice *Community Partners* through its Integrated Care Initiative. "In order to maximize the effectiveness of managed care," Elena Nicolella (January 28, 2013), the state's Medicaid Director, reported that "the scope of services needs to be broader and the impact at the provider level needs to be stronger." Critically, therefore, Medicaid beneficiaries enrolled in the state's new managed care options will receive the full range of Medicaid benefits, including long-term services and supports (EOHHS March 2013), a change strongly favored by community stakeholders, though some prefer stronger integration of behavioral health and substance abuse services into all Medicaid managed care programs as well (Hayward February 26, 2013; Neighborhood Health Plan of Rhode Island February 22, 2013).

The state's Waiver extension also includes a number of provisions intended to improve plan performance and beneficiaries' experiences at the point of service delivery, including promoting "patient-centered medical homes, integration of primary and behavioral health care, all payer collaboratives, cross provider teams, transition management and alignment of incentives in payment reform" (EOHHS March 2013). Under the Integrated Care Initiative, the state will contract with two or more managed care organizations to provide and coordinate all services under Rhody Health Options. Because Connect Care Choice lacks a central administrative authority—it consists of 17 separate physicians practices—the state will contract with a Coordinating Care Entity that will deploy a Community Health Team charged with coordinating all social supports and conducting data management, quality assurance, and quality improvement activities. Working closely with the nurse practitioners assigned to each physician practice and nurse care managers within EOHHS' Office of Community Programs, the Coordinating Care Entity will formulate and implement care plans and link with needed social supports.

The state also requests the authority to implement several pilot projects. One initiative would be the Delivery System Reform Incentive Payment program through which one or more hospitals and their affiliated community providers would become eligible for incentivize payments if certain performance-based targets are met. Another initiative would assign responsibility to a Community Health Team for providing a broad array of services and supports, including those not covered by the state plan, to Medicaid residents residing in a given geographic area and served by a defined network of primary care medical homes. The Community Health Team would be responsible for helping beneficiaries identify and access services appropriate to their conditions with the aim of improving population health and reducing preventable hospitalizations, emergency department visits, and nursing home stays. The Community Health Team may also conduct health education and nutrition counseling, facilitate access to housing stabilization and transportation, and coordinate with behavioral health. During the first year, the team would receive per member per month payments. This would continue during the second year at which point feedback on performance based on quality and utilization measures would also be provided. During years three through five, a portion of Team's payment would be withheld and allocated at the end of the contract year based on performance.

A major focus of the Waiver renewal is providing additional programs and services that improve quality of life and prevent future health care utilization by helping the most complex and high-risk cases "transition to the least restrictive setting, maintain independent community living, and maintain or improve health or wellness" (EOHHS March 2013). One example is the state's "Rhode to Wellness" program through which beneficiaries with one or more chronic conditions who receive primary care from a patient-centered medical home could qualify for additional benefits if they are willing to try alternative approaches to managing their conditions at the recommendation of their primary care practitioner. These additional benefits would include: disease/weight management classes, exercise/fitness programs, nutrition counseling, integrated pain management, tobacco cessation assistance, and assistance making/keeping preventive health appointments. Gift cards may also be awarded to incentivize ongoing participation and goal attainment. Another example is the provision of alternative benefits to certain qualified populations, including, for example, chiropractic care, acupuncture, and therapeutic massage for those suffering from chronic pain, and short-term recovery, detoxification, transitional, and/or referral services to the chronically inebriated.

DESIGN AND ADMINISTRATION OF HEALTH REFORM

There are a number of useful lessons that can be drawn from Rhode Island's experience with the Global Waiver regarding potential barriers and facilitators to designing and administering health care reform at the state level. Specific lessons include: ensuring sufficient levels of stakeholder input and transparency throughout the program design, approval, and implementation process; devoting adequate administrative and informational resources to program administration; and carefully considering the breadth and timing of the reform strategy put into place—factors that promote adoption, for example, may, in turn, impede implementation.

Ensuring Stakeholder Input and Transparency at All Stages

The U.S. Government Accountability Office has highlighted a lack of public input and transparency, both when states' Section 1115 waiver applications are developed and when they are approved by the federal government (U.S. Government Accountability Office July 12, 2002, July 24, 2007). Rhode Island's experience with the Global Waiver is certainly no exception. Development and approval of the Global Waiver was dominated by state officials working over a short period of time characterized by growing fiscal uncertainty. Thus, a common theme was the lack of opportunities for constructive input on the part of community stakeholders. This was evident both when program administrators designed the Global Waiver and when they negotiated approval from the federal government. Although some community forums and stakeholder meetings did in fact take place, the absence of specifics made it difficult for outside observers to provide feedback on what was being proposed.

Together, the lack of community input and transparency intensified stakeholder distrust and concern about the Global Waiver and its implications for the vulnerable populations Medicaid serves. This distrust, in turn, contributed to a more challenging implementation environment for program administrators than otherwise would have been the case. It also contributed to subsequent passage of oversight legislation, which required that all but simple administrative changes be approved by the General Assembly before being submitted for approval by the federal government. The result, somewhat paradoxically for the Waiver's architects, has been greater state legislative involvement in Medicaid program decision making than existed before the Global Waiver went into effect. Distrust, moreover, colored stakeholders' views about program administrators' intentions as the implementation process unfolded, a dynamic exacerbated by dissatisfaction with the Global Waiver Implementation Task Force. Most stakeholders did not believe that the Task Force operated well, at least initially, nor had much, if any, impact on the implementation process. Agendas were primarily set by the state, community leadership was mostly absent, and work group recommendations largely ignored.

In light of ongoing concerns about the lack of public input and transparency in Section 1115 waiver development and approval, the Affordable Care Act requires the U.S. Department of Health and Human Services to develop and issue regulations to ensure meaningful opportunities for public input (Alker March 2012). CMS issued its final regulations on February 22, 2012. The rules first establish a process states must follow when developing their waiver applications. This includes: a 30-day public notice and comment period; a comprehensive description "that contains sufficient level of detail to ensure meaningful input from the public" on the waiver proposal; a website on which pertinent materials are posted and at which interested parties can sign up for emails documenting progress; two public hearings at which the public can learn about and comment on the waiver application; and a final waiver application with specifics similar to the initial version made available to the public and which documents the public notice process that the state had undertaken and how it informed the final proposal.

The rules next establish a process that the federal government must follow when considering what a state has submitted. This includes: provision of a 15-day period during which the federal government must inform a state that it has received its waiver application, notice of which launches a 30-day federal comment period; posting of pertinent materials on the CMS website, including a notice of receipt, the waiver application, and an email address through which members of the public can comment publicly on the proposed application; and requirement that the federal government not make its final decision on a state's waiver application until at least 45 days after it has given a state notice that it has received the application. The final rule also addresses the post-approval period. Pertinent provisions include: opportunities for public feedback six months after implementation of the waiver has begun and annually thereafter, regular reviews of waiver implementation and compliance, and release of a publically available evaluation plan and annual reports.

CMS' rules regarding Section 1115 waiver program development, approval, and implementation are certainly a step in the right direction. However, it is important to recognize that what CMS has established are minimum requirements for community involvement. It is likely that stakeholder expectations regarding community participation in states' waiver program decisions will exceed the parameters lain out by CMS. Certainly, for example, community stakeholders in Rhode Island would have been even more dissatisfied than they already were if only two public hearings were held before the Global Waiver was sent to CMS, or if only one stakeholder meeting was held annually as implementation unfolded. Moreover, it is important to provide sufficient detail on proposed changes and to adopt mechanisms for public participation to not only keep community stakeholders informed and involved, but also to translate their input into program improvement, whether during the design, approval, or implementation stages of the policy process. This seems to be the approach taken by EOHHS with its Integrated Care Initiative and Waiver renewal request, thereby accounting, in part, for markedly greater stakeholder support for these initiatives than with the state's original Waiver application.

Rhode Island's experience suggests that pre-submission public forums can serve a useful role in informing community stakeholders about the state's intentions. However, a more productive purpose would be to acquire and incorporate public input into the state's plans as occurred with its Integrated Care and Waiver renewal proposals. Ideally, the Waiver development process should represent a collaborative approach whereby state officials integrate stakeholder feedback each step along the way, beginning with the initial concept paper, followed by the first draft, and then the actual waiver application itself. Such opportunities for feedback should continue into the federal approval process. Community stakeholders should not have to rely on their congressional delegation for information on the status of the state's negotiations with CMS. They should be able to count on state officials themselves.

Rhode Island's experience suggests that community forums such as the Global Waiver Implementation Task Force can serve as a useful conduit for informing community stakeholders about post-approval progress. Forums such as this, however, would be much more effective if community and state participants came to early agreement on the forum's mission; that is, whether it simply serves as an advisory body or as an active participant in the implementation process itself. Forums such as the Global Waiver Task Force would also be more effective if community leadership was established early on. Achieving a balance between representation of all pertinent stakeholder interests and the need to limit the size of such forums in order to make discussion and deliberation more manageable is important as well. So too is the provision of sufficient state administrative support, including integration of forum efforts with those being undertaken internally by the state. Although general brain storming can be helpful, stakeholder input can be obtained more productively if forum participants are asked to comment on and make suggestions for improving specific tasks or initiatives, as seems to have occurred more frequently later in the life cycle of the Global Waiver.

No matter the stage, it is advisable that community concerns be documented and acted upon in a timely manner and that reports and program updates clearly indicate how state policy decisions reflect the ongoing concerns and input of community members. It is also important that public input not be undertaken as a mere formality, but rather as a means to create a more effective partnership to ensure ongoing program improvement and success. In an open, democratic society, providing opportunities for community input is a desirable objective in and of itself. As a practical matter, however, it provides opportunities for program administrators to draw upon additional knowledge and expertise from among individuals representing those most intimately affected by the decisions being made, including beneficiaries and providers. It also provides opportunities for program administrators to obtain assistance with key implementation tasks, an important consideration among increasingly shorthanded state bureaucracies. Ultimately, the familiarity and trust that consultation and collaboration promotes should contribute to the creation of a less challenging environment, both politically, when new programs or initiatives are being designed, and administratively, when they are being implemented.

Devoting Sufficient Administrative and Informational Support to the Tasks at Hand

A state's capacity to undertake major endeavors is reflected in the concept of governing capacity, which has been defined as the "ability to formulate coherent, creative, plausible policy and carry it out efficiently, effectively, and accountably" (Thompson 1998). The capacity of states to govern has increased considerably over the last forty years—state legislatures have become more professional, for example (though Rhode Island's remains a part-term legislature), and administrative agencies have become better resourced and staffed (Thompson 1998). This general growth in capacity has increased confidence in the ability of states to tackle some of the nation's most pressing problems, particularly during periods in which federal action is not forthcoming. Health care is no exception.

"[The] American brand of pluralism," according to Richard Nathan (2006b), "with multiple points of access and maneuver, both horizontally and vertically, has produced cycles of activism alternating between the national government and the states, depending on the conditions and values in the society." Whereas the role of state governments as a source of innovation and spending tends to be enhanced during periods when conservative coalitions control the national government, the role of the federal government tends to be enhanced during more liberal periods (Nathan 2006a, 2006b). State intervention also tends to increase when gridlock exists at the federal level (Oliver 1991). Thus, prior to federal enactment of near universal health insurance coverage with the Affordable Care Act in 2010, it was states such as Massachusetts, Maine, Vermont, Oregon, Tennessee, and Hawaii that took the lead in expanding coverage to uninsured Americans, primarily with the aid of federal Medicaid waivers but also through initiatives such as employer and individual mandates (Hawaii and Massachusetts, respectively), insurance market reforms, and financial incentives targeted at expanding take-up in the small group health insurance market (Brodt et al. 2007; Trinity et al. 2008; Napel et al. January 2009).

Despite the significant role that state governments have played in the health sector, states' willingness and capacities to get things done vary considerably, both across states and over time. Thus, for example, growing fiscal pressures and changing political circumstances led states such as Tennessee and Oregon to ratchet back progress expanding access to coverage, while Massachusetts repealed its comprehensive but unimplemented 1988 health reform measure in 1996 only to pass it again in another form 10 years later (Emerson et al. 2012; Hurley 2006; McDonough et al. 2006; Oberlander 2007). Prior research reveals a strong positive association between state governing capacity and policy innovation in a broad range of areas (Barrilleaux and Miller 1988; Berry and Berry 1990, 2007; Miller 2004, 2005, 2006b; Miller and Wang 2009a; Schneider and Jacoby 1996). Particularly salient for programs such as Medicaid is a state's administrative capacity, or the level of resources accessible to state bureaucracies with which to influence policy, including the financial, intellectual, and personnel resources available to state agencies (Barrilleaux and Miller 1988; Derthick 1970; Schneider and Jacoby 1996; Miller 2006b; Miller and Wang 2009a; Miller et al. 2012; Walshe and Harrington, 2001).

Governors and state legislators mostly concern themselves with Medicaid program spending relative to spending on other priorities. This is in contrast to program administrators who must develop the particular policies that put proposed budget projections and spending objectives into effect. This division of labor makes particular sense for extremely complex and technical area such as Medicaid (Miller 2006a). Thus, while state bureaucrats contribute throughout the policymaking process, those contributions tend to be stronger with respect to the details of Medicaid program development and implementation than with respect to how much is spent overall.

Schneider, Jacoby, and Coggburn (1997) point out that federal law requires that a single administrative agency assume responsibility for Medicaid within each state, and that "these agencies are responsible for formulating all state-level Medicaid initiatives beyond the federally mandated provisions which are required." The authors also point out that informal norms and pressures due to the highly complex and technical nature of health-related issues further promotes bureaucratic responsibility. Lacking the time and expertise with which to deal with program details, elected officials "routinely defer to the judgments of administrators who are acknowledged experts in their fields." Greater administrative capacity is particularly important for developing and implementing major policy changes that require substantial financial resources, administrative wherewithal, technical expertise, and political support to put into place (Miller et al. 2009; Miller and Banaszak-Holl 2005).

Despite the importance of state administrative capacity for comprehensive health reform, "administrative expenses typically represent a small portion of the total costs of a program, and they often get shortchanged in the budgetary process" (National Academy of Public Administration and National Academy of Social Insurance 2009). Moreover, state and local governments have eliminated nearly 600,000 jobs since August 2008 while reducing investments in health, education, and other social welfare programs, largely as a result of the economic downturn (Williams, Leachman, and Johnson July 28, 2011). This has further limited states' ability to effectively implement major program changes. Rhode Island is emblematic.

EOHHS had to implement the Global Waiver at the same time its agencies had lost hundreds of employees due to changes in the state's retirement system meant to encourage such retirements, reductions that hit both central administrative personnel and frontline staff. The timing of these retirements was particularly problematic as the state's fiscal and economic environment increased the demand for Medicaid while slowing down the pace of new hires. The result was high levels of stress among program administrators, not only when performing day-to-day functions but also when administering the Global Waiver, including consulting with and incorporating input from community partners. The dearth of experienced leadership with a history of working collaboratively with community stakeholders only served to alienate potential allies in the provider and consumer communities even more.

Program administrators were further hampered by the data and informational architecture. Despite growing complexity in administering Medicaid and other public programs, Rhode Island relied on antiquated information systems that prevented timely access to the key data elements necessary to track and evaluate progress and that required the devotion of considerable time, energy, and money for maintenance and upkeep. Although the need to update the state's systems were widely recognized, modernization efforts did not begin until implementation of the Global Waiver had begun and not in earnest until after passage of the Affordable Care Act, including updating network, hardware and software resources, instituting data sharing across agencies, implementing centralized monitoring and reducing redundancy, and adopting a centralized portal for all programs. This was also true of stakeholder requests that the state track and make publicly available certain additional data elements over time, and that the state's evaluation plan look beyond spending and utilization to indicators of service scope and quality. It was not until the Rhode Island General Assembly explicitly requested release of some of these additional data elements were they made available on a regular basis.

Prevailing challenges in Rhode Island highlight the importance of ensuring the presence of sufficient numbers of experienced administrative personnel. Most obviously, this includes not undertaking significant endeavors such as the Global Waiver at the same time as other policy changes are being put into place to markedly reduce the size of the state's workforce. Such reductions not only make it more difficult to design and implement necessary changes but it also raises the costs as consultants must be contracted with to perform tasks that could otherwise be performed by state administrative personnel. It also includes not undertaking significant endeavors such as the Global Waiver when the ability to fill key positions is in doubt. In particular, the slow rate of new hires further spotlights challenges associated with implementing comprehensive reform during a fiscal crisis, even with the provision of substantial financial support from the federal government, most noteworthy of which included additional Medicaid matching dollars through the ARRA, the state's CNOM authority, and the Waiver's generous funding cap. Ideally, assessment should be made before implementation has been begun regarding: (1) the ability of state agencies to take on added functions and responsibilities without harming the administration of existing programs; (2) what types of, if any, additional personnel may be needed to effectuate the change desired; and (3) whether or not the requisite resources are available to fill in whatever gaps may exist.

Rhode Island's experience also highlights the need to retain or seek out agency leaders with both the management skills necessary to oversee comprehensive reform and the communication skills necessary to work productively and effectively with community stakeholders. The latter is particularly important in states such as Rhode Island with a history of making major programs changes in collaboration with community partners, though, of course, building support and cooperation is crucial for the successful development, adoption, and implementation of any major endeavor. Appointing trusted and experienced leaders who fit their roles well is a necessary precondition for that success, not only because administration is likely to go more smoothly but also because doing so is more likely to result in buy-in both on the part of internal agency personnel and on the part of external stakeholders, including state legislators, provider representatives, and program beneficiaries and their advocates.

Although it may not be possible to anticipate every conceivable need, it is crucial that the technology systems necessary to undertake all major programmatic tasks and to meet most reasonable data requests be put into place before implementation begins. The former includes program management and claims processing, clinical review and application processing, and eligibility determination and redetermination. Rhode Island has clearly made progress updating its information technology infrastructure in light of Affordable Care Act requirements requiring the adoption of streamlined and coordinated electronic eligibility determination processes. Indeed, the imposition of a tight time frame—an October 1, 2013, deadline—and the provision of federal funds at an enhanced 90% : 10% matching rate have spurred state efforts in this area where they once stagnated due to the high costs of technology and state budgetary limitations. By January 2013, 47 states had either applied for or received federal grants to upgrade their eligibility systems while 42 had already begun work on systems development (Heberlein et al. January 2013). Moreover, a growing number of states have instituted online applications (37) and renewals (28); a large majority (36) also now provides for online accounts.

When tracking performance, it is important that program administrators look beyond a general accounting of program activities and tasks and spending and utilization trends to indicators of service scope and quality—for example, number of applications and referrals; types, amount, and duration of services used across major program components and population groups; number of appeals and their outcomes; and indicators of beneficiary satisfaction, quality of life, and quality of care. Ultimately, the goal should be to keep track of and release that information necessary to assess impact, both for the state and federal governments and for program beneficiaries and providers, and to ensure the investment of sufficient resources to achieve program goals and to determine if and when modifications need to be made.

This objective would more readily be met if the federal government reemphasized the "research and demonstration" component of the 1115 waiver application process, making sure that states incorporated and executed detailed evaluation plans based on the most suitable social science techniques. Systematic assessment of waiver performance has not been the norm for nearly two decades. Although rigorous evaluations have indeed taken place, particularly in those instances where federal officials have hired independent contractors to perform such tasks, state evaluations of varying quality became the norm during the Clinton administration due to the imposition of smaller research budgets and rising workloads resulting from the growing numbers of waiver applications submitted and approved (Thompson and Burke 2007). This continued under the George W. Bush administration, where even less emphasis was placed on either the inclusion or execution of state evaluation plans (though some states nonetheless took this role seriously), and political appointees were reluctant to share whatever independent evaluation results were reported, not only to the general policy community but to professional staff within CMS. Overall, "the fact remains,"

Thompson and Burke (2007) report, "that the federal government did not systematically partner to assure rigorous evaluation of the 1115 demonstrations, the synthesis of major findings, and the vigorous dissemination of these results to other states and the broader policy community."

Transparency and public input are particularly important if policy learning is to take place both nationally and within and across states. Procedural, financial, and outcome data should be released voluntarily to the public on a regular basis without intervention on the part of the state legislature or other oversight body. These data should be released in a standardized and easily accessible format so that program performance can be accurately tracked and compared over time. Program administrators should be sure to incorporate the concerns of state legislators, advocates, providers, and other interested parties into their data tracking and evaluation processes, and choose measures that reflect these concerns. Program administrators should also notify community organizations as new program reports and data become available, say, through an email listserv to ensure broad data awareness and dissemination. Allowing for public input and transparency in this area should both improve the effectiveness of the state's data and information tracking processes and build trust between program administrators and their community partners, thereby contributing to a less challenging implementation, feedback, and modification environment than might otherwise be the case.

Carefully Considering the Breadth and Timing of Reform

Political scientists have long demonstrated that most policy change, whether as a characteristic of the budgetary process or policymaking more generally, is incremental (Berry 1990; Davis, Dempster, and Wildavsky 1966, 1974; Lindblom 1959, 1965; Wildavsky 1964). Recognizing that non-incremental policy change does indeed take place, however, leading theories of the policy process have sought to integrate the general tendency toward incrementalism into a broader perspective that accounts for this reality. Among the most noteworthy of these perspectives are the policy streams, punctuated equilibrium, and advocacy coalition frameworks (Kingdon 1995; Baumgartner and Jones 1993; Sabatier and Jenkins-Smith 1993). Together these theories provide insight into why Rhode Island was able to adopt its comprehensive overhaul of the Medicaid program when it did, whereas other states have continued along comparatively incremental trajectories.

Kingdon (1995) recognizes that while incrementalism may best characterize how most existing policy changes and new proposals are developed, interest in an issue does not typically build in a gradual or incremental fashion. Rather, " 'a subject rather suddenly hits,' 'catches on,' or 'takes off' " when a "window of opportunity" opens, thereby enabling three relatively independent streams—problems, policies, and politics—to come together. First, there is problem recognition in which problems come to capture the attention of people in and around government. Second, there is policy generation, in which potential solutions are formed and refined within communities of specialists. Last, there is politics, which is composed of such dimensions as the public mood, election results, and legislative and executive ideology. Although largely independent, with each having a life of their own, the three streams merge at critical times—known as policy windows—typically with the help of well-placed individuals or champions—often referred to as policy entrepreneurs who are willing to invest the time and resources necessary to promote a particular option and take advantage of windows of opportunity for policy change. Windows open for several reasons but primarily due to compelling problems or significant political events.

Baumgartner and Jones (1993) argue that most issues most of the time are under the control of monopolies of specialists and special interests. However, policy punctuations, or large-scale departures from existing policies occasionally occur as issues are defined in new ways and formerly uninvolved political actors and government institutions become involved. Particularly important are policy images and policy venues. Whereas policy images are simplified ways of explaining issues and the preferred alternatives to addressing them, policy venues are the institutional locations where authoritative decisions are made. Because any given policy area may be associated with competing policy images, and some venues may prove more amenable to certain images than others, major policy change can take place as actors manipulate the understandings of given policies in their search for those venues that will be most favorable to their interests (Baumgartner and Jones 1993). Shifts to more sympathetic venues may be facilitated by changes in prevailing socioeconomic and political conditions.

Sabatier and Jenkins-Smith (1993) propose that long-term policy change typically requires competition among two or more "advocacy coalitions," which consist of like-minded actors who exhibit a nontrivial degree of coordination in seeking to translate a particular set of values into public policy. Most policy change takes place gradually through a process of policy-oriented learning where coalition views and strategies are revised in light of experience and/or new information. Significant policy change can still occur, though, due to significant perturbations in social, political, and economic circumstances. This is because as long as the dominant coalition that champions a government policy remains in power, the core attributes of that policy are unlikely to change. By altering the distribution of resources among coalitions vying for influence, however, major shocks in broader, contextual conditions can promote the rise and fall of prevailing coalitions, which, in turn, lead to changes in government policies.

Each of the aforementioned policy process frameworks points to major perturbations in socioeconomic and political conditions as major stimulators of comprehensive change. Although the rising costs of Medicaid had long been a recognized problem, the onset of the fiscal downturn firmly placed the program at the forefront of policy discussions about how best to rein in the state's growing budget deficit. General recognition that Rhode Island relied primarily on expensive institutional care rather than cheaper noninstitutional services despite ongoing efforts to shift the locus of care to home- and community-based settings placed long-term care rebalancing at the center of the state's policy discussions in this area as well. It was during this period, therefore, that the predominant view of the state's Medicaid program shifted from a program that provided access to health and long-term care services to low-income Rhode Islanders to a growing drain on state resources. This is reflected in general consensus among elected leaders within Rhode Island regarding the seriousness of the fiscal problems that the state was facing and the potential for comprehensive Medicaid reform, including long-term care rebalancing to help solve it, not only with respect to the state's Republican Governor, Donald Carcieri, but also among Democratic legislators who ultimately committed themselves to the plan in the hopes of gaining tens of millions of dollars in savings for the state. While there was certainly sympathy among members of the state legislature for providers' and advocates' concerns about the potential impact of reform on beneficiary access and quality, the overriding imperative was the growing state budget deficit resulting largely from the state's rapidly deteriorating fiscal environment.

The political environment was also ripe for adoption of the Global Waiver given alignment of the political and ideological interests of Rhode Island's Republican administration with that of President George W. Bush, both of whom desired to restrain Medicaid program spending and to delegate further responsibilities to the states, and to rebalance long-term care away from institutions toward home- and community-based services, an issue over which there has been general bipartisan consensus. Moreover, as with the case of waivers more generally (Thompson and Burke 2007, 2009), Rhode Island's initiative provided President Bush, Governor Carcieri, and their administrations opportunities to exert leadership. Unable to convince Congress to block grant Medicaid, the Bush administration viewed the Global Waiver as a chance to demonstrate the potential success of this approach to reshaping Medicaid by recruiting a state willing to place an overall cap on federal expenditures. Unable either to slow the growth in state Medicaid spending or to rebalance long-term care despite ongoing efforts in both areas, Governor Carcieri and key appointees, including Gary Alexander, former Department of Human Services director and EOHHS Secretary, devoted considerable time, energy, and political capital to guiding the Global Waiver through the federal CMS and state legislative approval processes.

Clearly, Governor Carcieri and his subordinates served as policy entrepreneurs, taking advantage of prevailing economic and political circumstances and the resulting window of opportunity to promote a strategy for Medicaid reform broadly consistent with the strategy favored by the federal administration (Donnelly January 1, 2009). Both Governor Carcieri and Secretary Alexander considered the Global Waiver to be among their signature accomplishments. Thus, for example, the *Providence Journal* reported that at the end of his term in office, Governor "Carcieri says he leaves proud of all that he was able to accomplish in the years before and after 'the world collapsed' into a deep recession. He is also proud of having reduced the size of the state work force, pushed state workers into paying a portion of their health-insurance premiums and reined in pension costs. He's proud to have . . . won federal approval for a first-of-its-kind waiver giving the state flexibility in how it spends its Medicaid dollars on the poor, the elderly and the disabled" (Edgar and Gregg December 26, 2010). For his part, former EOHHS Secretary Gary Alexander later claimed that he and the Governor "took bold action to address the Medicaid issue" through "the most comprehensive attempt to fundamentally change the Medicaid system and end the current entitlement" and that "Rhode Island is the only state to act and achieve success, proving that bigger government and more money are not the solution. The Rhode Island experience is quietly being noticed as the mother of innovation and a model for the nation" (Alexander January 28, 2011).

Political and ideological alignment between the federal and state administrations is particularly important in areas such as Medicaid where the locus or venue for authoritative decision making has shifted over the last 20 years from Congress and the state legislatures to the executive branches of government. Gais and Fossett (2005) coined the term "executive federalism" to describe this new alignment, observing that "the President and [his] appointees have been able to produce significant changes in program management, coverage, and standards without new legislation. Even large policy changes depend less on major shifts in controls over Congress . . . and more on control of the presidency and governorships and the conditions facing the states." The upshot is that major change in how state Medicaid programs are run primarily reflects the outcome of discussions between federal and state officials rather than statutory changes enacted by Congress and/or the state legislatures.

Key to this shift has been exponential growth in the use of federal waiver authorities which, on the one hand, permit the President to fundamentally alter Medicaid without authorization from Congress, and, on the other hand, permits governors and their staffs to restructure their state's programs through negotiations and bargaining with their federal counterparts (Thompson and Burke 2007, 2009; Weissert and Weissert 2008). Negotiation and bargaining has been particularly important for 1115 waivers, which, because states typically seek to change Medicaid broadly, elicit strong views on the part of federal and state authorities (Thompson and Burke 2009). Moreover, like licenses, federal Medicaid waivers are approved for multiple years after which they are typically renewed indefinitely (Weissert and Weissert 2008). Barring fundamental changes in prevailing political and economic circumstances, the result, essentially, is permanent program changes largely insulated from broader democratic influences. Through December 5, 2012, CMS has granted 391 Medicaid waiver requests, just 48 of which have since expired (CMS 2012). This includes 44 current (15 expired) 1115 "research and demonstration" waivers; 25 current (5 expired) 1915(b) "managed care" waivers; and 273 current (27 expired) 1915(c) "home- and community-services" waivers.[3] The genesis of Rhode Island's Global Waiver is a paradigmatic example of executive federalism in action (Donnelly January 1, 2009).

In addition to prevailing fiscal challenges and political and ideological alignment between the Carcieri and Bush administrations, the relative weakness of the opposition proved critical to the successful promulgation of the Global Waiver. On the one hand, this was due to the lack of political clout generally held by Medicaid beneficiaries and their advocates although the program has increasingly been viewed as a middle-class entitlement rather than a poor persons' welfare program over time (Grogan and Gusmano 2007; Miller 2008; Miller and Banaszak-Holl 2005; Miller and Wang 2009a; Rosenbaum 2012; Thompson 2012). On the other hand, it was due to challenges Waiver opponents had in reacting to what was being proposed due to the tight time frame provided, the limited information made available, and uncontroversial generalities with which it was framed (e.g., ensuring the provision of "the right services at the right time in the right setting") (Donnelly January 1, 2009), in addition to the changing nature of what was being proposed—in particular, from a block grant with nearly unlimited state flexibility to a capped federal match with much more restricted state discretion. The opposition's weaknesses were also due to the breadth of the Global Waiver itself, which in touching virtually all aspects of the Medicaid program, made it difficult for affected beneficiaries, their advocates, and the providers that serve them to coalesce into an effective opposition despite the development of largely informal forums such as the Coalition for Responsible Medicaid Reform and the state's congressional delegation, both of which served as clearinghouses for information and grievances among consumer advocates and providers.

The limited impact of Rhode Island's Democratic Senators and Congressmen in opposing the Global Waiver highlights the varying interests of federal- and state-level officeholders. One would presume consistency in the views and positions of Democrat Party officials, no matter whether they served in federal or state government. The experience in Rhode Island clearly suggests that this need not be the case (Donnelly January 1, 2009). While Rhode Island's Democrat Party-dominated General Assembly must be responsive to their constituencies, they are also responsible for balancing the state budget, an imperative that can override what might otherwise be in their political and ideological interests, particularly during a severe economic downturn. This is in contrast to the state's congressional delegation which, because it is not responsible for the state budget, has greater freedom to pursue its political and ideological interests, at least as it relates to local constituencies.

The limited impact of consumer and provider representatives in opposing approval of the Global Waiver derived, in part, from considerable heterogeneity among the different groups that compete for Medicaid program resources, including the elderly, people with physical and developmental disabilities, the mentally ill, and children and families (Kronebusch 1997). Although ostensibly part of the same program, each group interacts differently with the political and administrative processes through which the program is designed and administered. These differences reflect variation in politics, needs, and economic constraints. "The political differences," according to Kronebusch (1997), "concern political participation and their relationships to political coalitions and electoral competition, the images of the groups in the eyes of other political actors, and the legacy of past and current public policy. The differing needs . . . concern the mix of medically and socially defined needs. Important constraints concern the political economy of labor markets and of government spending programs and the nature of the . . . providers' role in delivering services."

Unlike more limited reform efforts, the Global Waiver encompassed the entire Medicaid program, and, as such, included both acute and long-term care while engaging all populations served by the program and not a limited subset. Because of differences in the ways these groups interact with the Medicaid, the broad scope of the reform, in turn, made it more difficult to achieve consensus, both with regard to grievance and strategy, than if a more limited, homogeneous subset of Medicaid beneficiaries and providers had been affected. Although all parties were concerned about state flexibility and funding limits built into the proposal, for example, specific concerns varied depending on the particular population groups affected. There was a widely recognized need to rebalance long-term care for elders, though some still believed this goal could be achieved under the existing program framework despite the lack of progress to date. Alternatively, there were doubts about the need to do so for people with developmental disabilities and behavioral health/substance abuse problems, given that both populations already relied heavily on noninstitutional care settings at home and in the community. Advocates for children and families were especially fearful about the Waiver's implications for RIte Care, a successful program that might be financially compromised should savings deriving from state efforts to rebalance long-term care prove unsuccessful.

Interestingly, the same conditions that facilitated the adoption of the Global Waiver posed challenges for implementation. Adoption of the Global Waiver was clearly facilitated by the adverse implications of the economic crisis for the state budget, and the political and ideological alignment of the state's Republican administration with that of the federal government, both of which had sought to restrain Medicaid program spending in the past. This combination of fiscal and political imperatives, however, contributed to concern on the part of key stakeholder groups regarding the administration's commitment to the program, distrust that extended well into implementation of the Waiver's provisions, including the institution of a more stringent legislative oversight regime than had existed previously. The fiscal crisis also led to significant reductions in state administrative personnel, increased emphasis on cost control over programmatic improvement, and delayed implementation of important program elements, including planned increases in provider reimbursement and investments in key service supports (e.g., transportation, case management, personal spending allowances). These decisions have, in turn, slowed down progress and limited the level of financial savings achieved, particularly from long-term care rebalancing, an issue discussed in greater depth below. Overall, findings indicate that while poor fiscal environments may be the driving impetus behind reform, moving forward with significant program change during an economic downturn can affect state capacity and funding levels, thereby compromising implementation and leading to weaker than expected results.

Because the Global Waiver touches on most aspects of the Medicaid program, and because few details had been released to the general public, critics had a difficult time fomenting a clear and coherent opposition, particularly given substantial heterogeneity amongst the populations affected, thereby contributing to the Waiver's ultimate adoption, both by the federal government and the state legislature. But while potentially advantageous politically for the Waiver's proponents, the breadth of the Global Waiver made implementation far more challenging than if reform had been limited, say, to the state's system for providing long-term care for the elderly and people with physical disabilities. There were two key challenges in this regard. First, the large number and diversity of key stakeholder interests posed challenges for a shorthanded state bureaucracy charged with incorporating feedback from the multiple consumer advocacy and provider groups participating in the state's Global Waiver Implementation Task Force. While such interaction promoted greater cooperation and understanding across the various state agencies and provider and advocacy groups impacted, the scope of the task and degree of cross-sector learning required nonetheless proved daunting.

Second, and more importantly, continued imposition of organizational barriers across departments within the state bureaucracy has hampered implementation of the Global Waiver. Although increased communication, cooperation, and understanding is evident since the Waiver has gone into effect, development and implementation of a uniform, coherent policy affecting Medicaid continues to be inhibited by administration of the program across all EOHHS departments, whose coordination remains somewhat limited due to the weakness of the EOHHS Secretariat. Had the Global Waiver focused on elders and the physically disabled, then just EOHHS and two constituent departments—Human Services and Elderly Affairs—would have borne the brunt of implementation. Since the Global Waiver impacts all program populations, however, implementation of the Global Waiver has engaged staff in the Departments of Behavioral Healthcare,

Developmental Disabilities, and Hospitals, Children, Youth, and Families, and Health as well. The Lewin Group (2008) identified the Global Waiver as an opportunity to implement a coordinated Medicaid budgeting process and to reposition Medicaid as a cross-departmental leader and technical assistance resource. This has yet to happen, though the single state agency responsible for the Medicaid program has since shifted to EOHHS rather than the Department of Human Services. While placing the entire program under single waiver has helped break down the silo mentality, EOHHS continues to lack formal budget and administrative authority over its constituent departments, each of which reports directly to the governor and not the EOHHS director.

To promote coordination, program administration rules and incentives must be adopted to ensure the fidelity of each constituent implementing unit to the goals of reform. Agency theory suggests that if a department, as an agent, does not perfectly represent the interests of central administration, it is because that department's interests do not perfectly coincide with central administration's goals (Moe 1984; Pratt and Zekhauser, 1985). This implies more careful consideration of interagency flows of authority, closer monitoring, and aligning budgetary incentives so that constituent departments better conform to the interests of those leading reform. Transaction cost analysis highlights the costs of dealing with multiple departments, with the need to cross departmental boundaries contributing to "misunderstandings and conflicts that lead to delays, breakdowns, and other malfunctions" (Williamson, 1981). Efficiency within the transaction cost framework refers to the efficiency of organizational forms. This suggests the advantage of bringing all Medicaid functions under one authority rather than distributing those functions across multiple departments whose leaders and staff may not be sympathetic to what state leaders are trying to accomplish. Thus, to the extent possible, the goal should be to avoid agency problems and lower transaction costs by breaking down barriers that separate departments responsible for implementing Medicaid, including placing primary policy, budget, and management responsibilities in the hands of a single oversight agency. As long as Medicaid-funded services in Rhode Island are distributed across separate departments, each with its own priorities, constituencies, policies and staff, and director who reports independently to the Governor rather than to the state's EOHHS Secretary, reform is likely to fall short of its ultimate goals, programmatic or otherwise.

REBALANCING THE LONG-TERM CARE SYSTEM

Since a dominant focus of the Global Waiver was long-term care rebalancing, this study provides useful lessons for states looking to make progress in this area, particular given incentives contained within the Affordable Care Act aimed at spurring state action on the redistribution of Medicaid long-term care spending away from nursing homes and towards home- and community-based settings. Specific lessons include: understanding that progress toward rebalancing will be slow in states where nursing home spending has previously predominated, recognizing challenges to rebalancing posed by adverse fiscal circumstances, and prioritizing the documentation and promotion of sufficient provider capacity.

Rebalancing Occurs Slowly in States Where Nursing Home Care Currently Predominates

Nationally, there has been considerable growth in Medicaid home- and community-based services participants and expenditures, which have increased from 1.9 to 3.3 million and $17 to $50 billion, respectively, between 1999 and 2009 (Ng et al. December 2012; Howard, Ng, and Harrington, December 2011). Yet despite such progress, there is still a long way to go; in 2009, most Medicaid long-term care spending for the elderly and physically disabled continued to be directed toward institutional (64%) rather than noninstitutional (36%) services (Eiken et al. October 31, 2011). There is also considerable cross-state variation with the proportion of expenditures for the elderly and physically disabled directed toward noninstitutional care, ranging from 4.4% in Rhode Island and 10.2% in North Dakota to 62.1% and 78.7%, respectively, in Washington and New Mexico (Eiken et al. October 31, 2011). Although most Medicaid long-term care spending for the developmentally disabled was directed toward noninstitutional (66%) rather than institutional (34%) services in 2009, there was considerable cross-state variation in this area as well, ranging from 13.3% in Mississippi and 43.6% in Illinois to 99.1% and 99.2%, respectively, in Vermont and Michigan. Moreover, there is considerable cross-state variation in participants and per capita costs. Nationally, for example, Medicaid 1915(c) home- and community-based waiver expenditures per person served was $24,676 in 2009, but ranged from $10,343 in Mississippi to $57,326 in Maine (Ng et al. December 2012). That year, total participants in such programs reached 1,366,337 but ranged from less than 5,000 in Alaska, the District of Columbia, Delaware, Hawaii, Montana, North Dakota, Nevada, South Dakota, and Wyoming to more than 50,000 in California, Florida, Illinois, Minnesota, New York, Ohio, Pennsylvania, and Texas.

Rhode Island would seem to be an ideal state with which to make progress on rebalancing given so little use has traditionally been made of services provided in the home- and community-based sector. While many felt that the Global Waiver was unnecessary—that the state's existing 1915(c) waivers were enough—consolidation under a single authority did serve a useful role in placing the issue more firmly on the state's policy agenda. Thus, on the plus side, the Waiver has provided a framework that has served to organize discussions, consolidate initiatives, and spur progress on state efforts to rebalance the long-term care system, an area most felt the state had finally made tangible advancements on after years of limited gains. Indeed, the evidence cited above suggests that Rhode Island's rebalancing efforts have had some impact, though these trends largely began before the Global Waiver was implemented (The Lewin Group December 6, 2011; Allen, Gozalo, and Steinman June 30, 2011).

That overall spending has remained largely stagnant, however, suggests just how difficult it can be for laggard states that have historically spent substantially more on nursing homes to make more than marginal progress in this area, even with the provision of options and incentives that otherwise should promote rebalancing, including the relatively generous overall funding cap provided and the ability to draw in additional federal dollars for previously state-only funded programs under the Global Waiver's Costs Not Otherwise Matchable or CNOM authority. The slow progress made in Rhode Island despite the Global Waiver, Perry Sullivan Legislation, Real Choices Systems Change grants, and other measures does not bode well for the likely efficacy of the Affordable Care Act's rebalancing provisions, even among states, like Rhode Island, that seem highly motivated, either for cost or programmatic reasons, to shift spending from nursing homes to home- and community-based settings.

The Affordable Care Act seeks to address Medicaid's continuing institutional bias and to reduce prevailing interstate variation in this area by incentivizing and extending a number of Medicaid home- and community-based options. Most importantly, it provides additional financial incentives and options for states to expand home- and community-based services under Medicaid, including the State Balancing Incentive Payments program, which provides for enhanced federal matching payments from 2011 to 2015 for states increasing the proportion of spending in this area; a new Medicaid state plan option for attendant services and supports known as the Community First Choice Option; and modifications to the little used 1915(i) state plan option first promulgated under the Deficit Reduction Act of 2005. The Affordable Care Act also extends mandatory spousal impoverishment protections to community-based spouses of people receiving home- and community-based services, provides additional funding for Aging Disability and Resource Centers, and extends the Money Follows the Person Demonstration while shortening the length of nursing home residency required for participants to qualify for the program.

Harrington et al. (2012) argue that although providing important options and incentives for states to expand home- and community-based services under Medicaid, the impact of the State Balancing Incentive Payments program, Community First Choice Option; and 1915(i) state plan option will be limited. Most importantly, nursing home care continues to be a mandatory benefit and, as such, an entitlement all states must provide under Medicaid while home- and community-based services remains an optional benefit that states may offer at their discretion to a restricted number of participants, according to geographic location, target group, and/or the specific types of services required. In addition, the income level at which individuals can qualify for home- and community-based service benefits is often lower than the income level established for nursing home care, which is up to 300% of the Supplemental Security Income benefit in most states (Ng et al. December 2012).

While Medicaid pays for room and board for nursing home care, it may not do so for those receiving home- and community-based services, nor can room and board be counted as a medical expense for purposes of spending down to Medicaid eligibility as a result of the incurrence of large medical expenses under the medical needy programs adopted in 33 states and the District of Columbia (Watts and Young December 2012; Woodcock et al. June 14, 2011). Besides leaving investments in home- and community-based spending especially vulnerable to the vagaries of state budget and political processes (Harrington et al. 2012; Woodcock et al. June 14, 2011), the optional nature of these programs and the continuing absence of minimum standards and requirements to cover all geographic areas and target populations suggests persistent unmet need, both within and across states. This combined with varying dispositions for making the structural and administrative changes necessary to expand home- and community-based services and to qualify for additional federal matching support under the Affordable Care Act suggests the continuation of substantial cross-state variation in the amount of progress states make toward rebalancing long-term care under Medicaid.

Given disappointing progress despite the provision of additional options and incentives contained within the Global Waiver, Rhode Island is now seeking to bolster its rebalancing efforts through the provision of integrated care to Medicaid-only beneficiaries in need of long-term services and supports and to Medicaid beneficiaries who are also eligible for Medicare. Key to this effort will be participation in CMS' Financial Alignment Demonstration, through which the federal agency has sought to use its authority under the Affordable Care Act to improve care coordination, largely through the provision of appropriate and cost-effective services, including home- and community-based supports, to Medicare-Medicaid dual eligibles. Why the focus on the nation's 9.1 million duals? This group comprises an extremely poor population with especially complex service needs: many (55%) have multiple chronic conditions as well as physical (44%) and cognitive (54%) impairment (Jacobson, Neuman, and Damico April 4, 2012). This group is also comparatively expensive: Duals comprise only 20% of the Medicare population but constitute 31% of program expenditures; they comprise 15% of the Medicaid population but constitute 39% of its funding, with most of that (69%) going toward long-term services and supports (Jacobson, Neuman, and Damico April 4, 2012). Average spending for duals is nearly twice as high as for other Medicare beneficiaries. Combined federal and state spending on duals reached $320 billion 2011.

The focus on the high-cost dual population is not new; deficiencies in the care of dual eligibles are widely acknowledged (Grabowski 2007; Miller and Wiessert 2003, 2004). Duals often use a high volume of services from numerous provider types in a variety of settings. Inefficiency and fragmentation are rife: tests and procedures are often repeated, medications prescribed in ignorance, care transitions mishandled, and inter-provider communication nonexistent. Cost-shifting also occurs as both the state and federal governments have incentives to shift responsibility for high cost cases and providers have incentives to maximize reimbursement where possible, particularly when Medicare and Medicaid pay for the same modalities (e.g., nursing facility and home health care). High rates of preventable hospitalization and other indicators of poor quality suggest ample opportunities to improve care and save money.

Achieving system improvement is easier said than done. There is a long history of efforts to improve care coordination, and the variability of their success reflects the difficulty of the task. A primary cause of fragmentation is service delivery silos, which create incentives to reallocate costs (from nursing homes to hospitals, for example) and present logistical, informational, and cultural barriers to coordinating care. A potential solution to this problem is to give responsibility (and funding) for a bundle of services to a single entity—often, a managed care organization. This model is followed by several small programs, which, overall, enroll fewer than 2% of all duals nationally. The most notable example is PACE, which receives both Medicare and Medicaid capitation payments to deliver health and long-term services and supports by multidisciplinary care teams to individuals needing a nursing home level of care. The good news is programs such as PACE deliver high-quality care; the bad news is that they have never been shown to save money (Newman et al. 2012). The absence of net savings is also true of care coordination and disease management programs that attempt to improve care integration under traditional fee-for-service arrangements. Findings from the Medicare Coordinated Care Demonstration, for example, indicate that financial gains resulting from reduced rates of hospitalization were insufficient to offset costs associated with the interventions applied (Brown et al. 2012).

Prevailing experience therefore suggests that although the Affordable Care Act's attempts to better integrate care for dual eligibles is much-needed, success is not assured. Prior to the Affordable Care Act, legislation introduced Special Needs Plans for dual eligibles (D-SNPs), a type of Medicare Advantage plan. While some D-SNPs genuinely improve service delivery—often, by working with Medicaid-managed care organizations to deliver a coordinated package of care, including long-term services and supports—most have failed to do so, suggesting a lack of commitment to full integration (Grabowski 2012). Managing care for dual eligibles is challenging. To be effective, managed care organizations must demonstrate a willingness to work with this complex population, to develop an appropriate service delivery network (with providers who may need to change their work practices), and to invest the resources necessary to achieve organizational change and infrastructure development. Successful care coordination typically relies on a single entity (an individual or a team) able to manage the full bundle of Medicare and Medicaid services. This may be challenging when plans rely on subcontracts to other entities to deliver certain categories of services (e.g., mental health, long-term care), or where care managers must work effectively with multiple providers subject to their own particular incentives and rewards. The need to navigate separate regulatory requirements for Medicare and Medicaid, which remain imperfectly aligned, complicates matters even further.

It is likely most managed care organizations and managed fee-for-service programs participating in CMS' Financial Alignment Demonstration will lack the expertise in care coordination necessary to deliver high quality, cost-effective care to dual eligibles. What this often means, in practice, is inexperience working with the full range of services that this population needs–including long-term services and supports (Gold, Jacobson, and Garfield 2012). It also means an inability to cater service integration strategies to the diverse circumstances of particular duals; some are especially high cost to Medicare (e.g., heavy acute care users with multiple chronic conditions), Medicaid (e.g., frail and disabled individuals living in nursing homes), or both (Coughlin, Waidmann, and Phadera 2012). Given this inexperience and CMS requirement that plans demonstrate cost savings, there is concern that plans might resort to more reliable ways of cutting costs (via service denials and favorable selection, for example), rather than face the challenges and uncertain risks associated with service delivery innovation. Evidence on good practices in caring for dual eligibles exists: these share a focus on transitions among levels of care; ready access to patient information; attention to medication management; and care management which is team-based, involving participants across multiple settings. Potential savings, were these practices broadly implemented, could be as high as $125 billion to the federal government and $34 billion to the states over a 10-year period (Thorpe September 2011). Thus, although such an intensive approach might be costly, it could result in substantial savings.

Recognizing Challenges to Rebalancing Posed by Adverse Fiscal Circumstances

Adverse fiscal circumstances have slowed down progress toward long-term care rebalancing. Nationally, state waitlists for 1915(c) waiver services have grown in recent years. Just before the recession, from 2006 to 2007, the number of individuals on waitlists for 1915(c) waiver services declined by 7% (Ng et al. December 2012; Ng, Harrington, and Howard February 2011). At the start of the recession, however, from 2007 to 2008, the number of individuals on waitlists for 1915(c) waiver services increased considerably, by 17%; a year later, from 2008 to 2009, the number increased even more substantially, by 19%. Currently, there are more than 511,174 on waitlists for 1915(c) waiver services in 39 states, up from 428,571 the previous year, including 316,674 waiting for intellectual/developmental disability (I/DD) waiver services and 145,695 waiting for aged and disability waiver services (Ng et al. December 2012). Average waiting times now extend to more than two years (25 months), ranging from two months, on average, for mental health to 9, 15, and 40 months, respectively, for the age/disabled, aged, and I/DD waiver populations.

There have also been cutbacks to non-Medicaid-funded home- and community-based services and Medicaid-funded personal care services during the course of the latest economic downturn (Center on Budget and Policy Priorities January 28, 2010; Mollica 2009; Shishkin 2008; Walls et al. January 2011). As noted, nursing home care is a mandatory service under Medicaid, whereas most home- and community-based coverage is provided at a state's discretion. Thus, although general consensus exists about the desirability of rebalancing (Miller, Mor, and Clark 2010; Grabowski et al. 2010), home- and community-based options are at particular risk during periods of fiscal retrenchment. Thus, at the height of the recession, states continued to expand access to home- and community-based services, but the pace of expansion slowed while additional cost and utilization controls were added to the waitlists, enrollment caps, and coverage limits already in place (Smith et al. September 2010).

Home- and community-based providers are also at a comparative disadvantage in the competition for scarce resources. This is due, in part, to the nursing home industry's status as one of the most powerful lobbies in state government (Hrebenar and Thomas 1998–2007; Miller 2006a, 2006b; Miller and Wang 2009a, 2009b; Miller et al. 2012; Nownes, Thomas, and Hrebenar 2008). Perhaps this is best reflected in the Hrebenar–Thomas study where hospital and nursing home associations were ranked the fifth most influential interest across the fifty states in 2007 behind business, teacher, utility, and manufacturer interests. By contrast, senior citizens/AARP, perhaps the closest proxy for home- and community-based service providers given the strong preference for rebalancing among elder advocacy organizations, were thirty-ninth most influential, next to last on the list, just ahead of pro-tobacco interests (Nownes, Thomas, and Hrebenar 2008). Being heavily dependent on Medicaid for revenue, nursing homes are especially active in trying to influence policy in this area, with such activity being associated with increased likelihood of adoption of favorable Medicaid policies affecting nursing home spending, eligibility, enforcement, and reimbursement (Barrilleaux and Miller 1988; Grogan 1999; Harrington, Mullan, and Carrillo 2004; Miller 2008; Miller 2006a, 2006b; Miller and Wang 2009b; Miller et al. 2012).

Home- and community-based providers are also at a comparative disadvantage given the way annual increases in provider reimbursement are structured. Costs from which provider reimbursement levels are derived must be inflated forward to account for changes in market conditions. This can be accomplished through legislatively determined adjustments and/or nationally or locally derived indices previously written into statute or state regulation (Miller et al. 2009). This is an important distinction because annual legislative authorizations for inflation adjustment are quite different than building an inflation method into the law or regulation that will be applied regardless of a state's fiscal circumstances unless additional legislation is enacted. The latter, which is often indicative of state systems for reimbursing nursing home providers, tends to propel annual payment increases that, in turn, encourage steady growth in program spending (Woodcock et al. June 14, 2011). The former, which is often indicative of state systems for reimbursing home- and community-based providers, tends to retard annual payment increases that, in turn, discourage consistent growth in spending on such programs.

Home- and community-based services providers are also at a disadvantage in that most states (44) have adopted nursing home provider taxes, which enables them to draw in additional federal matching funds without concomitant increases in state expenditures, thereby helping bolster nursing home provider payments (Kaiser Family Foundation January 10, 2013; Miller and Wang 2009b). Provider tax arrangements involve the assessment of taxes on the gross revenue of nursing homes, hospitals, managed care organizations, residential care facilities, and other providers. A provider tax, also called a "fee" or "assessment," enables states to collect revenue from providers, which is then used to pay for services rendered to Medicaid recipients, thereby leveraging federal matching dollars without concomitant increases in state expenditures. Typically, states compensate providers for the cost of the tax through increases in the Medicaid reimbursement rate. To meet federal requirements, taxes must be "broad-based," meaning that the same tax rate must apply to all items or services within the same class of providers (e.g., nursing homes, hospitals, managed care organizations, etc.). They also must be uniform, meaning that they must be applied to all gross revenues, not just to those deriving from Medicaid. Moreover, providers cannot be "held harmless," meaning that states cannot guarantee return of 100 percent of providers' contributions under the tax, though taxes limited to six percent of providers' gross revenues could be returned without violating this prohibition. Few, if any states have adopted such taxes for purposes of boosting payments to home- and community-based services providers.

There are also challenges associated with the short-term investments necessary to get state home- and community-based services programs off the ground. In addition to policy changes at the federal-level, expansion of Medicaid home- and community-based services has been driven by state responses to consumer preferences to remain as long as possible in the least restrictive settings possible, typically at home, in a family member's home, or an assisted-living facility; rarely in a nursing home (typically <5% of those surveyed) (AARP April 2003; Kaiser Family Foundation December 2007; *The Los Angeles Times* October 2009). Expansion of home- and community-based services has also been driven by widespread belief among state policymakers that such programs are cost-effective as per capita Medicaid program costs are substantially lower for those receiving home- and community-based services rather than institutional care; a $44,000 per year difference, on average, according to one study (Kitchener et al. 2006; Wiener 2010). This belief that rebalancing saves money is prevalent despite evidence suggesting that expansion of home- and community-based programs can increase overall costs if services are not adequately targeted toward those who otherwise would have had entered a nursing home. Inadequate targeting combined with the presence of substantial unmet need within the community can result in large numbers of potential beneficiaries coming out of the "woodwork," a challenge long thought to hamper the cost-effectiveness of home- and community-based programs (Grabowski 2006; Weissert 1993). Recent research suggests that only when nursing home admissions are avoided does investment in home- and community-based services payoff from a cost-effectiveness perspective (Kaye, LaPlante, and Harrington 2009). It also suggests that expanding Medicaid home- and community-based services requires short-term increases in expenditures before institutional spending declines and long-term cost savings are achieved (Kay, LaPlante, and Harrington 2009; Mollica et al. March 2009).

Rhode Island has adopted a number of strategies with which to promote proper targeting. These include adoption of a new three-tier level of care eligibility determination system—"highest," "high," and "preventive, with only those deemed "highest" being entitled to nursing home care, though those deemed "high" had previously been eligible as well. These also include the creation of a central interagency mechanism—the so called Assessment and Coordination Organization—for making level of care determinations, supporting community-based placements, implementing consistent case management practices, and conducting high-cost case reviews. Tasking an onsite RN to collaborate with hospital social workers through the state's primary care case management program to identify Medicaid beneficiaries who might be discharged safely back into the community has contributed to the state's targeting efforts as well. In the future, Rhode Island intends to supplement these efforts with peer mentoring and expanding consumer assistance, among other initiatives.

The need to make short-term investments in the interest of obtaining subsequent longer term savings has proven somewhat problematic as Rhode Island sought to expand use of home- and community-based spending during the economic downturn. Indeed, there are several reasons to suspect that the Great Recession and slow recovery has posed challenges to implementing the Global Waiver by adversely impacting state capacity and funding levels. This, perhaps, is the major reason why the state did not make more progress rebalancing long-term care than it has to date. As noted, community stakeholders were especially concerned about substantial reductions in state administrative personnel, which while serving in part to address the state's short-term budget deficit, made implementation of the Global Waiver considerably more challenging than it might have been otherwise. Community stakeholders were also concerned about the state's decision to forgo a $400 increase in the amount of monthly income beneficiaries could keep to help pay for necessary housing, transportation, and other costs (Maigrett January 28, 2013). While perhaps making short-term budgetary sense, this decision hampered beneficiaries' ability to remain at home and in the community, a point the state seems to recognize with inclusion of a provision in its Waiver renewal application increasing the personal needs allowance for certain beneficiaries. Forgone increases in provider reimbursement, a common cost containment strategy during challenging fiscal circumstances, would seem to make short-term budgetary sense too, though if put into effect might otherwise have helped boost the state's limited capacity of home- and community-based services providers.

Although there are currently no waitlists in Rhode Island, the prevailing distribution of spending still overwhelmingly favors nursing homes, suggesting that the demand for home- and community-based services is far from being met. On the one hand, the lack of waitlists in Rhode Island could reflect insufficient identification of potential home- and community-based services clients, whether currently residing in the community or in a nursing home. On the other hand, the lack of waitlists could reflect use of federal CNOM and stimulus dollars to prevent service reductions that otherwise would have been made given the state of the economy. Thus, there remained concern that waitlists might be created in the future both for the "high" care recipients who would have been entitled to long-term care under the old leveling system and for the "preventive" care recipients who were not eligible under the old system should the state budgetary situation continue to deteriorate. This is a particular worry in light of continuing state fiscal challenges and the growing demand for services. Ultimately, Rhode Island's experience suggests the need for perseverance when seeking to expand home- and community-based services, particularly during tough economic times. Eventual savings take time to materialize but only over the long-term and with continued investments both to promote supply and to spur demand.

Documenting and Promoting Sufficient Provider Capacity

There is substantial variation in provider capacity and costs, both within and across states. Consider the assisted-living sector by way of example. According to Stevenson and Grabowski (2010), there are currently 11,276 assisted-living facilities containing 839,746 units in the United States, with an average of 74.5 units per facility and 22.9 facilities per 1,000 elderly people. Considerable differences exist across states, however, with the number of facilities per 1,000 elderly ranging from less than 10 in Connecticut

(4), Hawaii (2), and West Virginia (7) to more than 40 in Minnesota (104), Oregon (43), and Virginia (46). Considerable differences are also apparent within states with counties exhibiting higher assisted-living penetration being characterized by greater educational achievement, income, and home values, and lower poverty, unemployment, and minority representation. Assisted-living facilities are also more likely to be located in urban areas where they tend to be larger and more well-serviced, both in terms of amenities (privacy) and in term of professional staff (nurses) than their rural counterparts (Stevenson and Grabowski 2010). While the average cost of assisted living reached $3,550 per month or $42,600 per year in 2012, costs ranged from $2,751 per month in facilities offering five or fewer services to $3,789 for facilities offering 10 or more (Metlife Mature Market Institute November 2012). There was also substantial geographic variation in costs. Nationally, average costs ranged from $2,355 per month in parts of Arkansas to $5,923 per month in Washington, D.C. Costs differ considerably within states as well; for example, from $1,833 to $10,200 in Connecticut, $1,300 to $8,973 in California, and $780 to $4,471 in Kentucky.

As noted, federal Medicaid regulations do not permit the use of Medicaid funds to pay for room and board in assisted living, though some states nonetheless offer a combined rate that pays for both service and room and board costs (6 states) (Mollica September 2009). Most states, however, either cap room and board charges (23 states), supplement Supplemental Security Income payments for those living in a residential care setting (24 states), and/or permit family supplementation of residents' room and board payments (25 states). Because Medicaid does not explicitly pay for room and board, and because assisted-living facilities receive substantially less for serving Medicaid than private-pay clients, facilities (a) have less incentive to participate in the Medicaid program than, say, nursing homes, which receive payments that cover both service and room and board and (b) have less incentive to take a Medicaid client over a private-pay client even when they do participate (Carlson and Coffey November 2010; National Senior Citizens Law Center February 2011). The lack of incentive for assisted-living facilities to participate in the Medicaid program is in marked contrast to (a) the nursing home sector, which although involving considerable private contributions, either out-of-pocket (26.7%) or through private insurance (7.4%), relies heavily on Medicaid (40.6%) and Medicare (18.6%) and (b) the home health sector, which is weighted even more heavily toward government funding in the way of Medicaid (34.7%) and Medicare (41.2%) relative to out-of-pocket payments (10.1%) and private insurance (9.0%) (CMS 2010). Thus, although many of the people served in assisted living require levels of assistance comparable to those provided in other settings (Spillman, Liu, and McGilliard 2002; Zimmerman et al. 2003), the federal government exercises little to no oversight authority given the minor funding role. This is true even in the 41 states which, in 2009, relied on Medicaid to pay for home- and community services received by 131,208 assisted-living residents (74,970 through Section 1915(c) or 1115waiver programs; 56,238 through a state plan option), a figure up 43% since 2002 when only 34 states relied on Medicaid to pay for services provided to assisted-living residents (Mollica September 2009).[4]

Due largely to the fact that Medicaid coverage of assisted-living services is optional, the regulation of assisted living (and most Medicaid home- and community-based waiver services, for that matter) has been left largely up to the states, meaning even more variation in oversight than exists in other sectors (Mollica, Sims-Kastelein, and O'Keefe November 2007; Polzer 2011). This has resulted in substantial interstate differences in the types of providers considered to be assisted living and the kinds of services that may be offered, not to mention the types of individuals who may be served and the mechanisms put into place to protect them (Hawes et al. 2003, 2005; Stone and Reinhard 2007; Wilson, 2007; Zimmerman et al. 2003). It has also resulted in substantial variation in quality assurance and monitoring activities, not only with respect to assisted-living facilities but the nursing home and home health care sectors as well (Castle and Ferguson 2010; Harrington et al. 2011; Harrington, Mullan, and Carrillo 2004; Kelly, Lieberg, and Edwards 2008; Miller and Mor 2008; Miller, Mor, and Clark 2010; Mor 2005; Mor, Miller, and Clark 2010; Wiener, Freiman, and Brown 2007).

Rhode Island's experience suggests the importance of documenting and accounting for prevailing provider capacity, particularly if the goal is to markedly increase use of noninstitutional alternatives to nursing home placement. The lack of capacity among community providers to serve significantly greater numbers of clients resulting from nursing home diversions and transitions was one reason observers believed that the state had not progressed further rebalancing the long-term care sector. This is something that state officials would have been aware of and, perhaps, been able to address proactively had resource mapping been undertaken before rather than after beneficiaries started to be diverted and transitioned, and if more providers had elected to participate in the resource mapping exercise that eventually did take place. Clearly, prospectively documenting provider capacity is important because if the plan is to rely more on home- and community-based resources, it is critical that the extent to which those resources are able to meet the complex care needs of an increasingly larger service clientele be assessed. It is also critical that every effort be made to achieve as high a response rate as possible if survey methods are used, perhaps through some sort of financial incentive or other inducement.

In addition to the importance of resource mapping, Rhode Island's experience highlights the need to think broadly about the providers needed to successfully keep potential nursing home residents at home and in the community. This includes ensuring that there are sufficient numbers of high quality assisted-living facilities, adult day care centers, home care agencies, and other home- and community-based providers, both available and willing to participate in Medicaid. It also includes ensuring the availability of affordable housing and transportation options, both of which were lacking in Rhode Island but which the state's Waiver renewal application seeks to address. Prior research suggests just how important overcoming transportation barriers, both in terms of service scope and assistance, and limited housing options, both in terms of affordability and accessibility, can be to ensuring the success of initiatives to rebalance Medicaid long-term care away from institutional and toward noninstitutional settings (Farber et al. December 2011; Libson 2006; Robison et al. 2012; Rosenbloom 2009; Wardrip March 2010). Although still small, Rhode Island's shared-living program holds promise in this regard by permitting Medicaid beneficiaries to receive personal care, homemaker, transportation, and other services provided by a host caregiver/home, which may include a friend, relative, or neighbor other than a spouse or guardian.

Thinking broadly about providers further requires efforts on the part of policymakers to ensure the recruitment and retention of sufficient numbers of home health and personal care aides, whether they work independently or for an agency or facility, if the growing demand and need for care is going to be met. The paraprofessional workforce is particularly problematic given staff turnover rates of 44% to 65% and a growing gap in care capacity, with more than 522,000 home health aides and 477,000 personal aides projected to be needed over the next 10 years (PHI 2005; Seavey and Marquand December 2011; U.S. Bureau of Labor Statistics 2010). Challenges recruiting and retaining direct care staff derive from a number of factors, including: very low and stagnant wages, especially when compared to hospitals and even nursing home settings; inadequate or nonexistent benefits; poor public perception; an emotionally and physically demanding work environment; perceived lack of value and respect; insufficient training and autonomy; and limited opportunities for career advancement (CMS 2002; Fishman et al. May 24, 2004; Mickus, Luz, and Hogan April 2004; Miller and Mor 2007; Woodcock et al. June 14, 2011; Seavey and Marquand December 2011; Smith and Baughman 2007). Addressing the work force issue is particularly important for states, not only because it will otherwise be impossible to serve significantly more long-term care recipients in the home and community, especially as the population ages, but also because a larger body of research demonstrates a relationship between the type and quantity of staffing and quality of care received (Bostick et al. 2006; CMS 2002; Stone 2004). Perhaps the importance of the long-term care workforce issue is best reflected in the views of long-term care specialists who rank it as the most pressing challenge facing long-term care (Miller, Mor, and Clark 2010).

Thinking broadly about providers further requires efforts on the part of policymakers to ensure the necessary resources have been put into place to connect individuals and families to needed services and supports. Rebalancing long-term care increases the burden on already overburdened unpaid caregivers for, unlike nursing home care, very few home- and community-based programs pay for room and board or 24/7 care and supervision (Miller, Allen, and Mor 2008). As it is, the total estimated value of unpaid family caregiving, at $450 billion in 2009 (Feinberg et al. 2011), more than doubles the costs of all formal sources of long-term care combined ($207.9 billion in 2010) (The Scan Foundation January 2013).

Moreover, unlike nursing home care, few home- and community-based programs provide all the services necessary to meet individuals' needs. Instead, care recipients must typically find and coordinate services provided by multiple sources, a considerable challenge for individuals and families, particularly during periods of crisis. If the goal is to keep people out of nursing homes, the requisite resources must be put into place to connect people to necessary services and supports at home and in the community. Few know where to turn for advice and information should they or a family member need long-term care (Kaiser Family Foundation December 2007). To help people make informed choices, therefore, most (74.1%) long-term care specialists nationally feel that the adoption of formal care coordination services that explicitly link people to available long-term care options to be effective or very effective in improving system performance in this regard (Miller, Mor and Clark 2010). Most (67.0%) feel that counseling services that help people navigate the maze of available service options would be effective or very effective as well. Strategies adopted in Rhode Island to inform client decision making reflect this perspective. These include efforts to better educate hospital discharge planners and other long-term care referral sources about service and housing options in the community, including updates to the state's Rite Resources website, which provides up-to-date information on the services and supports available. Educating discharge planners is particularly important since hospitals are the principal entry points into long-term care. These also include efforts to improve the state's Aging Disability Resource Center, The Point, as a "one-stop-shop" where individuals and families might obtain the necessary information to make appropriate care decisions, in addition to plans to implement robust Consumer Assistance and Peer Mentoring Programs.

Rhode Island's experience further highlights the special importance of provider reimbursement. Some observers in Rhode Island felt that home- and community-based and assisted-living providers would rise to meet expected increases in demand independent of a rate increase, assuming that additional revenues resulting from a higher client caseload would prove sufficient to spur additional entries into the program. Most, however, felt that the market had, in fact, not responded, primarily because the level of reimbursement continued to remain low, especially in light of heightened acuity and complexity among the population served. This suggests that investing additional state dollars to build up the community network of providers may be especially important if growth in this sector is going to be driven primarily by nursing home diversions and transferees, although doing so may be difficult during challenging economic times. It also suggests the desirability of paying providers multiple rates or adjusting reimbursement for case-mix to better account for varying resource needs and, in so doing, promote access among the more difficult cases that otherwise would have entered nursing homes. Indeed, as we have seen, it is primarily issues associated with payment that explain why assisted-living facilities have chosen either not to participate in Medicaid or to restrict their level of participation if they do (Carlson and Coffey November 2010; National Senior Citizens Law Center February 2011).

A major concern in Rhode Island pertained to the ability of the state's Department of Health to monitor the quality of care provided by substantially greater numbers of home- and community-based providers. As noted, the number of state administrative personnel had been reduced markedly due to changes in the state's retirement policies. Moreover, the rate of new hires for key positions proceeded slowly due to the recession which, in turn, increased pressure on those who remained due both to rising case loads and to the added responsibilities associated with having a smaller workforce and the Global Waiver. Lack of sufficient numbers of experienced state personnel is particularly concerning where home- and community-services are concerned. There is the general perception that quality standards and measurement may not be as well developed in home care as they are in nursing homes (Miller, Clark, and Mor June 6, 2008; Mor, Miller, and Clark 2010). It is also substantially easier to monitor the quality of care provided to several hundred people being cared for in a single nursing home than the quality of care provided to the same number being cared for in their own homes by unsupervised staff.

Rhode Island's experience suggests that under certain circumstances the nursing home industry may come to accept, or at least not actively oppose, rebalancing. This finding is consistent with results deriving from a national survey of long-term care specialists where nearly half (45.7%) of nursing home providers surveyed supported rebalancing, a surprisingly high proportion though considerably lower than the proportion of the non-nursing home providers (80.1%) who reported doing so (Grabowski et al. 2010). Although Rhode Island's nursing home operators expressed some concern about the loss of Medicaid revenue, they nonetheless recognized that rebalancing was going to happen no matter whether they wished it or not given the marked spending imbalance in favor of nursing homes in the state. They also believed that there were limits to how much the industry could be downsized, both in light of population aging and because good transfer candidates would become increasingly scarce over time after residents with the lowest acuity levels and care needs were transferred first. Moreover, nursing homes in Rhode Island, like in other states, have begun to rely on alternative sources of revenue, including Medicare's skilled nursing facility benefit. Because nursing homes have increasingly been used for short-term post-acute and rehabilitative purposes, there has been growth in the overall volume of Medicare clients as residents are being discharged at an increasingly accelerated pace (Decker 2005). Thus, while the proportion of nursing home revenue deriving from Medicaid has declined with the growth of assisted living and other home- and community-based options to long-term nursing home placement, the proportion of nursing home revenue deriving from Medicare has risen.

Another important consideration for the nursing home sector is adjustment of nursing home reimbursement for resident acuity. Diverting or transferring relatively low-care cases from nursing homes leaves a frailer, more resource–intensive, long-stay population behind. Explicitly accounting for resident acuity in a state's reimbursement system, therefore, should help increase nursing home buy-in where rebalancing is concerned. Of course, the manner in which major reimbursement policy changes such as case-mix is instituted matters in this regard (Miller and Wang 2009a, 2009b; Miller et al 2012). Adopting case-mix typically benefits certain segments of the nursing home industry more than others with those serving disproportionately higher numbers of heavy-care residents tending to favor adoption and those serving less burdensome populations tending to be against it (Miller 2008; Miller and Banazak-Holl 2005). A certain degree of contention may therefore be unavoidable given that Medicaid constitutes such a large proportion of most nursing homes' revenue streams. Unless a state adopts a simultaneous increase in the base payments that nursing homes receive, an unlikely occurrence in the current fiscal climate, some conflict is inescapable. While Rhode Island's intention to ensure that no facility loses in the transition to acuity adjustment and that gains and losses in other aspects of the rate would be limited during this time period could prove helpful in this regard, the proposal to eliminate a planned $7.26 million rate increase in state FY 2014 will surely undermine the state's intentions (EOHHS 2013).

SUMMARY

As a capped federal match, the Global Waiver is not a model that supports the block grant approach to Medicaid reform. Moreover, the state did not receive unlimited discretion to administer the Global Waiver nor achieved nearly as much savings as has been claimed. Indeed, most of the savings obtained by Rhode Island during this time period derive not from the Global Waiver but from increased spending on the part of the federal government and from measures the state could have implemented independently of the Global Waiver authority negotiated. Although limited progress has been made rebalancing long-term services supports, efforts in this area have largely stagnated. Thus, in addition to implementing expedited eligibility, consumer assistance, housing and other supports, the state intends to further integrate its rebalancing and care coordination efforts, in part, by enrolling all Medicaid-only and Medicaid-Medicare dually eligible beneficiaries in need of long-term services and supports into managed care.

Independent of summative impact, the Global Waiver suggests several lessons for health and long-term care reform. When pursuing reform, it is important to ensure adequate levels of stakeholder input and transparency. This includes providing sufficient detail on proposed changes and adopting mechanisms for public participation during the design, approval, or implementation process. No matter the stage, it is advisable that community concerns be documented and acted upon in a timely manner and that reports and program updates clearly indicate how state policy decisions reflect the ongoing input of community members. It is also important that public input not be undertaken as a mere formality, but rather as a means to create a more effective partnership to ensure ongoing program improvement and success.

In an open, democratic society, providing opportunities for community input is a desirable objective in and of itself. As a practical matter, however, it provides opportunities for program administrators to draw upon additional knowledge and expertise from among individuals representing those most intimately affected by the decisions being made, including beneficiaries and providers. It also provides opportunities for program administrators to obtain assistance with key implementation tasks, an important consideration among increasingly shorthanded state bureaucracies. Ultimately, the familiarity and trust that consultation and collaboration promote should contribute to the creation of a less challenging environment, both politically, when new programs or initiatives are being designed, and administratively, when they are being implemented.

When undertaking major reform, it is critical that states ensure the presence of sufficient numbers of experienced administrative personnel. This includes not undertaking significant endeavors at the same time as other policy changes are being putting into place to markedly reduce the size of the state's workforce. It also includes not undertaking significant endeavors when the ability to fill key positions is in doubt, as occurs during major fiscal crises. Ideally, assessment should be made regarding: (1) the ability of state agencies to take on added functions and responsibilities without harming the administration of existing programs; (2) what types of, if any, additional personnel may be needed to effectuate the change desired; and (3) whether or not the requisite resources are available to fill in whatever gaps may exist.

Especially important is a state's ability to retain or seek out agency leaders with both the management and communications skills necessary to oversee comprehensive reform and to work productively with community stakeholders. It is also crucial that the requisite technology systems be put into place to undertake all major programmatic tasks and to meet most reasonable data requests, including timely access to the key data elements necessary to track and evaluate progress. Here, it is important to look beyond a general accounting of program activities and tasks and spending and utilization trends to indicators of service scope and quality. In the end, the goal should be to keep track of and release that information necessary to assess impact, and to ensure the investment of sufficient resources to achieve program goals and to determine if and when modifications need to be made.

Adoption of major Medicaid program change may be facilitated by prevailing economic conditions and ideological alignment between the state and federal governments. This combination of fiscal and political imperatives, however, may contribute to concern on the part of community stakeholders regarding the state's commitment to the program, distrust that may extend into implementation of the stages of the policy process, including, potentially, institution of a more stringent legislative oversight regime than had existed previously. Furthermore, while a poor fiscal environment may be a driving impetus behind reform, moving forward with significant program change during an economic downturn that adversely affects state administrative capacity and funding levels can compromise implementation, leading to weaker than expected results.

Reforms that touch on most aspects of the Medicaid program can make it difficult for critics to foment a clear and coherent opposition given substantial heterogeneity amongst the populations affected. While the subsequent ineffectiveness of the opposition can contribute to ultimate adoption, the breadth of such reform can make implementation far more challenging than if it was more limited. This is because the large number of populations impacted may pose challenges to shorthanded state bureaucracies charged with incorporating feedback from multiple stakeholder groups. It is also because the imposition of organizational barriers may preclude effective cooperation across the multiple state departments affected.

Although some forward movement has been made in expanding the use of home- and community-based services since implementation of the Global Waiver began, the distribution of long-term care spending in Rhode Island continues to be weighted heavily towards nursing home care. That overall spending has remained largely stagnant suggests just how difficult it can be for laggard states that have historically spent substantially more on nursing homes to make more than marginal progress even with the provision of options and incentives that otherwise should promote increased reliance on the home- and community-based sector. This does not bode well for the success of the Affordable Care Act's rebalancing provisions.

Most importantly, nursing home care will continue to be a mandatory benefit and, as such, an entitlement all states must provide under Medicaid while home- and community-based services remains an optional benefit that state's may offer at their discretion. Besides leaving investments in home- and community-based spending especially vulnerable to the vagaries of state budget and political processes, the optional nature of these programs and the continuing absence of minimum standards and requirements to cover all geographic areas and target populations suggest persistent unmet need, both within and across states. This combined with varying dispositions for making the structural, administrative, and service delivery changes necessary to expand home- and community-based services and to qualify for additional federal matching support suggests the continuation of substantial cross-state variation in the amount of progress states make toward rebalancing long-term care under Medicaid despite the provision of new options and incentives under the Affordable Care Act.

At the height of the recession, states continued to expand access to home- and community-based services, but the pace of expansion slowed while additional cost and utilization controls were added to the waitlists, enrollment caps, and coverage limits already in place. This is because home- and community-based providers are at a comparative disadvantage in the competition for scarce resources. Not only is nursing home care a mandatory service but the nursing home industry is one of the most powerful lobbies in state government while nursing homes are more dependent than noninstitutional providers on provider taxes and statutorily determined reimbursement adjustments that tend to promote steadier growth in spending.

That expanding reliance on home- and community-based services tends to entail short-term increases in spending before subsequent longer-term savings can be achieved is problematic, especially during economic downturns when the emphasis is more on achieving short-term fixes to state budgetary problems rather than long-term programmatic goals. States need to recognize that eventual savings take time to materialize, but only over the long-term and with continued investments that promote both the supply and demand for services.

A lack of capacity among community providers to serve significantly greater numbers of clients resulting from nursing home diversions and transitions can pose significant limitations on making progress rebalancing the long-term care sector. Clearly, prospectively documenting provider capacity is important because if the plan is to rely more on home- and community-based resources, it is critical that the extent to which those resources are able to meet the complex care needs of an increasingly larger service clientele be assessed. State officials need to ensure that there are sufficient numbers of home- and community-based providers, both available and willing to participate in Medicaid, in addition to affordable housing and transportation options, home health and personal care aides, and case management and other resources that connect clients to needed services and supports.

Increased reimbursement is especially important for attracting participating providers. So too is maintaining sufficient numbers of experienced state regulators since it is more difficult to monitor care quality for, say, 100 clients served separately in different homes than in a single nursing facility. Nursing home providers generally recognize that rebalancing is necessary but that there are limits to how much the industry can be downsized in light of population aging and that revenue from Medicare's skilled nursing facility benefit will increasingly substitute for that lost from Medicaid due to the rise of short-term, post-acute rehabilitative admissions. Adjusting payment for client acuity should help promote buy-in on the part of both institutional and noninstitutional providers given that rebalancing increases the relative complexity among clients served in both locations.

NOTES

1. The Lewin Group found that institutional services in Rhode Island's Medicaid program were assigned to one of five different claims categories: Eleanor Slater Hospital; Group Home; Behavioral Healthcare, Developmental Disabilities, and Hospitals services; Medicare CoPay; and Nursing Home services. Only that claims category directly impacted by the Waiver—Nursing Home services—was included in Lewin's analyses.
2. The Lewin Group assigned each home- and community-based service claim under Rhode Island's Medicaid program to one of eight service categories: Adult Day Care, Assisted Living Care, Home Health Aides, Personal Care Services, Assistive Devices/Home Modifications, Emergency Response Systems, Home Delivered Meals, and Behavioral Healthcare, Developmental Disabilities, and Hospitals Waiver Services. Members receiving home- and community-based services were also assigned to one of four recipient classification categories: Department of Elderly Affairs Members; Behavioral Healthcare, Developmental Disabilities, and Hospitals Members; Self-Directed Care Waiver; and the Home- and Community-Based Services Study Population (i.e., those not included in one of the other three categories). Since the former three groups were not impacted directly by the Global Waiver, only the latter was included in Lewin's analyses.
3. There is also one current (one expired) concurrent 1915(b) and 1915(c) waiver.
4. An additional 3,317 assisted living residents received home- and community-based services paid for by state general revenue programs in 2009.

9 Block Grants and Retrenchment

"If we could get a block grant today," Rhode Island State's Medicaid Director Elena Nicolella (October 22, 2012) asked rhetorically, "would we want one?" The answer is "no," both because the state is "not ready to give up on entitlement to health care" and because "federal involvement is both necessary and healthy." Indeed, at a November 26, 2012, Global Waiver Implementation Task Force meeting, Democratic EOHHS Director Steven Costantino reported that Rhode Island's Global Waiver would be rebranded simply as an 1115 Waiver (EOHHS November 26, 2012). He explained that "[p]ublications and media outlets have attempted to claim that Rhode Island's waiver is really a block grant. The new title of the Waiver will hopefully put this issue to rest." "The cap was set so high as to be meaningless for any other purpose," agreed Rhode Island Health Center Association President and CEO and former EOHHS Secretary Jane Hayward (February 26, 2013), "other than to allow those seeking to transform Medicaid into a block-grant program the opportunity to attempt to style the Global Waiver as such, or at least as a step towards that particular policy goal. There will be no practical change in spending or process either for the state or for the federal government by removing the spending cap and continuing the requirement of budget neutrality, and therefore it is the right thing to do at this point in time."

This chapter looks beyond Rhode Island to examine the ramifications of extant proposals to retrench Medicaid. It argues that block granting the program would do irreparable harm, resulting in marked reductions in state spending, beneficiary enrollment, and provider payments. It also highlights what role the Medicaid retrenchment debate will play as health care reform is implemented in today's hyper-partisan political environment.

SHARP REDUCTIONS IN SPENDING

In addition to Rhode Island's Global Waiver, conservatives have held up the Children's Health Insurance program (CHIP), the joint federal-state health insurance program for low-income children living in families with incomes too high to qualify for Medicaid, as a successful example of what might be achieved nationally if all states received block grants to run their Medicaid programs. As with the Global Waiver, however, there are flaws with this analogy. Like Medicaid, the federal government matches state spending under CHIP, though at higher levels. Unlike Medicaid, the total amount received is limited, with each state being provided with a capped allotment from the federal government. This is similar to the capped federal match Rhode Island has received under the Global Waiver. Moreover, in contrast to current block grant proposals, the federal government has sought to ensure that states have adequate resources to maintain and, ultimately, expand their CHIP programs. This includes funding CHIP at levels that exceeded states' needs during the programs first 10 years, redistributing federal funding from states with unused allocations to states with inadequate allocations, and appropriating additional CHIP funding when the total level of federal allocations proved insufficient (Broaddus June 28, 2011; Guyer, Heberlein, and Alker June 2, 2011).

The result has been that federal funding under CHIP has served more as a guarantee than as a constraint on state decision making. This has been especially true since 2009 when the program was reauthorized through 2013 with significant additional funding, a provision subsequently extended through 2015 under the Affordable Care Act. The result, according to the Congressional Research Service, has been substantial increases in federal allocations with post-reauthorization allotments increasing by an average of 96% across states, ranging from 14% in Delaware and 15% in Arizona to 359% and 426%, respectively, in Massachusetts and Rhode Island (Peterson January 14, 2009). It is expected that this increase in federal spending should, in turn, lead to a 4.1 million increase in the number of uninsured children enrolled in CHIP and Medicaid by September 2013 (Congressional Budget Office September 25, 2007). Indeed, 4.6 million children gained health insurance coverage under Medicaid or CHIP between 2007 and 2010 as the number with private health insurance declined, in contrast to the previous three years where the proportion of children with public coverage did not increase even as the number without private health insurance coverage grew (Kaiser Family Foundation July 2012a).

The generosity of both CHIP and Rhode Island's Waiver agreement is in marked contrast to proposals to block grant Medicaid, each of which would provide states with a fixed, markedly reduced allotment of federal funding in exchange for considerably greater flexibility over program eligibility, benefits, payments, and structure. Moreover, proposals to block grant Medicaid have become increasingly less generous over time. Federal allotments under a 1981 Reagan administration proposal would have equaled federal spending at FY 1981 levels plus 9%, adjusted in subsequent years for the Gross National Product's price deflator, an indicator of economic growth. Federal allotments under a 1995 House Republican proposal would have been determined by a complicated formula based on historical spending adjusted annually for state input costs, case mix, and number of poor people, subject to an overall, aggregate cap on federal Medicaid expenditures (Lambrew 2005). Under the 2003 Bush Administration proposal, spending levels in FY 2002 would have been used as the base from which federal allotments would be determined. These would have then been increased by 8.5% per year, the average Medicaid growth rate at the time.

The Romney plan did not indicate how allotments would be established during the first year but suggested that "Medicaid spending should be capped and increased each year by CPI +1%" (Romney 2012). Ryan's budget plans do not specify how baseline allotments would be established either but would limit increases to the CPI only and population growth (Ryan 2011, 2012, 2013). By contrast, his 2010 plan with Alice Rivlin would base the initial allotment on "the state's per capita low-income population based on the Federal Poverty Level with growth being limited to the GDP per capita plus one percentage point" (Rivlin and Ryan November 17, 2010). Perhaps the least generous proposal has been put forward by the House Republican Study Committee, which would establish block grants fixed at 2012 spending levels, with no subsequent adjustments for inflation or increases in health care costs (House Republican Study Committee 2012).

A variant on the block grant concept is a May 19, 2011 proposal introduced by Republican U.S. Senators Tom Coburn (Oklahoma), Richard Burr (North Carolina), and Saxby Chambliss (Georgia) that would essentially establish separate federal allotments, termed health grants, for pregnant women, children, and families, and for long-term care services and supports for elders and disabled persons for whom acute care funding would remain unchanged (Office of U.S. Senator Tom Coburn May 19, 2011). Initial grants would be based on the number of state residents below the Federal Poverty Level. Like the Ryan plan, increases in allotments would be based on the CPI and population growth.

Along with proposals to block grant Medicaid are Republican proposals to establish per capita limits on Medicaid program expenditure growth (Cassidy July 16, 2012; Upton and Hatch May 1, 2013). In contrast to a block grant, a per capita cap would not set a limit on overall spending; as enrollment rose, so too would the overall provision of federal funding. What a per capita limit would do is establish a preset amount that each state may receive for each beneficiary served. If, on average, a state spent less than the cap, then it would be able to keep all or part of the difference depending on how the program was structured. If, on average, a state spent more than the cap, then it would need to decide whether to use state funds to make up the difference or to cut back on program eligibility, benefits, and/or payments. The resulting incentives established by this dynamic should, according to proponents, spur states to adopt measures that promote efficiencies that reduce the rate of expenditure growth, typically facilitated by additional provisions providing states with more flexibility over program design and administration. Proponents argue that this approach represents a "middle ground" or "compromise" between the current Medicaid system and its out-of-control and inefficient spending and block grant proposals which would result in substantially more dramatic changes in the way the program was financed, including locking in total federal spending at a set amount even should enrollment rise (Cassidy July 16, 2012; Cassidy April 18, 2013; Upton and Hatch May 1, 2013).

Whereas one per beneficiary cap could be imposed on all Medicaid program recipients, recent proposals would establish separate caps for children, adult, elders, and the blind and disabled (Cassidy July 16, 2012; Upton and Hatch May 1, 2013), thereby accounting for marked variation in spending across groups but not within groups, say, between elders aged 65 to 74 years versus 85 years or older (Park May 8, 2013; Park and Broaddus October 4, 2012). Especially critical is the choice of initial per capita beneficiary amounts. As with block grants, setting initial amounts based on recent state experience would lock-in comparatively low levels of spending resulting from the proliferation of cost containment measures put into place as a result of the Great Recession and weak recovery. There is also the question about how to set initial amounts when there is little or no prior cost experience, as with childless adults with incomes below 138% of the Federal Poverty Level as per the January 1, 2014 expansion of Medicaid under the Affordable Care Act (Cassidy April 18, 2013). This is not an idle concern, as limiting per capita payments for this population may further discourage states from participating in the expansion in light of the U.S. Supreme Court's ruling that expanding Medicaid under the Affordable Care Act is, in fact, optional. That additional states may choose not to participate if federal financing is limited is reflected in fear in some circles regarding the ability of the federal government to meet its commitment to funding the expansion at promised levels—93%, on average, between 2014 and 2022, 90% thereafter—over the long term (Park May 8, 2013; Park and Broaddus October 4, 2012).

Also critical is the choice of growth factors. Linking growth in per capita amounts to the general CPI, for example, would neither account for changes in the composition of the population served, say, due to the aging of the "baby boom" generation, nor account for greater annual cost growth in the medical sector, including unexpectedly large increases resulting from technological advances (e.g., medical devices, prescriptions drugs) (Park and Broaddus October 4, 2012). Whether to apply the same initial per capita amounts and growth factors nationally or to establish separate amounts and growth factors for each state is an important decision as well. The latter is clearly preferable because it would account for substantial interstate differences in per beneficiary costs and cost growth. It would, however, be administratively more complex to calculate and enforce the numerous caps needed over time.

At first glance, per capita cap proposals are similar to requirements that federal waivers be budget neutral to the federal government; i.e., that federal costs per beneficiary not be any higher than they would have been without the Waiver. There are major differences, however (Park and Broaddus October 4, 2012). Under per capita cap proposals, the cap amounts and the rate at which they grow would be imposed on states by the federal government as per federal law or regulation; there would be no give-and-take between federal and state partners in determining parameters such as these. Under federal waiver agreements, by contrast, both the budget neutrality caps and growth rates derive from negotiations between state and federal officials in light of each waiver's particular circumstances, including the specific context within which it is situated and the specific way in which it is designed. Moreover, states can renegotiate their budget neutrality caps due to unforeseen cost increases, either while the waiver is in effect or after the demonstration period has run its course. They can also choose not to renew. None of these options would be available should per capita caps be adopted program-wide.

Looking forward, the Congressional Budget Office estimated that the Medicaid component of the Rivlin-Ryan plan to block grant Medicaid would reduce the federal budget deficit by $180 billion between 2011 and 2020 (Congressional Budget Office November 17, 2012). In addition, in 2011, the Congressional Budget Office estimated that federal Medicaid spending under Ryan's FY 2012 House budget proposal would fall 35% short of current projections for 2022 and 49% short of current projections for 2030 due to its block grant provisions (Congressional Budget Office April 5, 2011). A year later, the Congressional Budget Office reported that under Ryan's FY 2013 House budget proposal, federal Medicaid, CHIP, and health subsidy spending would fall 58.3%, 61.5%, and 75% short of current projections in 2023, 2030, and 2040, respectively (Congressional Budget Office March 2012a). It has also been estimated that the latest iteration of Ryan's proposal would reduce expected federal spending on Medicaid and CHIP from $578 billion to $347 billion in 2023 alone, with 40% of that reduction resulting from repeal of the Affordable Care Act and 60% from the proposed block grant (Adler, Akabas, and Collins March 12, 2013).

The Urban Institute estimated that Ryan's FY 2013 House budget plan proposal would reduce federal Medicaid spending by 22% or $810 billion between 2013 and 2022, independent of repealing the Affordable Care Act (Holahan et al. October 2012).[1] The impact of the House Republican Study Committee's proposal would be even more dramatic, decreasing total Medicaid spending by $1.1 trillion, or 30%, between 2013 and 2022, with federal Medicaid spending being 47% lower than it would be under current law by 2022 (Park and Broaddus March 28, 2012). Not surprisingly, there would be considerable differences in impact across states. In Rhode Island, Ryan's House budget plan would reduce Medicaid spending by 22%, or $4.3 billion, between 2013 and 2022. More generally, percent reductions in Medicaid spending from 2013 and 2012 due to the block grant would range from 20% in Louisiana to 25% in North Dakota and Wyoming.

Looking backward, the Center for Budget and Policy Priorities estimated that if the Ryan plan had went into effect in 2001, total federal Medicaid spending would have been $555.0 billion, or 31% less, between 2001 and 2010, with a $80.7 billion, or 37%, reduction experienced in 2010 alone (Park and Broaddus April 20, 2012). Moreover, the impact would have varied considerably across states, with North Dakota, for example, experiencing a 17% reduction in federal Medicaid spending during this time period as compared to an overall reduction of 61% in Arizona; the reduction in Rhode Island would have been 29%. In all, 33 states would have experienced reductions of at least 35% in 2010, six of which would have been over 50%.[2] Because annual growth in federal Medicaid allotments to states would only increase with population growth and inflation, it would grow at a much slower rate than otherwise expected. As a result, the gap between what the federal government provides and what states need to fund their programs would widen with each passing year. This dynamic is reflected in both the prospective and retrospective analyses of the Ryan proposal described here.

Doubts about the ability of block grants to account for changes in Medicaid program needs is also reflected in proposals made by the Reagan administration in 1981 and House Republicans in 1995. Both proposals included funding formulas later found to create a mismatch between proposed federal contributions and actual program costs. This is reflected in retroactive comparisons of Congressional Budget Office projections for spending under each proposal to actual program spending (Lambrew 2005). Under the Reagan administration's proposal, projected federal Medicaid spending under the cap would have been 6% lower than actual spending over five years and 26% lower than actual spending over 10. Moreover, the difference between projected and actual funding levels would have risen considerably over time, with projected spending levels under the cap being 2%, 27%, and 53% lower than actual levels in 1984, 1988, and 1991, respectively.

Under the 1995 House Republican proposal, projected federal Medicaid spending under the cap would have been 3% higher than actual spending over five years and 2% lower than actual spending over seven. Again, the difference between actual and projected funding levels would have varied considerably over time, with the amount by which projected levels would have exceeded actual levels declining from 7% in 1997 to 2% in 1998, after which projected spending levels under the cap would have been lower than actual spending; for example, 3%, 8%, and 16% in 2000, 2001, and 2002, respectively. It should be noted that national figures such as these mask substantial differences across states. Thus, in 2002, projected spending levels under the House Republican plan ranged from 15% and 5% above actual spending in West Virginia and Texas, respectively, to 45% below actual spending in Arkansas. Nationally, this reduction in spending would have resulted in 6 million people losing Medicaid coverage that year if states addressed the entire shortfall by tightening program eligibility.

Prior experience suggests just how difficult it is to create a suitable and fair formula to determine funding levels for a Medicaid block grant. The Bush administration's proposal, for example, set yearly allocations by using spending in FY 2002 as a base rate, and increasing this amount yearly by 8.5%, the average Medicaid growth rate. This is far more generous than the House budget proposals put forward by Congressman Ryan, which would simply increase the federal allocation using the CPI and the House Republican Study Committee, which would not include future any inflation adjustments at all. Even if the goal was to establish funding formulas that adequately met future program needs, doing so is extremely challenging as economic, demographic, and medical inflation trends can be highly variable and unpredictable. Perhaps this is best reflected in comparison of actual federal Medicaid spending to projections made by the Congressional Budget Office (Lambrew 2005). Results indicate that the accuracy of three-year projections made for the years 1990 through 2002 ranged from 28% above actual spending in 1996 to 31% below in 1992. Results also indicate that the accuracy of five-year projections made for the years during this time period ranged from 44% above spending in 1998 to 37% below in 1992. Together, these findings suggest that spending projections and funding formulas are very difficult to establish and are likely to result in funding shortfalls and service cuts, especially over the long term.

Republican proposals are in marked contrast to the Obama administration's FY 2014 budget proposal which (of course) keeps the Affordable Care Act intact, proposes some minor program enhancements, including extension of the Transitional Medical Assistance and Qualified Individual Programs through 2014, and seeks to achieve $22.1 billion in net program savings from FY 2014 to FY 2023 through such initiatives as strengthening program integrity efforts, limiting durable medical equipment reimbursement, and clarifying Medicaid drug rebate and payment policies (U.S. Department of Health and Human Services April 10, 2013). Instructively, the Obama administration removed provisions included in earlier budget proposals that would have resulted in substantially greater total federal Medicaid savings, in the $100 billion or more range, over 10 years, to avoid discouraging state participation in the Medicaid expansion, which previously had been mandatory but now was optional due to the U.S. Supreme Court (Park and Solomon June 24, 2011; Park May 8, 2013). Provisions excised include imposing a combined federal matching rate on Medicaid and CHIP and limiting the use of provider taxes which, as noted previously, enable states to draw in additional federal matching funds without concomitant increases in state expenditures. Republican proposals are also in stark contrast to Washington State Democrat and Senate Budget Committee Chairman Patty Murray's budget proposal, which would retain the Affordable Care Act and makes only about $10 billion in unspecified reductions in non-Medicare health programs over the course of the next decade; overall, non-Medicare health spending would be $2.5 trillion more under Senator

Murray's budget than Congressman Ryan's budget over this time period (Adler, Akabas, and Collins March 15, 2013).

It is unlikely that states could overcome marked reductions in federal spending through increased efficiencies. Critics argue that Medicaid is already a lean program with both per capita spending and per capita spending growth lagging behind the private health insurance market (Cassidy April 18, 2013; Park May 8, 2013; Park and Broaddus October 4, 2012). Indeed, states already aggressively pursue cost containment under the existing Medicaid program framework, including reducing provider payments, limiting the scope of benefits, eliminating optional services, contracting with managed care plans, instituting pharmaceutical management tools, and restricting eligibility in areas exempt from the Affordable Care Act's maintenance of effort provisions[3] (Feder and Van de Water March 18, 2013; Holahan and McMorrow 2012; Johnson, Oliff, and Williams February 9, 2011; Rosenbaum 2012; Williams, Leachman, and Johnson July 28, 2011; Smith et al. October 2012). Cost containment has been driven, in part, by marked reductions in state revenues in the aftermath of the Great Recession and by the political desirability or need to fund competing priorities under such circumstances. Thus, although average annual Medicaid expenditure growth is expected to reach 8.5% over the next decade, growth in per enroll spending is expected to continue at a relatively modest 3.6%, with the remaining portion of projected growth in spending resulting from increases in enrollment (Holahan and McMorrow 2012). This suggests that there is little more states can do to wring additional savings out of the program. Unable to further reduce per enrollee costs, states would be left with one of two options should the program be turned into a block grant or other significant federal retrenchment occur, either funding their programs at existing levels but making up the difference through increased state spending, or, more likely, contracting their programs considerably by severely ratcheting back on enrollment and/or markedly reducing provider payments beyond already low levels.

ADVERSE CONSEQUENCES FOR PROVIDERS

Although states have a variety of different strategies with which to restrain Medicaid spending, freezes and reductions in provider payments often proven politically more palatable than cuts in benefits and eligibility, especially during hard economic times when people need Medicaid most (Miller 2002; Smith et al. 2012). As a result, according to Thompson (2011), "payment rates have traditionally been the Achilles' heel of Medicaid, trailing those of Medicare or employer insurance." This suggests that marked reductions in federal spending associated with block granting or other Medicaid program retrenchment would have adverse implications not only for state budgets but also Medicaid providers and, in turn, access to and the quality of care received by program beneficiaries.

The Urban Institute estimated that Ryan's FY 2013 House budget plan would reduce total hospital and nursing home payments by $363.8 and $220.2 billion, respectively, between 2013 and 2022 (Holahan et al. October 2012). Reductions in hospital payments would range from less than $1.0 billion in eight states[4] to approximately $20.0 billion in Florida, Illinois, and Texas and more than $40 billion in California and New York. Reductions in nursing home payments would range from less than $1.0 billion in 13 states[5] to approximately $20.0 billion in California and Pennsylvania and more than $30.0 billion in New York. In Rhode Island, the House budget plan would decrease hospital and nursing home payments by $1.5 and $2.2 billion, respectively.

Such major reductions in payments could compromise the fiscal viability of already financially stressed safety net providers while reducing incentives for others to participate in the Medicaid program, or to serve fewer Medicaid beneficiaries if they do participate, thereby compromising access and quality. The impact on urban hospitals, nursing homes, and other providers that depend heavily on Medicaid revenue would be particularly dramatic. Medicaid, for example, is the primary purchaser of nursing home care in the United States, accounting for 32.8% of total nursing home spending in 2009, followed by out-of-pocket payments (29.1%), Medicare (20.4%), private insurance (7.7%), and other sources (10.0%) (CMS 2011). According to the National Nursing Home Survey, nearly all nursing home beds—98.5%—are Medicaid certified (Jones et al. 2009). Furthermore, whereas Medicaid served as the primary source of payment for more than one-third of nursing home admissions (34.8%), it paid for all or part of the care received by nearly 60% of residents at the time the National Nursing Home Survey was conducted (59.7%). Overall, two in three nursing home residents are paid for, all or in part, by Medicaid (67%) (U.S. Government Accountability Office October 2003).

Evidence from the nursing home sector suggests just how important the level of payment and type of methodology chosen is, not just for access but also for quality of care (Feng et al. 2008, 2010; Harrington, Swan, and Carrillo 2007; Intrator and Mor 2004; Mor et al. 2011). Due largely to differentials in reimbursement, nursing home care in the U.S. has been "driven to tiers," with the lowest quality facilities—those with the fewest nurses, most deficiencies, and lowest occupancy rates—being those serving predominately Medicaid residents (Mor et al. 2004). The most poorly performing facilities are also more likely than their better performing counterparts to serve African Americans and Hispanics and to be located in poor counties and rural areas (Fennell et al. 2010; Kang, Meng, and Miller 2011; Mor et al. 2004; Smith et al. 2007).

Low levels of reimbursement, delays in payment, and other administrative burdens are the reasons why many doctors have either elected not to participate in Medicaid or have limited the extent of their participation to a restricted number of clients, thereby leaving many beneficiaries to seek care from hospital emergency rooms, federally qualified health centers, or other safety-net providers (Cunningham and Nichols 2005; Cunningham and O'Malley 2009; Zuckerman et al. 2004). Perhaps the challenges that Medicaid beneficiaries face is best reflected in a 2011 national survey where nearly one-third of all physicians (31%) reported that they did not plan to take any new Medicaid patients as compared to less than 20% who reported that they would not accept any new Medicare beneficiaries (17%) or private pay patients (18%) (Decker 2012). Physicians working in smaller practices and in metropolitan areas were even more likely than others to avoid new Medicaid patients; those practicing in states with higher Medicaid-to-Medicare fee ratios were significantly more likely to do so. This latter finding, in particular, suggests just how important the level of reimbursement can be in influencing provider decision making in this regard.

Recognizing challenges recruiting providers due to low payment levels, the Affordable Care Act increases payments to primary care physicians under Medicaid to Medicare levels, with the difference between the amount paid by a state as of July 1, 2009 and the pertinent Medicare rate being financed entirely by the federal government. This change, however, will only last two years—2013 and 2014—and, as such, may have minimal impact on improving Medicaid beneficiary access to primary care over the long run. Given the history in this area and the lingering effects of the fiscal crisis, it is highly unlikely that states will maintain Medicare-level reimbursement rates unless the federal government picks up the tab, an even more remote possibility should Medicaid's financing structure be turned into a block grant or per capita cap.

Because Medicaid is the single largest revenue source for safety-net providers, the impact of fiscal retrenchment, including block granting, on the limited revenue streams of public hospitals and entities that serve large numbers of low income patients is especially concerning. Medicaid constituted 35% of $47 billion in net revenues received by public hospitals in 2010, followed by commercial insurance (27%), Medicare (21%), and other federal, state, and local subsidies (13%) (Kaiser Family Foundation 2013). During the same year, Medicaid constituted 38% of the $12.7 billion in operating revenues received by health centers, again, the largest third-party payment source. Evidence is mixed about the quality of care provided to patients served in safety-net hospitals relative to other hospitals, with the majority of analyses demonstrating worse quality (Chatterjee et al. 2012; McHugh, Kang, and Hasnain-Wynia 2009; Werner, Goldman, and Dudley 2008) but some demonstrating few, if any differences in the quality of care provided (Genther and Gourin 2012; Marshall et al. 2011; McHugh, Kang, and Hasnain-Wynia 2009). There is little doubt, however, that safety-net hospitals provide Medicaid and uninsured patients access to higher quality care than otherwise would be the case. That this is likely true is reflected in the results of one recent study which, in finding improved survival among low income surgical cancer patients in safety-net hospitals (SNHs) relative to other settings, concluded that "even if SNHs have lower quality on certain measures, low-income or underserved patients may fare better when treated in a safety net setting than they would without access to an SNH and affiliated resources" (Sabik and Bradley 2012). It is also reflected in findings from another study that found that communities with well-structured safety net systems are able to provide large proportions of low income, uninsured residents with access to basic medical care at reasonable cost (Hall, Hamacher, and Johnson 2012; Hall, Hwang, and Jones 2011). Safety-net providers will continue to play an important role after health care reform goes into effect, not only in serving the larger proportion of Americans covered by Medicaid but in continuing to serve the more than 20 million individuals expected to remain uninsured, including undocumented immigrants, individuals given an affordability exemption from the individual mandate, and those eligible for but not enrolled in Medicaid or the Children's Health Insurance program (Buettgens and Hall March 2011).

Provisions contained within the Affordable Care Act reducing disproportionate share hospital (DSH) payments under both Medicaid and Medicare could pose a particular challenge to the nation's safety net system. The Medicaid DSH program enables states to provide additional reimbursement to providers who disproportionately serve low income individuals who are more likely to be uninsured or on Medicaid. The Medicare DSH program also serves this purpose in addition to maintaining access for Medicare beneficiaries more generally. In all, federal Medicaid and Medicare DSH payments total $11.3 billion and $10.3 billion per year, respectively, according to the most recent data (Davis July 2012). The Affordable Care Act markedly reduces DSH payments under both programs while directing more equitable distribution of what is provided to the financially least well off hospitals located in the neediest areas.

On the Medicaid side, the U.S. Department of Health and Human Services (DHHS) Secretary is directed to reduce DSH allotments by $500 million in FY 2014 and $600 million in both FY 2015 and FY 2016, and by $1.8, $5.0, $5.6, and $4.0 billion, respectively, in FY 2017, FY 2018, FY 2019, and FY 2020 (Mitchell December 18, 2012). Together with a subsequent one-year extension equal to the FY 2020 reduction plus the percent change in the CPI (Congressional Budget Office January 1, 2013; Mitchell December 18, 2012),[6] the total estimated reduction in Medicaid DSH payments will be $26.3 billion through FY 2022.

On the Medicare side, the Secretary of DHHS is directed to reduce base Medicare DSH payments by 75% in FY 2014, though hospitals treating large numbers of uninsured patients will receive higher payments beginning that year, with overall payments projected to be 28% lower relative to existing law through 2019 (Davis July 2012). Moreover, the Affordable Care Act also reduces overpayments to Medicare Advantage plans for an estimated 10 year savings of $135 billion, in addition achieving an estimated 10 year savings of $157 billion by reducing the rate of growth in payments to hospitals, nursing homes, home health agencies, physicians, and other Medicare providers (Moon 2012). Combined with other provisions, the result is expected to be $716 billion in Medicare savings from 2013 to 2022 (Davis and Stremikis August 23, 2012).

A major goal is to direct savings obtained from reducing provider payments under Medicare toward improving program benefits, investing in public health, and subsidizing Medicaid and private health insurance coverage for the uninsured (Davis and Stremikis August 23, 2012). The latter justification is especially important for providers as one reason most did not actively oppose the Affordable Care Act was the expectation that the Medicaid expansion together with increased access to subsidized private coverage obtained through the health insurance exchanges would, along with increased efficiencies, compensate for lost revenues resulting from reductions in DSH and other public payment sources (Dorn et al. March 2013; Jost and Rosenbaum 2012; Moon 2012; Oberlander 2012). It has been estimated that, on the one hand, hospitals will receive $239.9 billion more between 2013 and 2022 with rather than without the Medicaid expansion (Dorn et al. March 2013). On the other hand, it is estimated that patient shifting from private insurance to Medicaid coverage under the expansion would result in losses of $113.6 billion during this time period due to Medicaid's traditionally low reimbursement rates. Still, hospitals should benefit overall with each dollar in private revenue lost corresponding with $2.59 in Medicaid revenue gained. It is no wonder that hospitals have been among the strongest advocates for expanding Medicaid coverage as governors and state legislatures debate whether to do so or not under the U.S. Supreme Court's ruling making the Medicaid expansion under the Affordable Care Act optional (The Advisory Board December 12, 2012, February 4, 2013, April 15, 2013; Dorn et al. March 2013).

Safety-net providers are particularly concerned about the Medicaid expansion since many "have not focused on effective management, cost control, quality improvement, or services that attract [privately] insured patients" (Kane et al. 2012). Instead, they will need to compete for those newly insured under Medicaid. This suggests that those safety net providers located in states that choose not to expand Medicaid coverage or to aggressively pursue enrollment of potential eligibles if coverage is expanded[7] will have fewer resources to care for their patients than they had previously given the concomitant reduction in federal subsidies made available. The experience in Massachusetts, which achieved near universal coverage and served as the model for the federal health reform legislation, is instructive in this regard. Here, the diversion of funds from the state's uncompensated care pool toward subsidizing Medicaid and private health insurance coverage together with reductions in the amount of money paid to providers, particularly in light of the state's growing budget deficit, led to large negative operating margins among the state's safety net hospitals, thereby leading to staff and service reductions among the affected facilities (Felland and Stark

November 2012; Kane et al. 2012). Safety-net providers also fear the loss of other funding sources (Felland and Stark November 2012). This includes the elimination of provider taxes, which as noted, enable states to draw in additional federal Medicaid matching dollars without concomitant increase in state contributions, in addition to the drying up of local funding streams as political will erodes due to perceptions that prevailing access problems have been solved, and because of a lack of support for assisting those who remain uninsured, say, because they are undocumented immigrants.

Resulting fiscal pressures could, in turn, limit the provision of uncompensated care, increase bad debt, and result in closures of critical safety-net institutions while adversely impacting access to and quality of care. It has been demonstrated, for example, that Medicaid payment pressures adversely impacted the provision of uncompensated care by core safety-net hospitals in the years following implementation of the Balanced Budget Act of 1997 (Bazzoli et al. 2006). It has also been demonstrated that the most profitable safety net hospitals in the years preceding the recession received more generous local taxpayer subsidies (e.g., property tax transfers) and Medicaid supplemental payments than their less well subsidized counterparts (Kane et al. 2012). This suggests that the ability of safety-net providers to serve their missions has declined as "the economic downturn, slow recovery, and politics of deficit reduction have eroded the ability of [state and] local governments to support the safety net" (Kane et al. 2012), even as the demand for services has risen due to the large number of Americans that lost private health insurance coverage during the recession (Bazzoli et al. 2012; Jones and Sajid 2010; Mobley, Kuo, and Bazzoli 2011). Subsequent closures and for-profit conversions among safety-net hospitals has, in turn, resulted in longer travel times (Bazzoli et al. 2012) and delays in access to care as measured by changes in hospital admissions for ambulatory care sensitive conditions (Mobley, Kuo, and Bazzoli 2011). Clearly, the adverse consequences associated with this dynamic would extend even more broadly should substantial reductions in federal Medicaid spending be enacted as per proposals to block grant the program and to reduce the rate of expenditure growth to, say, one percentage point above the CPI, as the resources available for paying providers would decline and fewer states would choose to participate in the Medicaid expansion while many of those that had chosen to participate would likely withdraw (Rosenbaum 2012).

ADVERSE CONSEQUENCES FOR BENEFICIARIES

Marked reductions in federal spending associated with block granting Medicaid would have especially adverse implications for beneficiaries. There are several reasons. As noted, subsequent reductions in provider payments would lead to considerable fiscal pressures that would lead to reductions in the number of participating providers while compromising access and quality. Moreover, restrictions on the number and scope of benefits would be put into place along with increases in beneficiary cost-sharing. The latter is particularly problematic. Extant research indicates that increasing cost-sharing through premiums, co-pays, and deductibles cause people to disenroll and/or reduce use of needed services, especially among the low-income populations Medicaid primarily serves (Wu and Wachino July 7, 2005; Artiga and O'Malley May 2005). It also indicates that cost sharing disproportionately disadvantages the chronically ill and those who have more frequent need of health care services.

Even more fundamental, considerably more stringent restrictions on program eligibility would be adopted while investments in education and outreach aimed at enrolling otherwise eligible individuals would decline or cease. This, in turn, would impact a majority of Americans, 51% of whom report some degree of personal connection to the program, either because they, a family member, or friend have received some level of health and long-term care support (Kaiser Family Foundation May 2011). The Urban Institute estimates that Ryan's FY 2013 House Budget Plan would result in 14.3 to 20.5 million fewer persons on the Medicaid rolls by 2022, a 25% to 35% reduction, with states needing to increase spending by $164.2 to $273.0 billion, or 46% to 77%, to avoid this decrease (Holahan et al. October 2012).[8] Nationally, enrollment decreases would range from 21% to 22% in Alaska to 31% to 46% in New Jersey, with state spending increases required to avoid expected reductions in enrollment ranging from 34% to 61% in New Hampshire ($0.5 to $0.9 billion) to 79% to 131% in Mississippi ($1.7 to $2.7 billion). Rhode Island would be expected to serve 46,000 to 69,000 fewer enrollees, a 24% to 35% reduction, by 2022, with state spending needing to increase from $0.9 to $1.5 billion, or 40% to 68%, if this reduction was going to be averted.

Most of those removed from the Medicaid rolls would become uninsured. The number of uninsured Americans increased markedly from 43.4 to 49.2 million between 2007 and 2010 with the decline in employer-based coverage stemming from rising levels of unemployment and declining family incomes during the late recession and slow recovery (Kaiser Family Foundation September 2012). However, this figure would have been far higher without Medicaid and CHIP, both quintessential countercyclical programs that currently provide coverage to 17.6% of the under 65 population and that kick into higher gear during hard economic times when the demand for government-subsidized assistance grows. It has been estimated that every percentage point increase in the unemployment rate is associated with both a 1.1 million increase in uninsured and a 1.0 million increases in Medicaid enrollment (Dorn et al. April 2008). Thus, from December 2007 to June 2010, the number of Medicaid enrollees increased by 7.6 million, or 17.8%, as the unemployment rate rose from 5.0 to 9.5% nationally (Kaiser Family Foundation February 2011). Moreover, despite increases in the overall number of uninsured, the number of children without insurance actually decreased by 600,000 due to 4.6 million additional children acquiring Medicaid or CHIP coverage during this time period (Kaiser Family Foundation July 2012c).

Now consider the Affordable Care Act, which could expand Medicaid to all non-Medicaid eligible individuals under age 65 with family incomes up to 138% of the FPL or $15,856 for an individual and $32,499 for a family of four in 2013.[9] Because it requires states to provide coverage for 10 categories of essential health benefits, most new Medicaid enrollees would receive more comprehensive coverage than that made available in a typical employer-based health insurance plan.[10] The Medicaid expansion is set to go into effect in 2014, at which point the federal government will pay for 100% of the costs of the expansion for three years, after which the proportion of costs paid for by the federal government will gradually decrease, so that from 2020 onward it will pay for 90% of the expansion's costs and the state's will pay for 10%. Individuals with incomes between 100% and 138% on up to 400% of the FPL will also be eligible for federally-subsidized private health insurance coverage through the health insurance exchanges, with maximum premium payments made toward the cost of coverage ranging from 2.0% to 9.5% of income for those at 100% and 400% of the FPL, respectively, and limits on cost-sharing ranging from 6.0% of the actuarial value of the plan for those at 100% of the FPL to 30.0% at 400%.

It was expected that the Medicaid expansion would result in greater uniformity in Medicaid eligibility nationally, with an additional 17 million Americans obtaining health insurance coverage as a result of the expansion by 2022 (Congressional Budget Office March 2012b), a figure recent analyses place at 21.3 million, 41% above expected enrollment levels without the Affordable Care Act (Holahan et al. November 2012). As noted, however, in a surprise move, the U.S. Supreme Court, while upholding the individual mandate and other aspects of the Affordable Care Act, basically made the Medicaid expansion optional for states in its June 28, 2012, decision in *National Federation of Independent Business v. Sebelius* (Jost and Rosebaum 2012).[11] The Court found that the Medicaid expansion was an unconstitutionally coercive exercise of the Constitution's Spending Clause because it made continued receipt of all federal Medicaid matching dollars contingent upon participating in the expansion (Muscumeci July 2012). In view of the decision, the impact of the expansion has been revised downward; it is now only expected to result in 11 million additional enrollees (Congressional Budget Office July 2012).

To qualify for the expansion, state residents must have incomes below 138% of the FPL. To qualify for subsidies to purchase private health insurance coverage through the exchanges, residents would need to have incomes between 100% and 400% of the FPL. That there is no overlap between the public and private coverage groups for those with incomes up to 100% of the FPL suggests that of the lowest income people living in states that either elect not to expand Medicaid coverage under the Affordable Care Act or to pull back on the expansion should the program be capped or block granted would be ineligible for subsidies through the exchanges and, as such, would remain uninsured. In turn, those losing coverage would face considerable obstacles to obtaining needed care with adverse implications for health and well-being. Evidence from a randomized trial in Oregon provides strong evidence in this regard (Allen et al. 2010; Baicker et al. 2013; Baicker and Finkelstein 2011; Finkelstein et al. 2012).

Results from the first year indicate that those enrolled in Medicaid after being randomly selected to apply had a higher probability of prescription drug, outpatient care, and inpatient hospital use but no difference in emergency department use than those who remained disenrolled but on a waitlist for the program (Baicker and Finkelstein 2011; Finkelstein et al. 2012). First-year results further indicate that those enrolled in the program were more likely to have a usual source of care and to use preventive services, including cholesterol screening, diabetes screening, mammograms, and pap smears. Increased use of health care services provided both health and financial benefits. Health-wise, Medicaid coverage increased the probability of reporting being happy and in better self-reported health while decreasing the likelihood of being screened for depression. Financially, Medicaid coverage reduced the likelihood of having to borrow money or to skip payments on other bills to pay for medical expenses, in addition to lowering the probability that unpaid bills would be referred to a collection agency.

Second-year results also demonstrate increased use of prescription drugs, office visits, and preventive services such cholesterol monitoring, pap smears, prostate screening, and mammograms; a higher likelihood of having a usual source of care; and near elimination of catastrophic medical costs and other forms of economic distress (Baicker et al. 2012). Second-year results demonstrate lower rates of depression and increased rates of diabetes detection and management as well (Baicker et al. 2012). Medicaid coverage did not significantly improve physical health outcomes after two years, however, including blood-pressure, cholesterol, or blood sugar levels, nor impacted the diagnosis and treatment of high blood pressure and cholesterol. These latter findings suggest several possibilities, either no effect of Medicaid coverage on the physical health outcomes measured, study limitations (e.g., small sample size, lack of baseline data), or too short a follow-up period to permit the physical-health benefits of coverage to accumulate.

Although less methodologically rigorous than the Oregon Experiment, findings from this unique randomized trial are broadly consistent with numerous other investigations that demonstrate access, health, and financial improvements associated with Medicaid and CHIP coverage, particularly when compared to being uninsured (Coughlin et al. May 2013; Institute of Medicine May 21, 2002; Kaiser Family Foundation October 2012, March 1, 2013; Ku and Ferguson June 2011). The 2010 Commonwealth Fund Health Insurance Survey, for example, which compared the experience of people covered by different types of health insurance, found that in comparison to people without insurance, Medicaid recipients were less likely to report having access or financial problems due to the cost of medical care and more likely to report having a medical home, afterhours access, and a higher quality experience, all at levels that did not differ significantly from privately insured individuals (Davis et al. 2012). Similarly, analysis of the 2012 National Health Interview Survey indicates that compared to people without health insurance, Medicaid/other public insurance recipients were considerably more likely to report having a usual source of care and less likely to postpone seeking or going without needed care due to cost (Kaiser Family Foundation October 2012). Moreover, analysis of data pooled from the 2003 to 2009 Medical Expenditure Panel Surveys indicates that other than similar rates of emergency department use, Medicaid beneficiaries would be substantially less likely to use most health services, including prescription drugs, specialist visits, primary care visits, and inpatient hospital care, and to have a usual source of care while facing substantially greater out-of-pocket costs if uninsured (Coughlin et al. May 2013). Moreover, other than high rates of emergency department use and lower rates of specialist visits, Medicaid beneficiaries would experience similar levels of access to other health care services if covered by employer-sponsored insurance but at substantially higher costs. Medicaid beneficiaries would experience substantially higher out-of-pocket expenditures if covered through the employer-based market as well.

Still other studies find psychological and survival benefits associated with coverage. The psychological benefits associated with insurance is reflected in findings deriving from eight focus groups with a diverse array of uninsured individuals residing in four major cities throughout the U.S. (Perry et al. 2012). Despite physical and mental health problems and a desire for health insurance, participants reported that no affordable options were available. They also reported experiencing physical and emotional pain as a result of going without and delaying needed care, and acquiring large medical debts when care was, in fact, received. Among the most common words used to describe being uninsured included "scary," "vulnerable," "frustrated," "worried," "horrible," and "sucks." Among the most common words used to describe the prospect of obtaining health care coverage included "relief," "less stress," "security," "happy," "spectacular," and "peace of mind."

The survival benefits associated with coverage is reflected in a study that compared three states—New York, Maine, and Arizona—that expanded adult Medicaid eligibility since 2000 to neighboring states that did not expand coverage. Results indicate that expansion was associated with a significant reduction in mortality, particularly among older adults, minorities, and residents of poor counties, increased rates of Medicaid coverage and decreased rates of lack of insurance, lower rates of delayed care, and improvements in self-reported health (Sommers, Baicker, and Epstein 2012). The mortality benefit, in particular, is consistent with the conclusions of an influential Institute of Medicine's report that the uninsured not only receive too little care too late and receive poorer care when it is received, but are sicker and die earlier, including an estimated 18,314 deaths resulting from a lack of coverage in 2000 (Institute of Medicine May 21, 2002). Subsequent analyses by the Urban Institute place the number of deaths resulting from the lack of coverage between 2000 and 2006 in the 137,000 to 165,000 range (Dorn January 2008).

MEDICAID REFORM IN A HYPER-PARTISAN AGE

How exactly would particular states respond if the Medicaid program was block granted? The answer will depend largely on a combination of political and economic considerations. States "face different incentives" in how they respond to Medicaid program changes promulgated by the federal government "depending on their overall budgetary situation, their current thresholds for Medicaid eligibility, the amounts that they and their local governments spend to provide health care to uninsured people or to pay providers for uncompensated care, the number of people likely to enroll in the program after [a prospective change has gone into effect], the federal contributions toward the cost of their care, and many other factors" (Congressional Budget Office July 2012). Block granting the program would greatly increase state discretion over Medicaid program design and administration beyond the considerable levels states already possess in this regard. Because policy necessarily evolves and adapts to local conditions, the way in which a block granted program would be implemented and the challenges state officials and affected providers and populations would face in doing so would vary nationally.

Traditionally, states of all types—rich and poor, conservative and liberal—have responded reliably to financial incentives promulgated by the federal government under Medicaid (Kaiser Family Foundation August 2012). More than half implemented the program in 1966, the year in which federal funding first became available. All but Alaska (1972) and Arizona (1982) implemented their programs within four years of this date. Thereafter, states responded to federal incentives to expand Medicaid to both newly mandatory and optional populations, including pregnant women, infants, and children. Moreover, during FY 1998, the first year in which enhanced federal fiscal support became available under CHIP, virtually all states (45) expanded coverage to low and moderate income children and families, with all remaining states doing so within the next year or two.

Federal matching grants such as Medicaid both increase the recipient government's income and lower the price of the public good that is being provided (Miller 2004). Whereas states with a 50% FMAP, for example, pay for half of Medicaid program costs (e.g., New York, California), those with a 67% FMAP pay for one-third (e.g., Georgia, Michigan), and those with a 75% FMAP pay for just one-fourth (i.e., Mississippi). The result is that poor, largely conservative states should have even greater incentives than financially well off states to increase spending beyond what otherwise would have been the case, a dynamic missing with block grants, which have an income effect only and therefore tend to be much less simulative in their impact. This suggests that the gap in coverage between rich and poor states would surely widen if a block grant strategy was pursued.

Today's hyper-partisan political environment further suggests that those states that might be most adversely impacted if the program were block granted may, in fact, be most supportive if the federal government pursued this approach to Medicaid reform. Consider some pertinent public opinion data. A May 2011 survey found that 35% of Americans preferred that Medicaid be changed so that the federal government gave states a fixed amount of money with each state deciding who to cover and what services to pay for, while 60% preferred the status quo (Kaiser Family Foundation May 2011). The proportion preferring to block grant the program, however, increased from 18% among Democrats to 36% among Independents and 57% among Republicans (Kaiser Family Foundation May 2011). This basic public opinion structure has remained largely intact over the last 15 years. In particular, a July 1996 survey found that 47% of Americans favored proposals to turn over responsibility for Medicaid to the states, while 43% opposed such a proposal (Kaiser Family Foundation July 30, 1996). The proportion preferred turning the program over, however, increased from 34% among Democrats to 47% among Independents and 63% among Republicans. When asked whether each state should be given a fixed amount of federal dollars along with flexibility to decide how to spend it, considerably fewer respondents—29%—now favored turning the program over to the states with a much higher proportion—57%—opposing. Again, however, the proportion favoring doing so increased progressively from Democrats (16%) to Independents (30%) and Republicans (48%) (Kaiser Family Foundation July 30, 1996). Together, these two polls strongly suggest that conservative states dominated by Republican officials should exhibit substantially stronger support for block grants and other strategies for devolving Medicaid program functions since such proposals began to hit their stride in conservative circles nearly 30 years ago.

The role of governors as Medicaid power brokers largely accounts for the varying support that blocking granting the program has received over time (Thomson and Burke 2007, 2009; Thompson 2012). Thompson and Burke (2009) explain that "[t]wo primary attributes have defined Medicaid as an entitlement. First, the program features an open-ended funding commitment by the national government, which agrees to match at varying rates whatever states choose to spend. Second, once a state determines eligibility, service packages, and provider payment rates (subject to minimum requirements established by the national government), they are obligated to subsidize these services for all Medicaid recipients until such time as they modify state law." Block grants eliminate both aspects of the Medicaid entitlement.

Not only do they provide states considerably more discretion in determining program attributes, though some federal requirements would undoubtedly remain, but they also eliminate the federal government's open-ended commitment to funding the program. Governors of both parties have long sought to obtain as much flexibility administering Medicaid as possible, thereby contributing to interstate variation in program coverage and benefits nationally. At the same time, they have typically sought to maintain and even expand the federal government's opened-ended funding commitment, which, in addition to federal underwriting of incremental improvements in program benefits and eligibility, include successfully lobbying for enhanced federal matching support during the last two economic downturns. This includes the provision of $10 billion in additional Medicaid funds provided by the Jobs and Growth Tax Relief Reconciliation Act of 2003, and $87 billion in additional Medicaid funds with the American Recovery and Reinvestment Act of 2009. This bipartisan consensus toward enhancing the federal government's open-ended funding commitment has broken down, however, during periods of "intense, asymmetrical partisan polarization" when republican leaders at the state level have viewed themselves as part of a broader ideological movement to vitiate government programs such as Medicaid, thereby contributing to potential retrenchment in federal financial support (Thompson 2012). The first such instance occurred during the "devolution revolution" of the mid-1990s; the second, which continues to the present day, began with the Tea Party and the election of President Barack Obama. In between, President George W. Bush failed to garner sufficient gubernatorial support to turn the Medicaid program into a block grant despite Republican control of the Presidency, both Houses of Congress, and the majority of governorships at that time.

Medicaid was not on House Speaker Newt Gingrich's radar until a taskforce of 10 Republican governors set in motion the Congressional majority's MediGrant proposal, a policy change that 25 of 30 Republican governors eventually supported (Thompson 2012). Had it not been for President Clinton's veto of the Balanced Budget Act of 1995, Medicaid's open-ended funding commitment would have been eliminated and replaced with a block grant at substantially reduced levels of funding, particularly for Midwestern and Northeastern states, which would not have fared nearly as well as their faster growing, lower income counterparts in the South and West under the federal financing formula adopted. For its part, the Clinton administration advocated expanded state discretion and enhanced budgetary control through a per capita limit on expenditure growth but otherwise kept Medicaid's basic structure intact. The National Governor's Association, which represents the interests of all governors—Democratic and Republican—sought to reconcile the two approaches by proposing a resolution combining a fixed allocation as per Congress' MediGrant strategy with the provision of additional "umbrella funds" should enrollment rise faster than anticipated while increasing state discretion over program administration and reducing the proportion paid for by the states (Feder, Lambrew, and Huckaby 1996; Rowland March 6, 1996). This, too, failed to gain contraction. Subsequently, when the Clinton administration once again proposed a per capita cap on program spending, the National Governors Association released a letter signed by 41 governors, including those that had originally supported the block grant proposal, opposing any federal limit on Medicaid spending (Thompson 2012).

A few years before the George W. Bush administration unveiled its proposal to block grant Medicaid, the National Governors Association issued a 2001 proposal to restructure the program (Holahan 2001; Kaiser Family Foundation July 2001). The goal of this bipartisan proposal was to enhance the federal government's financing commitment while granting states considerably more flexibility over program administration. If enacted, this proposal would have required states to maintain mandatory services for mandatory eligibility groups at the existing federal matching rate. Beyond that, it would have granted states substantially more discretion in defining program eligibility and benefits, including optional benefits for mandatory eligibility groups and mandatory and optional benefits and, potentially, cost sharing requirements up to 5% of family income for optional eligibility groups. States providing optional benefits to mandatory groups and benefits resembling the CHIP package to optional groups would have received an enhanced federal matching rate, 30% higher than the normal rate. Otherwise, it was proposed that states be permitted to cover any beneficiaries or benefits at the existing federal matching rate independent of federal guidelines.

The National Governors Association's 2001 proposal was consistent with the general predilection of governors of both parties to seek greater administrative flexibility while maintaining and, perhaps, even enhancing federal fiscal support for the program. So, too, has been marked growth in federal approval of both 1115 "research and demonstration" and 1915(c) home- and community-based services waivers which, as noted previously, proliferated under both the Clinton and George W. Bush administrations. "Through the Medicaid waiver process, Thompson and Burke (2007) explain, "governors could increasingly have their cake and eat it, too; they gained impressive new power to shape their state programs without having to forego the national government's open ended funding commitment." Due, in part, to states' ability to use existing waiver authorities to make significant program changes without risking the federal government's open-ended funding commitment, the Bush administration had trouble recruiting governors to support its 2003 proposal to block grant the program (Thompson 2012; Thompson and Burke 2007, 2009). Three Republican governors, however, agreed to promote the administration's proposal within the National Governors Association, including Jeb Bush (Florida), Bill Owens (Colorado), and John Rowland (Connecticut). This contributed to the formation of a 10-member bipartisan taskforce that produced general principles for reform, which although largely consistent with the Bush administration's proposal, included provisions exempting mandatory program requirements from the block grant: it would only apply to the two-thirds of Medicaid program spending directed toward optional populations and benefits, protecting states' from the financial risk posed by the federal funding cap and transferring sole responsibility for the costs of caring for the most expensive population—Medicaid beneficiaries that are also eligible for Medicare, to the federal government (Park et al. June 5, 2003). Possibly because these latter two requirements were unlikely to be included in any subsequent federal legislation, and because of pressure from Democratic congressional leaders and the Republican administration's focus on other priorities, the tentative bipartisan consensus stalled and the block grant proposal was abandoned (Lambrew 2005; Thompson 2012).

Prevailing evidence strongly suggests that as was the case in 1995, partisanship will play a prominent, if not determinative role in informing state decision making regarding Medicaid in the present political environment, even more so than fiscal or programmatic concerns. After all, it was Republican-led states, including those with the highest proportion of uninsured residents, that delayed accepting federal stimulus money, including $87 billion in additional Medicaid funding, despite the largest state budget deficits since the Great Depression (Miller and Blanding 2012). It was also Republican-led states that challenged the constitutionality of the Affordable Care Act and elected not to form their own health insurance exchanges. In all, 25 states sought to have the Affordable Care Act overturned while 12 supported the law, two—Washington and Iowa—both supported and opposed the law due to the varying positions of their governors and attorney generals, and 12 took no position. All but one of the states challenging health care reform—Colorado—had a Republican governor. All but one of the states supporting the law—New Mexico—were led by a Democrat. Similarly, 27 states indicated that they will default to a federally facilitated exchange as compared to 17 that plan to establish a state-based exchange and seven that will establish an exchange but in partnership with the federal government (Kaiser Family Foundation May 10, 2013). All but two of the states defaulting to the federal exchange—Missouri and Montana—have a Republican Governor. All but three states electing to establish a state-based exchange—Nevada, Idaho, and New Mexico—are led by a Democrat.

Not surprisingly, it is Republican-led states that have declined to participate in the Affordable Care Act's Medicaid expansion, a position seemingly shared by rank-and-file Republicans. According to an April 2013 survey, 50% of Americans would prefer to expand Medicaid while just 41% would like to keep the program as it is (Kaiser Family Foundation April 2013). But whereas 72% of Democrats and 47% of Independents would like to see the program expanded as compared to 21% and 42% who would prefer no changes, 68% of Republicans surveyed would prefer the status quo as compared to 21% who would like to broaden eligibility to cover more low-income uninsured adults. That the federal government will pay 100% of the costs during the first three years and at least 90% thereafter while eliminating almost all uncompensated care costs and providing health coverage to millions more Americans suggests just how good a deal the expansion is for state governments no matter what their particular political, economic, or programmatic circumstances (Rosenbaum and Westmoreland 2012; Angeles July 25, 2012). Whereas the Congressional Budget Office estimates that the expansion will increase state Medicaid costs by just 2.8% between 2014 and 2022 relative to current law, the Urban Institute and Lewin Group project increases of just 1.4% and 1.1%, respectively, between 2014 and 2019 (Angeles July 25, 2012). In a more recent analysis, the Urban Institute projects that if all states expanded the program, state costs would be just 0.3% or $8 billion higher between 2013 and 2022 relative to current law as compared to an increase of 21% or $800 billion for the federal government (Holahan et al. November 2012). Moreover, states can expect a net decrease in costs of $10 billion as a result of an expected reduction of $18 billion in state and local uncompensated care costs.

Ten states had already chosen not to participate in the Medicaid expansion by January 15, 2013 and an additional five were leaning toward not doing so, each with a Republican governor (The Advisory Board Company January 15, 2013).[12] This is in contrast to four Democratic-led states and one Republican-led state that were leaning towards participating at that time and 18 states and the District of Columbia which had chosen to do so, all but four of which—Rhode Island (Independent) and Arizona, Nevada, and New Mexico (Republican)—had a Democratic governor.[13] Other Republican governors eventually came on board, including those in Michigan, North Dakota, Ohio, and Florida. Thus, by May 13, 2013, 28 states had governors supporting expansion, including 19 led by Democrats, one by an Independent, and eight by Republicans. There was also one state leaning towards expanding coverage—New York, a Democratic-led state. By contrast, 15 states had governors who announced their positions opposing the expansion with five more leaning towards not doing so, all Republican led (The Advisory Board Company January 15, 2013).

In short, those governors that were quickest to declare that their states would not participate (i.e., by January 15, 2013) led states that would have benefited more from the expansion than those governors that were quickest to declare that their states would participate. This is reflected in the finding that, on average, states declining to expand by January 15 would have experienced a 20.3% increase in total Medicaid spending, primarily due to the provision of additional federal financial support, between 2013 and 2022, as compared to a 13.8% estimated increase for states that agreed to do so by that date.[14] It is also reflected in the finding that, on average, states declining to expand would have experienced an estimated incremental reduction of 24.5% in the number of uninsured residents during this time period as compared to an estimated reduction of 17.4% for states that had already agreed to expand coverage under the program.

By May 13, 2013, most governors had a made a decision one way or the other. On average, states declining to expand by May 13 would have experienced an 18.4% increase in total Medicaid spending between 2013 and 2022, as compared to a 14.1% estimated increase for states that agreed to do so by that date. On average, states declining to expand would have experienced an estimated incremental reduction of 22.6% in the number of uninsured residents during the period analyzed as compared to an estimated reduction of 19.5% for states that had already agreed to expand. Including those states leaning one way or the other, results indicate that non-expansion states would have experienced an 18.2% estimated increase in total Medicaid spending and 22.1% estimated reduction in the number of uninsured residents, on average, as compared to 16.1% and 18.8%, respectively, for expansion states. Overall, it is estimated that between 2013 and 2022, Republican-led states, which had the most difficult time, at least politically, in deciding whether or not to participate in the expansion, could expect a 19.3% increase in Medicaid expenditures and 21.5% reduction in the number of uninsured as a result of the expansion as compared to a 14.1% increase in expenditures and 18.8% reduction in the number of uninsured for states led by Democrats.

Importantly, the Obama administration has indicated that it will not permit states to implement partial expansions, say, for example, by enrolling those with incomes up to100% of the FPL into Medicaid with those between 100% and 138% being left to obtain federally-subsidized private health insurance coverage in the exchanges. However, the administration has expressed a willingness to consider alternative strategies as long as the number gaining coverage is the same. Thus, the administration has reacted favorably to Democratic Governor Mike Beebe's proposal to use Medicaid dollars to enroll Arkansas' expansion eligible population in private health insurance plans obtained through the state's health insurance exchange at the same federal match as other expansion programs (i.e., 100% for three years down progressively to 90% after 2020). Beebe's request is not unique. There is currently 47 premium assistance programs in 39 states authorized by various federal statutory authorities and funded by Medicaid, CHIP, or both (U.S. General Accountability Office January 29, 2010). At less than 1% of total Medicaid and CHIP spending in 2008–2009, these programs tend to be quite small, largely due to challenges achieving cost effectiveness, including limited access to employer-sponsored coverage available to the low-income populations eligible for such programs (Alker March 2013). Federal approval of Arkansas and Iowa's Section 1115 waiver applications to expand Medicaid coverage via premium assistance plan have not been approved yet and will depend on a number of factors, not least of which include the state's ability (a) to keep costs down—it costs considerably less, on average, to insure someone under Medicaid than through a private health insurance plan and (b) to reconcile private plan design with core Medicaid program requirements—strict limitations on beneficiary cost-sharing, for example (Hancock May 1, 2013).

Governor Beebe made his proposal largely to overcome Republican resistance in the state legislature. Thus, it should not be surprising that a number of Republican governors (e.g., in Iowa) have expressed interest in seeking federal approval for alternative approaches to covering Medicaid-eligible uninsured residents come 2014 to better satisfy partisan demands (The Advisory Board April 1, 2013; Kliff March 18, 2013). Using Medicaid dollars to purchase health insurance in the private market is ideologically more palatable to conservative politicians either because: (a) they wrongly perceive it to be more efficient—as noted, Medicaid is in fact substantially cheaper while providing more generous coverage and comparable levels of access on most though not all measures or (b) doing so benefits key constituencies, including commercial carriers and for-profit medical companies. But regardless of the merits, permitting states to expand coverage via premium assistance may prove to be an effective means of overcoming political resistance to increasing access to health insurance coverage in otherwise recalcitrant states.

The Obama administration has indicated that it may be willing to grant a limited number of waivers permitting states to experiment with alternative strategies to increasing coverage with Medicaid expansion funds with additional approvals in future years being contingent on lessons learned. That this strategy may attract additional support for extending coverage is reflected in the position of Republican governors such as Iowa's Terry Branstad and Tennessee's Bill Haslam who have linked expansion in their states to federal willingness to allow enrollment of the expansion population into private plans (The Advisory Board May 13, 2013).

That this strategy may not bear fruit is evidenced by failure of the Florida state legislature to pass a budget including the expansion (even as premium assistance), despite endorsement by Republican Governor Rick Scott, a major health reform opponent and former chief executive of Columbia/HCA, the largest for-profit health care company in the country (Anonymous May 6, 2013; Kliff May 5, 2013). Should this decision stand, Florida will have given up approximately $66.1 billion in additional federal matching funds over the course of a decade, while 869,000 who otherwise would have gained coverage through the expansion would remain uninsured (Holahan et al. November 2012).

Rick Scott is not the only Republican Governor to face this dilemma. A number of otherwise supportive Republican chief executives have seen their efforts to achieve passage of legislation authorizing expansion of Medicaid lose momentum and stall (The Advisory Board May 6, 2013; Cheney and Millman May 2, 2013; Somashekhar May 2, 2013). In Arizona, for example, Republican Governor Jan Brewer, another health reform opponent turned Medicaid expansion advocate (or realist, depending on one's point-of-view) lost patience and threatened to veto all bills until the state legislature made progress passing the state budget and Medicaid expansion. Soon thereafter, the Governor vetoed five bills, indicating that her threat was far from idle (Wrigley May 24, 2013). For their part, Republican state legislators promised to dig in their heels with Arizona Senate President Andy Biggs claiming that "he will do 'everything in my power' to keep a vote on Medicaid from even coming to the floor" and Arizona House Appropriations Committee Chairman, John Kavanagh, claiming that "he would 'like nothing better than it not even come to a vote' " (Wrigley May 24, 2013). Governor Brewer ultimately won this standoff. For good measure, the Texas state legislature passed a proposal explicitly preventing implementation of the Medicaid expansion by requiring that state officials provide no one medical assistance after December 31, 2013, unless they would have met state eligibility levels in effect on that date even though the state's Republican Governor, Rick Perry, had already announced his opposition to the expansion (MacLaggan May 26, 2013). What does such intransigence cost? Arizona would have given up approximately $10.7 billion in additional federal matching funds over the course of a decade to provide Medicaid coverage to 52,000 uninsured people (Holahan et al. November 2012). Texas will give up approximately $65.6 billion in additional federal matching funds over the course of a decade to provide Medicaid to 1.2 million currently without coverage.

"For states," observed Harold Pollack (2013), "[the Supreme Court ruling making the expansion optional] brings both new flexibility and new accountability. Conservative legislators who have traditionally railed against Medicaid while accepting large subsidies will now have to actively accept or reject billions of dollars in federal resources made possible through this program." It seems that many of these legislators have chosen partisan and ideological purity consistent with their own beliefs and the highly conservative districts that elected them, rather than giving President Obama, the Democratic Party, and their constituencies a "win" by expanding Medicaid coverage to previously uninsured individuals at a far superior federal matching rate. Even the Oregon Health Experiment, which used a randomized controlled trial, the "gold standard," to examine the impact of Medicaid coverage on the well-being of enrollees, has been interpreted through a partisan lens. Thus, despite generally positive findings regarding depression diagnosis, diabetes detection and management, having a usual source of care, preventive screening, and fiscal distress, Avik Roy (May 2, 2013), a conservative commentator and contributor to *The Apothecary* blog, concluded that the results, which found no significant improvement in physical health outcomes over two years, "calls into question the $450 billion a year we spend on Medicaid, and the fact that Obamacare throws 11 million more Americans into this broken program." Similarly, the Cato Institute's director of health policy Michael Cannon, argues that the study "throws a huge stop sign in front of the Medicaid expansion. . . . The benefits are highly questionable" (Kliff May 1, 2013).

Just as the Affordable Care Act passed Congress without a single Republican vote, House Budget Committee Chairmen Paul Ryan's FY 2012 and FY 2013 budget proposals, which included provisions block granting Medicaid, passed the House of Representatives strictly along party lines before failing to make any progress in the Democratically controlled Senate. This proposal was strongly favored by the nation's Republican governors. In a letter to Congressman Ryan endorsing his "bold FY 2012 budget proposal," the leadership of the Republican Governor's Association, including Chairmen Ricky Perry (Texas), Vice Chairman Bob McDonnell (Virginia), Policy Chairman Haley Barbour (Mississippi), and Vice Chairman Chris Christie (New Jersey), wrote that "Medicaid reform is welcome and the Republican Governors overwhelmingly support the creation of a Medicaid block grant program. This well established approach will give states the freedom to innovate, share best practices, and create cost-effective ways to deliver quality health care to our most vulnerable populations" (Republican Governors Public Policy Committee April 5, 2011). Subsequently, 29 republican governors sent a letter to Congress, which although not explicitly endorsing the approach lain out by Congressmen Ryan, contained seven principles, including permitting "states and territories . . . to innovate by using flexible, accountable financing mechanisms that are transparent and that hold states accountable for efficiency and quality healthcare. Such mechanisms may include a block grant, a capped allotment outside of a waiver, or other accountable and transparent financing approaches" (Republican Governor's Association June 13, 2011). A later proposal sought to operationalize these basic principles with 31 solutions that continued to acknowledge the potential desirability of block granting the program but focused more on holding states accountable for meeting certain goals in exchange for an expedited federal review process and seemingly unlimited flexibility over program design and administration (Republican Governors Public Policy Committee August 30, 2011).

Not surprisingly, the nation's Democratic governors have a substantially different view. Perhaps this is best illustrated by a letter sent to the Congressional leadership in which 17 Democratic governors "strongly oppose[d] a congressionally-mandated block grant of federal Medicaid spending, which would shift costs and risk to states," but "continue[d] to seek greater flexibility to improve . . . Medicaid in ways that work for . . . individual states." Thus, Democratic governors were open to negotiation about beneficiaries' entitlement to program services but not states' entitlement to federal fiscal support in contrast to Republican governors, who were open to negotiating radical departures in both areas. As with the Medicaid expansion, those states reportedly in favor of blocking granting the program—that is, Republican led states, would be more adversely impacted by doing so than those states rejecting this approach to Medicaid reform—that is, Democratic led states. This is reflected in the finding that new state spending required to avoid enrollment cuts resulting from the House Republican block grant proposal varies across Republican and Democratic governorships, with the former being affected more, on average, than the latter although they have advocated strongly for this approach to reform. Thus, it is estimated that in 2022, Republican-led states would have to increase spending by 53.7% to 89.6% on average, as compared to 49.0% to 81.6% in states led by Democrats, to prevent enrollment cuts that would otherwise result from blocking granting the program.[15]

Of course, neither block granting Medicaid nor repealing the Affordable Care Act is going to happen anytime soon in light of President Obama's electoral triumph. Furthermore, the Budget Control Act of 2011, enacted August 2, 2011, to end the debt ceiling crisis, excludes Medicaid as well as Social Security, veterans, civilian and military employee pay, and Medicare (beyond provider payments) from automatic budget sequestration—that is, $1.2 trillion in across the board spending cuts from 2013 to 2012—if Congress and the President do not agree on deficit reduction equal to this amount. The Act, however, does not prevent Congress and the President from including Medicaid in a deal should negotiations to either prevent or ameliorate the effects of sequestration prove successful.

At 7%, Medicaid is the third largest domestic program in the federal budget, behind Medicare and Social Security, at 17% and 23%, respectively (Kaiser Family Foundation March 2013). Furthermore, the Congressional Budget Office projects that between 2012 and 2023, federal Medicaid spending will increase by an average annual rate of approximately 8%, from $251 to $572 billion during this time period, with enrollment rising from 67 to 84 million (Kaiser Family Foundation March 2013). Both Democrats and Republicans agree that, as a major contributor to the long-term federal budget deficit, growth in federal health care spending needs to be restrained.[16] Where they disagree is how best to achieve this objective with, according to Rosenbaum (2012), "Democrats emphasiz[ing] transformation of the health care system through payment reform and organizational restructuring and Republicans favoring tougher limits on federal spending that might galvanize deep downstream changes on the part of health care providers and consumers." It is likely, therefore, that block grants and other strategies to significantly retrench the Medicaid program will continue to be proposed by Republican officials, both in future budget proposals and presidential party platforms.

CONCLUSION

Medicaid has remained remarkably durable over time, overcoming concerted efforts on the part of Republican presidents and Congressional majorities to implement block grants and other forms of major retrenchment (Thompson 2012). Although it now serves as the backbone of the nation's health reform efforts, continued vigilance will be necessary to promote expansion to the low-income uninsured in recalcitrant states. Continued vigilance will also be necessary to ensure that sufficient resources are deployed to the requisite education and outreach required to identify and to recruit potentially eligible participants. In this context it is critical that examples purported to support the block grant approach to Medicaid reform be fully vetted. Claims that Rhode Island's Global Waiver resulted in $100 million in savings over 18 months has led conservative politicians and commentators to hold up the Waiver as a successful example of what block granting the Medicaid program could achieve nationally. The Global Waiver, however, is not a model that supports the block grant approach to Medicaid reform.

Most fundamentally, the Global Waiver is not a block grant but a capped federal match. Moreover, the state did not receive unlimited discretion to administer the Global Waiver nor achieved nearly as much savings as has been claimed. Indeed, most of the savings obtained by Rhode Island during this time period derive not from the Global Waiver but from increased spending on the part of the federal government and from measures the state could have implemented independently of the Global Waiver authority negotiated with CMS. Furthermore, the generosity of the Waiver agreement received by Rhode Island is in marked contrast to most block grant proposals, which would substantially reduce the level of federal fiscal support, nor permit states to back out via a Global Waiver-like escape clause should the fiscal situation become untenable. Such a marked reduction in federal spending would have devastating consequences, not only for state budgets but for provider reimbursement, beneficiary access and quality, and program benefits and eligibility. The number of uninsured Americans would increase dramatically if the block grant strategy were put into place, contrary to progress currently being made with the implementation of health care reform. If the Medicaid program is to meet the needs of vulnerable Americans—low income children and families, the mentally ill, the developmentally disabled, the physically disabled, a growing population of elders in need of long-term services and supports, its basic entitlement—both for states and beneficiaries—must remain intact. Program performance must continue to improve as well, perhaps informed by lessons drawn from state health reform efforts, including the Global Waiver implemented in Rhode Island.

NOTES

1. See Holahan et al. (2011) for an earlier version of this analysis.
2. States with estimated reductions between 35% and 49% in 2010 include: Arkansas, Colorado, the District of Columbia, Florida, Georgia, Hawaii, Illinois, Indiana, Iowa, Maryland, Michigan, Minnesota, Mississippi, Missouri, Montana, North Carolina, Ohio, Oklahoma, Oregon, Pennsylvania, South Carolina, Tennessee, Texas, Utah, Vermont, Virginia, and Wisconsin. Those with reductions of 50% or greater include: Alaska, Arizona, Delaware, Idaho, Nevada, and New Mexico.

3. Areas exempt from the Affordable Care Act's maintenance of effort provisions include expiring waivers and, in states certifying a budget deficit, coverage for adults above 138% of the federal poverty level (Smith, Gifford, and Ellis October 2012).
4. Eight states with reductions in hospital payments of less than $1.0 billion: Alaska, Maine, Montana, New Hampshire, North Dakota, South Dakota, Vermont, Wyoming.
5. Thirteen states with reductions in nursing home payments of less than $1.0 billion: Alaska, Delaware, the District of Columbia, Hawaii, Idaho, Montana, Nevada, New Mexico, North Dakota, South Dakota, Utah, Vermont, Wyoming.
6. Enacted with the Middle Class Tax Relief and Job Creation Act of 2012 (P.L. 112–96) and the American Taxpayer Relief Act of 2012.
7. Currently, for example, more than 70% of uninsured children are potentially eligible for Medicaid or CHIP (Kaiser Family Foundation March 1, 2013).
8. The range in enrollment reductions is based on the application of two potential scenarios. The first assumes that states maintain per person spending growth equal to GDP per capita plus 1.6%, the pre-Affordable Care Act baseline. The second assumes that states exhibit strong control over costs, thereby maintaining per person spending growth equal to the GDP per capita (Holahan et al. October 2012).
9. The 138% FPL limit reflects the Affordable Care Act's 133% FPL eligibility threshold combined with a five percentage point FPL income disregard also included in the Act (Kaiser Family Foundation July 2012b). It should also be noted that the Affordable Care Act replaces states disparate disregards and income counting methods with a uniform standard for determining Medicaid financial eligibility based on Modified Adjusted Gross Income (MAGI). States will be required to apply this new standard to pregnant women, children, parents, and newly qualifying adults as of July 1, 2014. It will not apply to the elderly or people with disabilities.
10. Categories of essential health benefits include: ambulatory patient services; emergency services; hospitalization; maternity and newborn care; mental health and substance use disorder services, including behavioral health treatment; prescription drugs; rehabilitative and habilitative services and devices; laboratory services; preventive and wellness services and chronic disease management; and pediatric services, including oral and vision care (see http://www.healthcare.gov/glossary/e/essential.html).
11. 567 U.S.____ (2012).
12. Those Republican-led states choosing not to participate in the Medicaid expansion as of January 15, 2013 included: Alabama, Georgia, Idaho, Louisiana, Maine, Mississippi, Oklahoma, South Carolina, South Dakota, and Texas. Those Republican-led states leaning towards not participating in the Medicaid expansion at that time included: Iowa, Nebraska, New Jersey, Virginia, and Wyoming. By February 20, 2013, three additional Republican led states—North Carolina, Pennsylvania, and Wisconsin—had decided to eschew the expansion as well. By May 13, 2013, Republican governors in Alaska and Iowa had also placed their states in the no column. Thus, as of that date, states electing not to participate included: 15 Republican-led states: Alabama, Alaska, Georgia, Idaho, Iowa, Louisiana, Maine, Mississippi, North Carolina, Oklahoma, Pennsylvania, South Carolina, South Dakota, Texas, and Wisconsin. There were also five additional Republican-led states leaning towards not doing so, including Kansas, Nebraska, Utah, Virginia, Wyoming (The Advisory Board Company January 15, 2013, February 20, 2013; May 13, 2013).

13. Those Democratic-states choosing to participate in the Medicaid expansion as of January 15, 2013 included: Arkansas, California, Colorado, Connecticut, Delaware, the District of Columbia, Hawaii, Illinois, Maryland, Massachusetts, Minnesota, Missouri, Montana, Vermont, and Washington. Those republican led-states choosing to participate as of January 15, 2013 included: Arizona, New Mexico, and Nevada. Rhode Island, an Independent-led state, had chosen to do so as well. Those leaning toward participating in the Medicaid expansion at that time included four Democratic-led states—Kentucky, New Hampshire, New York, and Oregon, and one Republican-led state—North Dakota. By February 20, 2013, two additional Democratic-led states (New Hampshire and Montana) and four Republican-led states (Florida, Michigan, North Dakota, and Ohio) had pledged their participation. By May 13, 2013, Republican and Democratic governors in New Jersey and West Virginia, respectively, had pledged to do so as well. Thus, as of that date, participating states included: 19 Democratic-led states (Arkansas, California, Colorado, Connecticut, Delaware, the District of Columbia, Hawaii, Illinois, Maryland, Massachusetts, Minnesota, Missouri, Montana, New Hampshire, Montana, Oregon, Vermont, West Virginia, and Washington), 1 Independent-led state (Rhode Island), and 8 Republican-led states (Arizona, Florida, Michigan, New Jersey, New Mexico, Nevada, North Dakota, and Ohio). New York is highly likely to participate as well (The Advisory Board Company January 15, 2013, February 20, 2013; May 13, 2013).
14. These and subsequent figures reported in this paragraph derive from analysis of data reported in Holahan et al. November 2012. Reported findings reflect the change in expenditures under the Affordable Care Act with all states expanding Medicaid to expenditures under a no Affordable Care Act baseline. Results are similar when the baseline reflects expenditures under the Affordable Care Act with no states expanding Medicaid. In this case, results indicate that states declining to expand would have experienced a 17.8% increase in total Medicaid spending, again, primarily due to an increase in federal dollars, between 2013 and 2022, as compared to a 9.9% estimated increase for states that have already agreed to participate.
15. These figures derive from data reported in Holahan et al. October 2012. Reported findings reflect new state spending required in 2022 to avoid enrollment cuts due to block granting Medicaid relative to baseline expenditures in which the Affordable Care Act had been repealed. The range reflects different estimated growth rates based on the GDP and GDP plus 1.6%.
16. However, Republicans feel more strongly in this regard than Democrats. This is reflected in a May 2011 survey that found that just 13% of Americans favor major reductions in Medicaid as part of a deal to reduce the federal budget deficit; 30% favor minor reductions; and 53% no reductions at all (Kaiser Family Foundation May 2011). But whereas most Democrats (69%) and Independents (54%) favor no reductions, a majority of Republicans favor some level of reduction, either minor (44%) or major (20%).

References

AARP. 2003. *Beyond 50.03: A Report to the Nation on Independent Living and Disability.* Washington, D.C.: AARP. Accessed January 2, 2012. http://assets.aarp.org/rgcenter/il/beyond_50_il.pdf.

AARP. 2009. *Long-Term Care in Rhode Island.* Washington, D.C.: AARP. Accessed October 28, 2012. http://assets.aarp.org/rgcenter/health/state_ltcb_09_ri.pdf.

Adler, Loren, Shai Akabas, and Brian Collins. 2013, March 12. *Paul Ryan's Fiscal Year 2014 Budget: The Details.* Washington, D.C.: Bipartisan Policy Center. Accessed May 25, 2013. http://bipartisanpolicy.org/blog/2013/03/ryan-fy14-budget.

———. 2013, March 15. *Patty Murray's Fiscal Year 2014 Budget: The Details.* Washington, D.C.: Bipartisan Policy Center. Accessed May 25, 2013. http://bipartisanpolicy.org/blog/2013/03/senate-dems-budget.

The Advisor Board Company. 2012, December 12. *In Red States, Hospitals Push Leaders to Expand Medicaid: Nevada Governor is First Republican Governor to Pledge Participation.* Accessed May 24, 2013. http://www.advisory.com/Daily-Briefing/2012/12/12/Hospitals-push-red-states-to-expand-Medicaid.

———. 2013, January 15. *Where Each State Stands on ACA's Medicaid Expansion: A Roundup of What Each State's Leadership Has Said about Their Medicaid Plans.* Accessed January 8, 2013. http://www.advisory.com/Daily-Briefing/2012/11/09/MedicaidMap#lightbox/1/.

———. 2013, February 4. *S. C. Hospitals: We'll Pay for the Medicaid Expansion: Gov. Haley Has Opposed the Proposal.* Accessed May 24, 2013. http://www.advisory.com/Daily-Briefing/2013/02/04/SC-hospitals-We-pay-for-the-Medicaid-expansion.

———. 2013, February 20. *Where Each State Stands on ACA's Medicaid Expansion: A Roundup of What Each State's Leadership Has Said about Their Medicaid Plans.* Accessed February 22, 2013. *http://www.advisory.com/Daily-Briefing/2012/11/09/MedicaidMap.*

———. 2013, March 12. *Florida Lawmakers Veto Medicaid Expansion, Eye Arkansas Model: Scott Had Proposed a Three-Year Expansion for the Sunshine State.* Accessed May 24, 2013. http://www.advisory.com/Daily-Briefing/2013/03/12/Florida-lawmakers-veto-Medicaid-expansion.

———. 2013, April 1. *HHS: With Permits, States Can Privatize Medicaid Expansion: Announcement May Allow More States to Follow Arkansas's Lead.* Accessed May 24, 2013. http://www.advisory.com/Daily-Briefing/2013/04/01/HHS-With-permits-states-can-privatize-Medicaid-expansion.

———. 2013, April 15. *In Ohio, Hospitals Get 'Aggressive' in Push for Medicaid Expansion: 'We're Not Going to Give Up on This,' Cleveland Clinic Official Says.* Accessed May, 2013. http://www.advisory.com/Daily-Briefing/2013/04/15/In-Ohio-hospitals-get-aggressive-in-push-for-Medicaid-expansion.

———. 2013, May 6. *Governors Run into Legislative Walls on the Medicaid Expansion: WSJ-Interparty-Squabbles-Could-Leave-Millions-Uninsured.* Accessed May 25, 2013. http://www.advisory.com/Daily-Briefing/2013/05/06/Governors-run-into-legislative-walls-on-the-Medicaid-expansion.

———. 2013. "Fla. Legislature Adjourns Without Medicaid Expansion Deal." *Kaiser Health News,* May 6. Accessed May 24, 2013. http://www.kaiserhealthnews.org/Daily-Reports/2013/May/06/medicaid-expansion.aspx.

———. 2013, May 13. *Where Each State Stands on ACA's Medicaid Expansion: A Roundup of What Each State's Leadership Has Said about Their Medicaid Plans.* Accessed May 23, 2013. http://www.advisory.com/Daily-Briefing/2012/11/09/MedicaidMap.

Alexander, Gary D. 2010. *Modernization 21st Century.* Cranston, Rhode Island: Executive Office of Health & Human Services.

———. 2011, January 28. *Rhode Island Medicaid Reform Global Consumer Compact Waiver: A National Model for Medicaid Reform.* Accessed July 30, 2012. http://www.galen.org/assets/RIMedicaidReform.pdf.

Alker, Joan C. 2008, August 5. *Rhode Island's Global Compact Waiver.* Washington, D.C.: Georgetown University Health Policy Institute. Accessed November 6, 2010. http://ccf.georgetown.edu/wp-content/uploads/2012/03/RI-testimony.pdf.

———. 2012, March. *The New Review and Approval Process Rule for Section 1115 Medicaid and CHIP Demonstration Waivers.* Washington, D.C.: The Henry J. Kaiser Family Foundation. Accessed November 12, 2012. http://www.kff.org/medicaid/upload/8292.pdf.

———. 2013, March. *Premium Assistance in Medicaid and CHIP: An Overview of Current Options and Implications of the Affordable Care Act.* Washington, D.C.: The Henry J. Kaiser Family Foundation. Accessed May 24, 2013. http://kaiserfamilyfoundation.files.wordpress.com/2013/03/8422.pdf.

Allen, Heidi, Katherine Baicker, Amy Finkelstein, Sarah Taubman, Bill J. Wright, and the Oregon Health Study Group. 2010. "What the Oregon Health Study Can Tell Us About Expanding Medicaid." *Health Affairs* 29 (8): 1498–1506.

Allen, Susan M., Pedro Gozalo, and Bernard A. Steinman. 2011, June 30. *Change in the Characteristic of Rhode Island Medicaid Population in Nursing Homes, 2008–2010.* Providence, Rhode Island: Center for Gerontology and Health Care Research, Brown University. Accessed October 26, 2012. http://www.dhs.ri.gov/Portals/0/Uploads/Documents/Public/Reports/Change_in_Characteristics_of_RI_Medicaid_Pop_June_2011.pdf.

Angeles, January. 2012, July 25. *How Health Reform's Medicaid Expansion Will Impact State Budgets.* Washington, D.C.: Center for Budget and Policy Priorities. Accessed November 19, 2012. http://www.cbpp.org/files/7–12–12health.pdf.

Arno, Peter S. 2006. *Prevalence, Hours and Economic Value of Family Caregiving: Updated State-by-State Analysis of 2004 National Estimates.* Washington, D.C.: National Family Caregivers Association and Family Caregiver Alliance. Accessed November 22, 2012. http://www.caregiver.org/caregiver/jsp/content/pdfs/State_Caregiving_Data_Arno_20061107.pdf.

Artiga, Samantha. 2009, March. *The Role of 1115 Waivers in Medicaid and CHIP: Looking Back and Looking Forward.* Washington, D.C.: The Henry J. Kaiser Family Foundation. Accessed October 28, 2012. http://www.kff.org/medicaid/upload/7874.pdf.

Artiga, Samantha, and Molly O'Malley. 2005, May. *Increasing Premiums and Cost Sharing in Medicaid and SCHIP: Recent State Experiences.* Washington, D.C.: The Henry J. Kaiser Family Foundation. Accessed October 28, 2012. http://www.kff.org/medicaid/loader.cfm?url=/commonspot/security/getfile.cfm&PageID=53261.

Baicker, Katherine, and Amy Finkelstein. 2011. "The Effects of Medicaid Coverage—Learning from the Oregon Experiment." *The New England Journal of Medicine* 365 (8): 683–85.

Baicker, Katherine, Sarah L. Taubman, Heidi L. Allen, Mira Bernstein, Jonathan H. Gruber, Joseph P. Newhouse, Eric C. Schneider, Bill J. Wright, Alan M. Zaslavsky, and Amy N. Finkelstein for the Oregon Health Study Group. 2013. "The Oregon Experiment—Effects of Medicaid on Clinical Outcomes." *The New England Journal of Medicine* 368 (18): 1713–1722.

Balla, Steven J. 2001. "Interstate Professional Associations and the Diffusion of Policy Innovations." *American Politics Research* 29: 221–45.

Barrilleaux, Charles J., and Mark E. Miller. 1988. "The Political Economy of State Medicaid Policy." *American Political Science Review* 82: 1089–1107.

Baucus, Max, John D. Rockefeller IV, Jack Reed, and Sheldon Whitehouse. 2008, June 19. *Secretary of the DHHS*. Accessed October 26, 2012. http://www.finance.senate.gov/newsroom/chairman/release/?id=f939060e-a664–41e5-a32b-5124ed7839bc.

Baumgartner, Frank, and Bryan D. Jones. 1993. *Agendas and instability in American politics*. Chicago: The University of Chicago Press.

Bazzoli, Gloria J., Woolton Lee, Hui-Min Hsieh, and Lee R. Mobley. 2012. "The Effects of Safety Net Hospital Closures and Conversions on Patient Travel Distance to Hospital Services." *Health Services Research* 47 (1, Pt. 1): 129–50.

Bazzoli, Gloria J., Richard C. Lindrooth, Ray Kang, and Romana Hasnain-Wynia. 2006. "The Influence of Health Policy and Market Factors on the Hospital Safety Net." *Health Services Research* 41 (4 Pt. 1): 1158–1180.

Beckwith, Jill. 2008, September 15. *How to Take Action on the Global Medicaid Waiver*. Providence, Rhode Island: Rhode Island Kids Count. Accessed November 6, 2010. http://www.rikidscount.org/matriarch/documents/What%20you%20can%20do_Global%20Waiver.pdf.

———. 2013, March 1. *Comments in Response to the Proposed Extension Request for the 1115 Waiver*. Providence, Rhode Island: Rhode Island Kids Count. Accessed May 18, 2013. http://www.ohhs.ri.gov/documents/documents13/Comments_RI_KIDS_COUNT.pdf.

Berry, Frances S., and William D. Berry. 1990. "State Lottery Adoptions as Policy Innovations: An Event History Analysis." *American Political Science Review* 84 (2): 395–415.

———. 2007. "Innovation and Diffusion Models in Policy Research." In *Theories of the Policy Process*, edited by Paul A. Sabatier, 223–260. Boulder, Colorado: Westview Press.

Berry, William D. 1990. "The Confusing Case of Budgetary Incrementalism: Too Many Meanings for a Single Concept." *Journal of Politics* 52:167–96.

Bostick, Jane E., Marilyn Rantz, Marcia Flesner, and C. Jo Riggs. 2006. "Systematic Review of Studies of Staffing and Quality in Nursing Homes." *Journal of the American Medical Directors Association* 7 (6): 366–76.

Braybrooke, David, and Charles E. Lindblom. 1963. *A Strategy of Decision*. New York: Free Press.

Broaddus, Matt. 2011, June 28. *CHIP's Success Not an Argument for Block-Granting Medicaid*. Washington, D.C.: Center for Budget and Policy Priorities. Accessed November 8, 2012. http://www.cbpp.org/files/6–29–11health.pdf.

Brodt, Amanda, Alice Burton, Donald Cohn, Brynnan Cox, Amanda Folsom, Isabel Friedenzohn, Enrique Martinez-Vidal, and Margaret Trinity. 2007, January. *State of the States: Building Hope, Raising Expectations*. Washington, D.C.: AcademyHealth. Accessed November 17, 2012. http://www.statecoverage.org/files/SCI%20State%20of%20the%20States%202007.pdf.

Brown, Randall S., Deborah Peikes, Greg Peterson, Jennifer Schore, and Carol M. Razafindrakoto. 2012. "Six Features of Medicare Coordinated Care Demonstration Programs that Cut Hospital Admissions of High-Risk Patients." *Health Affairs* 31 (6): 1156–1166.

Bryant, Elizabeth B. 2008, August 5. *Testimony RE: Global Medicaid Waiver*. Providence, Rhode Island: Rhode Island Kids Count. Accessed November 6,

2010. http://www.rikidscount.org/matriarch/documents/Global%20Waiver%20 Hearing%208–5-08%20Testimony_EBB%281%29.pdf.
Buettgens, Matthew, and Mark A. Hall. 2011, March. *Who Will Be Uninsured After Health Insurance Reform?* Washington, D.C.: The Urban Institute. Accessed December 28, 2012. http://www.urban.org/UploadedPDF/1001520-Uninsured-After-Health-Insurance-Reform.pdf.
Caffrey, Robert J. 2013, January 28. *1115 Waiver Extension Forum Testimony.* Woonsocket, Rhode Island: Homefront Health Care. Accessed May 18, 2013. http://www.ohhs.ri.gov/documents/documents13/WrittenPublicComment012813.pdf.
Carcieri, Donald L. 2004, February 5. *Fiscal Fitness: Improving State Government Finding and Recommendations.* Providence, Rhode Island: Office of the Governor. Accessed October 28, 2012. http://www.fiscalfitness.ri.gov/documents/GovernorsFiscalFitnessReport.pdf.
———. 2009, January 5. *Global Waiver Q & A.* Providence, Rhode Island: State of Rhode Island Department of Elderly Affairs. Accessed January 5, 2009. http://www.dea.ri.gov/Global%20Medicaid%20Waiver/index.php.
"Carcieri urges lawmakers to approve Medicaid overhaul." 2009. *The Associated Press,* February 18. Accessed November 21, 2010. http://www2.turnto10.com/news/2009/jan/09/carcieri_urges_lawmakers_to_approve_medicaid_overh-ar-49376/.
Carlson, Eric, and Gene Coffey. 2010, November. *Medicaid Payment for Assisted Living: Preventing Discrimination against Medicaid-Eligible Residents.* Washington, D.C.: National Senior Citizens Law Center. Accessed November 22, 2012. http://www.nsclc.org/wp-content/uploads/2011/06/Medicaid-Payment-for-AL-White-Paper-11.17.10.pdf.
Cassidy, Amanda. 2013. "Health Policy Briefs: Per Capita Caps in Medicaid." *Health Affairs* April 18. Accessed May 26, 2013. http://healthaffairs.org/healthpolicybriefs/brief_pdfs/healthpolicybrief_90.pdf.
Cassidy, Bill. 2012, July 16. *Overview of Medicaid Accountability and Care Act.* Washington, D.C.: Office of U.S. Congressman Bill Cassidy. Accessed May 26, 2013. http://cassidy.house.gov/cassidy-in-the-news/overview-of-medicaid-accountability-and-care-act.
Castle, Nicholas G., and Jamie C. Ferguson. 2010. "What is Nursing Home Quality and How is it Measured?" *The Gerontologist* 50 (4): 426–42.
Center on Budget and Policy Priorities. 2010, January 28. *Recession Still Causing Trouble for States: Federal Economic Recovery Funds Providing Some Relief.* Accessed January 2, 2013. http://www.cbpp.org/files/policy-points10–20–08.pdf.
Centers for Medicare and Medicaid Services. 2002. *Appropriateness of Minimum Nurse Staffing Ratios in Nursing Homes Phase II Final Report.* Baltimore, Maryland: Centers for Medicaid and Medicare Services.
———. 2010. *National Health Expenditure Projections: 2009–2019.* Baltimore, Maryland: Centers for Medicare and Medicaid Services. Accessed April 12, 2010. www.cms.gov/NationalHealthExpendData/ downloads/proj2009.pdf.
———. 2011. *National Health Expenditure Projections: 2010–2020.* Baltimore, Maryland: CMS. Accessed August 3, 2011. www.cms.gov/NationalHealthExpendData/downloads/proj2010.pdf.
———. 2011, April. *Number of Medicare-certified Home Health Agencies and Hospices, as of April 21, 2011.* Baltimore, Maryland: Centers for Medicare and Medicaid Services. Accessed November 21, 2012. http://www.nahc.org/Facts/2011hhas.pdf.
———. 2012. *Waivers.* Baltimore, Maryland: Centers for Medicare and Medicaid Services. Accessed December 5, 2012. http://www.medicaid.gov/Medicaid-CHIP-Program-Information/By-Topics/Waivers/Waivers.html.

———. 2012, July 1. *Rhode Island Demonstration Proposal, Comments*. Baltimore, Maryland: Centers for Medicare and Medicaid Services. Accessed May 19, 2013. http://www.financialalignmentproposalcomments.org/default.aspx.

———. 2013, May 10. *Financial Alignment Demonstration*. Baltimore, Maryland: Centers for Medicare and Medicaid Services. Accessed May 19, 2013. http://www.cms.gov/Medicare-Medicaid-Coordination/Medicare-and-Medicaid-Coordination/Medicare-Medicaid-Coordination-Office/FinancialModelstoSupportStatesEffortsinCareCoordination.html.

Chafee, Lincoln. 2011. *Budget: Fiscal Year 2012*. Providence, Rhode Island: Office of the Governor. Accessed May 20, 2013. http://www.budget.ri.gov/Documents/Prior%20Year%20Budgets/Operating%20Budget%202012/ProgramSupplement/HS/1_Office%20of%20Health%20and%20Human%20Services.pdf.

Chatterjee, Paula., Karen. E. Joynt, John Orav, and Ashish K. Jha. 2012. "Patient Experiences in Safety-Net Hospitals: Implications for Improving Care and Value-Based Purchasing." *Archives of Internal Medicine* 172 (16): 1204–1210.

Cheney, Kyle, and Jason Millman. 2013. "Medicaid Expansion Stalls in Red States." *Politico* May 2. Accessed May 24, 2013. http://www.politico.com/story/2013/05/medicaid-expansion-stalls-in-red-states-90878.html.

Coffey, Gene. 2009. *Rhode Island LTC Plan Still Comes Up Short*. Washington, D.C.: National Senior Citizens Law Center. Accessed November 6, 2010. http://familiesusa2.org/conference/health-action-2009/conference-materials/saturday-handouts/rhode-island-ltc-plan-coffey.pdf.

Congressional Budget Office. 2007, September 24. *Letter to Honorable John D. Dingell*. Washington, D.C.: Congressional Budget Office. Accessed November 8, 2012. http://www.cbo.gov/sites/default/files/cbofiles/ftpdocs/86xx/doc8655/hr976.pdf.

———. 2010, November 17. *Preliminary Analysis of the Rivlin-Ryan Health Care Proposal*. Washington, D.C.: Congressional Budget Office, November 17. Accessed November 7, 2012. http://www.cbo.gov/sites/default/files/cbofiles/ftpdocs/119xx/doc11966/11–17-rivlin-ryan_preliminary_analysis.pdf.

———. 2011, April 5. *Long-Term Analysis of a Budget Proposal by Chairman Ryan*. Washington, D.C.: Congressional Budget Office. Accessed October 28, 2012. http://www.cbo.gov/sites/default/files/cbofiles/ftpdocs/121xx/doc12128/04–05-ryan_letter.pdf.

———. 2012a, March. *The Long-Term Budgetary Impact of Paths for Federal Revenues and Spending Specified by Chairman Ryan*. Washington, D.C.: Congressional Budget Office. Accessed October 28, 2012. http://cbo.gov/sites/default/files/cbofiles/attachments/03–20-Ryan_Specified_Paths_2.pdf.

———. 2012b, March. *Updated Estimates for the Insurance Coverage Provisions of the Affordable Care Act*. Washington, D.C.: Congressional Budget Office. Accessed October 28, 2012. http://www.cbo.gov/sites/default/files/cbofiles/attachments/03–13-Coverage%20Estimates.pdf.

———. 2012, July. *Estimates for the Insurance Coverage Provisions of the Affordable Care Act Updated for the Recent Supreme Court Decision*. Washington, D.C.: Congressional Budget Office. Accessed November 14, 2012. http://www.cbo.gov/sites/default/files/cbofiles/attachments/43472–07–24–2012-CoverageEstimates.pdf.

———. 2013, January 1. *Detail on Estimated Budgetary Effects of Title VI (Medicare and Other Health Extensions) of the American Taxpayer Relief Act of 2012*. Washington, D.C.: Congressional Budget Office. Accessed January 2, 2012. http://www.cbo.gov/sites/default/files/cbofiles/attachments/SenateHR8-TitleVI.pdf.

Costantino, Steven. M. 2011. *Letter to the 2011 Global Waiver Taskforce*. Accessed August 8, 2012. http://www.eohhs.ri.gov/documents/documents11/EOHHS_Secretary_letter.pdf.

Coughlin, Tesesa A., Sharon K. Long, Lisa Clernans-Cope, and Dean Resnick. 2013, May. *What Differences Does Medicaid Make?: Assessing Cost Effectiveness, Access, and Financial Protection Under Medicaid for Low-Income Adults.* Washington, D.C.: The Henry J. Kaiser Family Foundation. Accessed May 25, 2013. http://kaiserfamilyfoundation.files.wordpress.com/2013/05/8440-what-difference-does-medicaid-make2.pdf.

Coughlin, Teresa A., Timothy A. Waidmann, and Lokendra Phadera. 2012. "Among Dual Eligibles, Identifying the Highest-Cost Individuals Could Help in Crafting More Targeted and Effective Responses." *Health Affairs* 31 (5): 1083–1091.

Courtot, Brigette, and Teresa Coughlin. 2012, November. *Cross-Cutting Issues: Progress in Implementing Selected Medicaid Provisions of the Affordable Care Act: A 10-State Analysis.* Washington, D.C.: The Urban Institute. Accessed May 16, 2013. http://www.urban.org/UploadedPDF/412697-Progress-in-Implementing-Selected-Medicaid-Provisions-of-the-Affordable-Care-Act.pdf.

Cross-Call, Jesse. 2012, March 16. *Claimed State Savings from Rhode Island's Medicaid Cap Heavily Overblown, Report Shows.* Washington, D.C.: Center on Budget and Policy Priorities. Accessed October 26, 2012. http://www.cbpp.org/files/3–16–12health.pdf.

Cross-Call, Jesse, and Judith Solomon. 2011, March 22. *Rhode Island's Global Waiver Not a Model for How States Would Fare Under a Medicaid Block Grant.* Washington, D.C.: Center on Budget and Policy Priorities. Accessed May 5, 2011. http://www.cbpp.org/cms/index.cfm?fa=view&id=3428.

Crowley, Jeffrey. S., and Molly O'Malley. 2008, November 17. *Vermont's Choices for Care Medicaid Long-Term Services Waiver: Progress and Challenges as the Program Concluded its Third Year.* Washington, D.C.: The Henry J. Kaiser Family Foundation. Accessed October 28, 2012. http://www.kff.org/medicaid/7838.cfm.

Cunningham, Peter J., and Ann S. O'Malley. 2009. "Do Reimbursement Delays Discourage Medicaid Participation by Physicians?" *Health Affairs* 28 (1): 17–28.

Cunningham, Peter. J., and Len M. Nichols. 2005. "The Effects of Medicaid Reimbursement on the Access to Care of Medicaid Enrollees: A Community Perspective." *Medical Care Research & Review* 62 (6): 676–96.

Davidson, Stephen. M. 1997. "Politics Matters! Health Care Policy and the Federal System." *Journal of Health Politics, Policy and Law* 22 (3): 879–896.

Davis, Corey. 2012, July. *Q & A: Disproportionate Share Hospital Payments and the Medicaid Expansion.* Washington, D.C.: National Health Law Program. Accessed December 27, 2012. http://www.apha.org/NR/rdonlyres/328D24F3–9C75–4CC5–9494–7F1532EE828A/0/NHELP_DSH_QA_final.pdf.

Davis, Karen, and Kristof Stremikis. 2012, August 23. *Medicaid Works: Public Program Continues to Provide Access to Care and Financial Protection for Society's Most Vulnerable.* New York: The Commonwealth Fund. Accessed December 27, 2012. http://www.commonwealthfund.org/~/media/Files/Publications/Blog/2012/Aug/Davis_Medicaid_works_blog_08232012_v2.pdf.

Davis, Karen, Kristof Stemkis, Michelle M. Doty, and Mark A. Zezza. 2012. "Medicare Beneficiaries Less Likely to Experience Cost- and Access-Related Problems than Adults with Private Coverage." *Health Affairs* 31 (8): 1866–1875.

Davis, Marion. 2008. "Medicaid Waiver May Fall Short." *Providence Business News* December 1. Accessed November 6, 2010. http://povertyinstitute.org/matriarch/documents/12.2.08%20Providence%20Business%20News%20Medicaid%20Waiver%20May%20Fall%20Short.pdf.

Davis, Otto A., M. A. H Dempster, and Aaron Wildavsky. 1966. "A Theory of the Budgetary Process." *American Political Science Review* 60: 529–547.

———. 1974. "Towards a Predictive Theory of Government Expenditure: U.S. Domestic Appropriations." *British Journal of Political Science* 4: 419–52.

Davis, P. 2008. "Health System Revamp Defended." *The Providence Journal* November 11. Accessed November 6, 2010. http://www.projo.com/news/content/MEDICADE_WAIVER_11-11-08_3NC82I6_v12.3c724fc.html.

Decker, Frederic. H. 2005. *Nursing Homes, 1977–99: What Has Changed, What Has Not?* Hyattsville, MD: National Center for Health Statistics. Accessed November 22, 2012. http://www.cdc.gov/nchs/data/nnhsd/nursinghomes1977_99.pdf.

Decker, Sandra. L. 2012. "In 2011 Nearly One-Third Of Physicians Said They Would Not Accept New Medicaid Patients, But Rising Fees May Help." *Health Affairs* 31 (8): 1673–1679.

Department of Human Services. 2010, January. *FY 2010 DHS—Medicaid Budget Savings Initiatives.* Cranston, Rhode Island: Department of Human Services. Accessed December 6, 2010. http://www.eohhs.ri.gov/documents/documents10/DHS_2010_Savings_Initiatives_Jan2010.pdf.

———. 2010, January–2013, February. *Rhode Island Global Consumer Choice Compact 1115 Waiver Demonstration 11W-00242/1: Section 1115 Quarterly Progress Reports, July 1, 2009-September 30, 2009 to October 1, 2012-December 31, 2012.* Accessed May 5, 2013. http://www.eohhs.ri.gov/reports/index.php.

———. 2010, April. *Shared Living Fact Sheet.* Accessed November 22, 2012. http://www.eohhs.ri.gov/documents/documents10/SL_fact_sheet_4_23_10.pdf.

Derthick, Martha. 1970. *The Influence of Federal Grants.* Cambridge, Massachusetts: Harvard University Press.

Dingell, John D., Frank Pallone Jr., Patrick Kennedy, and James R. Langevin. 2008, August 21. *Letter to HHS Secretary Regarding Rhode Island Medicaid Waiver Request.* Accessed November 6, 2010. http://www.highbeam.com/doc/1P3-1537558711.html.

Donnelly, Kevin P. "The Rhetoric of Reform: Examining the Role of Political Language in Rhode Island's Health Care Debate." PhD diss., Northeastern University, 2009. Accessed May 20, 2013. http://iris.lib.neu.edu/cgi/viewcontent.cgi?article=1005&context=pub_int_aff_diss.

Dorn, Stan. 2008, January. *Uninsured and Dying Because of It: Updating the Institute of Medicine Analysis on the Impact of Uninsurance on Mortality.* Washington, D.C.: The Urban Institute. Accessed December 30, 2012. http://www.urban.org/UploadedPDF/411588_uninsured_dying.pdf.

Dorn, Stan, Bowen Garrett, John Holahan, and Aimee Williams. 2008, April. *Medicaid, SCHIP and Economic Downturn: Policy Challenges and Policy Responses.* Washington, D.C.: The Henry J. Kaiser Family Foundation. Accessed December 31, 2012. http://www.kff.org/medicaid/upload/7770.pdf.

Dorn, Stan, Bowen Garrett, John Holahan, and Caitlin Carroll. 2013, March. *The Financial Benefit to Hospitals from State Expansion of Medicaid.* Accessed May 24, 2013. http://www.urban.org/uploadedpdf/412770-The-Financial-Benefit-to-Hospitals-from-State-Expansion-of-Medicaid-Summary.pdf.

Edgar, Randal. 2012, December 13. "Former R.I. health and human services secretary, now working in Pennsylvania, draws attention for long commute." *The Providence Journal.* Accessed May 20, 2013. http://news.providencejournal.com/politics/2012/12/former-rhode-island-health-and-human-services-secretary-now-working-in-penn.html.

Edgar, Randal, and Katherine Gregg. 2010. "R.I. Gov. Carcieri reflects on 8 years in office." *The Providence Journal* December 26. Accessed April 25, 2011. http://www.projo.com/news/content/CARCIERI_12-26-10_S3LK83S_v103.2d579e0.html.

"Editorial: Waiting for a Waiver." 2008. *The Providence Journal*, July 29. Accessed July 29, 2008. http://pqasb.pqarchiver.com/projo/access/1520257521.html?FMT=CITE&FMTS=CITE:FT&date=Jul+29%2C+2008&author=Anonymous&pub=The+Providence+Journal&edition=&startpage=B.4&desc=Waiting+for+a+waiver.

Eiken, Steve, Kate Sredl, Brian Burwell, and Lisa Gold. 2011, October 31. *Medicaid Spending for Long-Term Services and Supports 2011 Update*. Cambridge, MA: Thomson Reuters. Accessed November 25, 2012. http://www.balancingincentiveprogram.org/sites/default/files/Thomson_Reuters_2011LTSSExpenditures_Update_Final.pdf.

Emerson, Janice S., Pamela C. Hull, Van A. Cain, Meggan Novotny, Rodney E. Stanley, and Robert S. Levine. 2012. "TennCare Disenrollment and Avoidable Hospital Visits in Davidson County, Tennessee." *Journal of Health Care for the Poor and Underserved* 23 (1): 425–45.

Executive Office of Health and Human Services. 2007, October. *The Future of Medicaid*. Cranston, Rhode Island: Executive Office of Health and Human Services. Accessed November 6, 2010. http://www.eohhs.ri.gov/reports/documents/RIFutureofMedicaidFinal%20Report-10–07.pdf.

———. 2008, August 7. *The Rhode Island Global Consumer Choice Compact Waiver*. Cranston, Rhode Island: Executive Office of Health and Human Services. Accessed May 28, 2010. http://www.ohhs.ri.gov/global/documents/pdf/TheRIGlobalConsumerCompactGlobalWaiverFinal082808.pdf.

———. 2009, May 12. *Rhode Island Global Consumer Choice Compact 1115 Demonstration Waiver External Task Force Meeting, Agenda and Minutes*. Cranston, Rhode Island: Executive Office of Health and Human Services. Accessed November 21, 2010. http://www.eohhs.ri.gov/taskforce/documents/TFagenda_5_12_09.pdf and http://www.eohhs.ri.gov/taskforce/documents/TaskforceMay12mtgmin.pdf.

———. 2009, October 7. *Modernization Steering Committee Minutes*. Accessed November 21, 2010. http://www.dhs.ri.gov/Portals/0/Uploads/Documents/Public/Modernization/M_Steer_Comm_%20mm_10_7_09.pdf.

———. 2009, December 2. *Modernization Steering Committee Minutes*. Cranston, Rhode Island: Executive Office of Health and Human Services. Accessed November 21, 2010. http://www.eohhs.ri.gov/documents/documents09/Mod_mm_12_2_09.pdf.

———. 2009, December 21. *Global Waiver Implementation Task Force Agenda and Minutes*. Accessed November 21, 2010. http://www.eohhs.ri.gov/documents/documents10/GW_TF_agenda_12_21_09.pdf & http://www.eohhs.ri.gov/documents/documents10/GW_TF_mm_12_21_09.pdf.

———. 2010, January 25. *Global Waiver Implementation Task Force Agenda and Minutes*. Cranston, Rhode Island: Executive Office of Health and Human Services. Accessed December 6, 2010. http://www.eohhs.ri.gov/documents/documents10/GW_TF_%20agenda_1_25_10.pdf & http://www.eohhs.ri.gov/documents/documents10/GWTF_mm_1_25_10.pdf.

———. 2010, February 22. *Global Waiver Implementation Task Force Agenda and Minutes*. Cranston, Rhode Island: Executive Office of Health and Human Services. Accessed December 6, 2010. http://www.eohhs.ri.gov/documents/documents10/GWTF_agenda_2_22_10.pdf & http://www.eohhs.ri.gov/documents/documents10/GWTF_mm_%202_22_10.pdf.

———. 2010, June 28. *Global Waiver Implementation Task Force Meeting Agenda and Minutes*. Cranston, Rhode Island: Executive Office of Health and Human Services. Accessed: December 6, 2010. http://www.eohhs.ri.gov/documents/documents10/GWTF_%20agenda_6_28_10.pdf & http://www.eohhs.ri.gov/documents/documents10/GWTF_mtg_6_28_10.pdf.

———. 2011, January–2013, April. *Report to the Rhode Island General Assembly Senate Committee on Health and Human Services: Designated Medicaid Information July 1, 2009–December 31, 2009 to July 1, 2012–September 30, 2012*. Cranston, Rhode Island: Executive Office of Health and Human Services. Accessed May 13, 2013. http://www.eohhs.ri.gov/reports/index.php.

———. 2011, May 5. *Global Waiver Implementation Task Force Agenda and Minutes*. Cranston, Rhode Island: Executive Office of Health and Human Services. Accessed May 5, 2011. http://www.eohhs.ri.gov/documents/documents11/Agenda_1_24_11.pdf. http://www.eohhs.ri.gov/documents/documents11/GWTF_mtg_1_24_11.pdf.

———. 2011, May 23. *Global Waiver Implementation Task Force Meeting Agenda and Minutes*. Cranston, Rhode Island: Executive Office of Health and Human Services. Accessed October 23, 2012. http://www.eohhs.ri.gov/documents/documents11/GWTF_agenda_5_23_11.pdf and http://www.eohhs.ri.gov/documents/documents11/GWTF_mtg_min_6_27_11.pdf

———. 2011, June. Rhode Island Annual Medicaid Expenditure Report—State Fiscal Year *2010*. Cranston, Rhode Island: Executive Office of Health and Human Services. Accessed October 23, 2012. www.eohhs.ri.gov/documents/documents11/RI_Medicaid_Expend_SFY2010_FINAL.pdf.

———. 2011a, November 28. *Global Waiver Implementation Task Force Agenda and Minutes*. Cranston, Rhode Island: Executive Office of Health and Human Services. Accessed October 26, 2012. http://www.eohhs.ri.gov/documents/documents11/GWTF_agenda_11_28_11.pdf & http://www.eohhs.ri.gov/documents/documents11/GWTF_mtg_11_28_11.pdf.

———. 2011b, November 28. *Rite Resources Web Site*. Cranston, Rhode Island: Executive Office of Health and Human Services. Accessed October 28, 2012. http://www.eohhs.ri.gov/documents/documents11/RIte_Resources_presentation.pdf.

———. 2011, December 19. *Global Waiver Implementation Task Force Agenda and Minutes*. Cranston, Rhode Island: Executive Office of Health and Human Services. Accessed October 28, 2012. www.eohhs.ri.gov/documents/documents11/GWTF_agenda_12_19_11.pdf & www.eohhs.ri.gov/documents/documents11/GWTF_mtg_min_12_19_11.pdf.

———. 2012, September 7. *Responses to Public Comments from Stakeholders, 9/7/12 (excel document format)*. Cranston, Rhode Island: Executive Office of Health and Human Services. Accessed May 18, 2013. http://www.eohhs.ri.gov/integratedcare/resources/.

———. 2012, October. *Monitoring Quality and Access in RIte Care & Rhody Health Partners*. Cranston, Rhode Island: Executive Office of Health and Human Services. Accessed May 22, 2013. http://www.eohhs.ri.gov/documents/documents12/Monitoring_Quality_Access_10_2012.pdf.

———. 2012, November. *Rhode Island Global Consumer Choice Compact 1115 Demonstration Waiver External Task Force Meeting, Agenda and Minutes*. Cranston, Rhode Island: Executive Office of Health and Human Services. Accessed May 15, 2013. http://www.ohhs.ri.gov/documents/documents12/GWTF_agenda_11_26_12.pdf &http://www.ohhs.ri.gov/documents/documents12/GWTF_mtg_min_11_26_12.pdf.

———. 2013. *EOHHS SFY 13–14 Budget Initiatives*. Accessed May 15, 2013. http://www.ohhs.ri.gov/documents/documents13_2ndQ/EOHHS_Medicaid_Initiatives.pdf.

———. 2013, January 18. *The Request to Extend the Rhode Island 1115 Research and Demonstration Waiver Project No. 11-W-00242/1*. Cranston, Rhode Island: Executive Office of Health and Human Services. Accessed May 17, 2013. http://www.eohhs.ri.gov/documents/documents13/1115_Waiver_No_11_W_00242_1.pdf.

———. 2013, March. *The Request to Extend the Rhode Island 1115 Research and Demonstration Waiver Project No. 11-W-00242/1*. Cranston, Rhode Island: Executive Office of Health and Human Services. Accessed May 13, 2013. http://www.eohhs.ri.gov/documents/documents13/1115_Waiver_Demonstration.pdf.

———. 2013, March 18. *RI Medicaid Section 1115 Waiver Extension Request: Public Process and Public Comments*. Cranston, Rhode Island: Executive Office of Health and Human Services. Accessed May 17, 2013. http://www.eohhs.ri.gov/documents/documents13/Public_Comments_PartI_and_II_03152013.pdf.

Fahrenthold, David A. 2013. "House Votes to Repeal Obamacare for 37th Time." *The Washington Post,* May 16. Accessed May 25, 2013. http://articles.washingtonpost.com/2013–05–16/politics/39306992_1_house-republicans-repeal-health-care-law.

Farber, Nicholas, Douglas Shinkle, Jana Lynott, Wendy Fox-Grage, and Rodney Harrell. 2011, December. *Aging in Place: A State Survey of Livability Policies and Practices.* Denver, Colorado: National Conference of State Legislatures. Accessed November 21, 2012. http://www.ncsl.org/documents/transportation/Aging-in-Place-2011.pdf.

Feder, Judy, and Paul N. Van de Water. 2013, March 18. *Financing Medicare and Medicaid.* Testimony before the Subcommittee on Health, Committee on Energy and Commerce, U.S. House of Representatives. Accessed May 24, 2013. http://www.urban.org/UploadedPDF/904579-Financing-Medicare-and-Medicaid.pdf.

Feinberg, Lynn. F., Sandra L. Newman, Leslie Gray, and Karen N. Kolb. 2004. *The State of the States in Family Caregiver Support: A 50 State Study.* San Francisco, CA: Family Caregiver Alliance. Accessed November 21, 2012. http://www.caregiver.org/caregiver/jsp/content/pdfs/50_state_report_complete.pdf.

Feinberg, Lynn, Susan C. Reinhard, Ari Houser, and Rita Choula. 2011. *Valuing the Invaluable: 2011 Update, The Growing Contributions and Costs of Family Caregiving.* Washington, D.C.: AARP. Accessed May 20, 2013. http://assets.aarp.org/rgcenter/ppi/ltc/i51-caregiving.pdf.

Felland, Laurie. E., and Lucy Stark. 2012. *Local Public Hospitals: Changing with the Times.* Washington, D.C.: Center for Studying Health System Change. Accessed December 28, 2012. http://www.hschange.com/CONTENT/1326/1326.pdf.

Feng, Zhanlian, David C. Grabowski, Orna Intrator, Jacqueline Zinn, and Vincent Mor. 2008. "Medicaid Payment Rates, Case-Mix Reimbursement, and Nursing Home Staffing—1996–2004." *Medical Care* 46 (1): 33–40.

Feng, Zhanlian, Yong S. Lee, Sylvia Kuo, Orna Intrator, Andrew Foster, and Vincent Mor. 2010. "Do Medicaid Wage Pass-Through Payments Increase Nursing Home Staffing?" *Health Services Research* 45 (3):728–747.

Fennell, Mary. L., Zhanlian Feng, Melissa A. Clark, and Vincent Mor. 2010. "Elderly Hispanics More Likely to Reside in Poor-Quality Nursing Homes." *Health Affairs* 29 (1): 65–73.

Finkelstein, Amy, Sarah Taubman, Bill Wright, Mira Bernstein, Jonathan Gruber, Joseph P. Newhouse, Heidi Allen, Katherine Baicker, and Oregon Health Study Group. 2012. "The Oregon Health Insurance Experiment: Evidence from the First Year." *The Quarterly Journal of Economics* 127 (3): 1057–1106.

Fishman Michael. E., Burt Barnow, Asaph Glosser, and Karen Gardiner. 2004, May 21. *Recruiting and Retaining a Quality Paraprofessional Long-Term Care Workforce.* Washington, D.C.: U.S. Department of Health and Human Services. Accessed December 5, 2011. aspe.hhs.gov/daltcp/reports/ natwis.pdf.

Flynn, Bill, and Maureen Maigret. 2012, June 30. *Re: Rhode Island Capitated Financial Alignment Demonstration Proposal for Medicare-Medicaid Enrollees.* Accessed May 18, 2013. http://www.financialalignmentproposalcomments.org/default.aspx.

Freyer, F. J. 2011. "Is the Rhode Island's Famous 'Global Waiver for Medicaid Working?" *The Providence Journal*, April 11.

Gais, Thomas, and James Fossett. 2005. "Federalism and the Executive Branch. "In *The Executive Branch*, edited by Joel D. Aberbach, and Mark A. Peterson, 486–522. New York: Oxford University Press.

Genther, Dane J., and Christine G. Gourin. 2012. "The Effect of Hospital Safety-Net Burden Status on Short-Term Outcomes and Cost of Care after Head and

Neck Cancer Surgery." *Archives of Otolaryngology—Health & Neck Surgery* 138 (11): 1015–1022.

Gibson, Mary. J. 2003, April. *Beyond 50.03: A Report to the Nation on Independent Living and Disability.* Washington, D.C.: AARP Public Policy Institute. Accessed November 25, 2012. http://assets.aarp.org/rgcenter/il/beyond_50_il_1.pdf.

Glaser, Barney. G., and Anslem L. Strauss. 1967. *The Discovery of Grounded Theory*. New York: Aldine De Gruyter.

Gold, Maureen R., Gretchen A. Jacobson, and Rachel L. Garfield. 2012. "There is Little Experience and Limited Data to Support Policy Making on Integrated Care for Dual Eligibles." *Health Affairs* 31 (5): 1176–1185.

Gold, Rachel. B. 2004, August. *Different Paths, Same Goal: End Medicaid as We Know It.* The Guttmacher Report on Public Policy. Accessed October 28, 2012. http://www.guttmacher.org/pubs/tgr/07/3/gr070304.html.

Goodnough, Abby. 2009. "Rhode Island to Test Medicaid Spending Gap." *The New York Times,* January 22. Accessed November 21, 2010. http://www.nytimes.com/2009/01/22/us/22deal.html?pagewanted=all.

Grabowski, David C. 2006. "The Cost-effectiveness of Non-institutional Long-term Care Services: Review and Synthesis of the Most Recent Evidence." *Medical Care Research and Review* 63 (1): 13–28.

Grabowski, David C. 2007. "Medicare and Medicaid: Conflicting Incentives for Long-Term Care." *The Milbank Quarterly* 85 (4): 579–610.

Grabowski, David C. 2012. "Care Coordination for Dually Eligible Medicare-Medicaid Beneficiaries Under the Affordable Care Act." *Journal of Aging & Social Policy* 24 (2): 221–232.

Grabowski, David C., Rebecca O. Cadigan, Edward A. Miller, David G. Stevenson, Melissa A. Clark, and Vincent Mor. 2010. "Supporting Home- and Community-Based Long-Term Care: Views of Long-Term Care Specialists." *Medical Care Research and Review* 67 (Supp. 4): 82S-101S.

Graham, John R. 2011, January. *In the Nick of Time: Rhode Island's Medicaid Waiver Shows How States Can Save Their Budgets from Obamacare's Assault.* San Francisco, California: The Pacific Research Institute. Accessed May 20, 2013. Available at: http://heartland.org/sites/all/modules/custom/heartland_migration/files/pdfs/30379.pdf.

Gregg, Katherine. 2008. "Cut in Benefits Thins Ranks of State Workers." *The Providence Journal,* October 1. Accessed November 6, 2010. http://www.projo.com/news/content/retirement_deadline_10–01–08_80BP8HQ_v20.1c095a7.html.

———. 2009. "As the Assembly Convenes, Hints Emerge of Carcieri's Plan to Curb Massive Budget Deficit." *The Providence Journal,* January 7. Accessed November 21, 2010. http://www.projo.com/news/content/general_assembly_opens_01–07–09_FACS42B_v37.3c7ac86.html.

———. 2009. "Lucas Group Bid for Job as Medicaid Consultant". *The Providence Journal*, January 9. Accessed November 21, 2010. http://www.projo.com/news/content/lucas_group_01–09–09_CSCT7TN_v25.6489e1.html.

———. 2009. "Senate Abruptly Puts Alexander's Nomination on Hold." *The Providence Journal*, May 21. Accessed November 21, 2010. http://www.projo.com/generalassembly/NEW_ALEXANDER_HEARING__05–21–09_EGEEUG7_v7.3b03113.html.

———. 2009. "Nominee's Claims Disputed." *The Providence Journal*, June 9. Accessed November 21, 2010. http://www.projo.com/generalassembly/lucas_06–09–09_6QELEND_v18.3db78c9.html.

———. 2009. "Alexander Posting is Confirmed by Senate." *The Providence Journal*, June 10.

———. 2009. "State to Pay Lucas Group $370,000 for Work Previously Called 'Voluntary'." *The Providence Journal*, June 13. Accessed November 21, 2010.

http://www.projo.com/news/content/lucas_group_settlement_06-13-09_NDEN4IO_v13.3db53db.html.
———. 2009. "Probe Sought on Lucas Group Payment." *The Providence Journal*, June 16. Accessed November 21, 2010. http://www.projo.com/news/stategovernment/content/Lucas_group_06-16-09_72ENTK8_v15.3cda6a2.html.
Gregg, Katherine, and Phillip Marcelo. 2011. "Cuts, Changes in RIte Care Under Examination: General Assembly." *The Providence Journal*, June 7, A8.
Grogan, Colleen. M. 1999. "The Influence of Federal Mandates on State Medicaid and AFDC Decision-Making." *Publius* 29 (3): 1–30.
Grogan, Colleen. M., and Michael K. Gusmano. 2007. *Health Voices, Unhealthy Silence: Advocacy and Health Policy for the Poor.* Washington, D.C.: Georgetown University Press.
Guyer, Jocelyn. 2003, May. *Bush Administration Medicaid/SCHIP Proposal.* Washington, D.C.: The Henry J. Kaiser Family Foundation. Accessed October 28, 2012. http://www.kff.org/medicaid/loader.cfm?url=/commonspot/security/getfile.cfm&PageID=14347.
———. 2006, April. *Vermont's Global Commitment Waiver: Implications for the Medicaid Program.* Washington, D.C.: The Henry J. Kaiser Family Foundation. Accessed October 28, 2012. http://www.kff.org/medicaid/upload/7493.pdf.
Guyer, Jocelyn, Martha Heberlein, and Joan Alker. 2011, June 2. *CHIP: Not a Model for a Medicaid Block Grant.* Accessed November 8, 2012. http://ccf.georgetown.edu/wp-content/uploads/2012/03/Federal%20medicaid%20policy_CHIP-not-a-model-for-block-grant.pdf.
Hall, Mark. A., Linda Hamacher, and James J. Johnson. 2012. "The Costs and Adequacy of Safety Net Access for the Uninsured in Genesee County, Michigan." *Journal of Health Care for the Poor and Underserved* 23 (1): 327–338.
Hall, Mark. A., Wenke Hwang, and Alison S. Jones. 2011. "Model Safety-Net Programs Could Care for the Uninsured at One Half the Cost of Medicaid or Private Insurance." *Health Affairs* 30 (9): 1698–1707.
Hall, Megan. 2011. "Former DHS director published unauthorized report on global waiver." *The Pulse,* January 20. Accessed July 30, 2012. http://wrnihealthcareblog.wordpress.com/2011/01/20/what-happened-to-gary-alexander/.
Hancock, J. 2013. "The Arkansas Medicaid Model: What You Need to Know About the 'Private Option.'" *Kaiser Health News,* May 1. Accessed May 25, 2013. http://www.kaiserhealthnews.org/Stories/2013/May/02/Arkansas-Medicaid-Private-Option-FAQ.aspx.
Harrington, Charlene, Beverly Granda, Helen M. Carrillo, Jamaie Chang, Brandee Woleslagle, James H. Swan, Kathy Dryer, Brenda Woodford, W. N. Orakpo, and Janice Gill. 2008, June. *State Data Book on Long Term Care, 2007: Program and Market Characteristics.* San Francisco, California: Department of Social & Behavioral Sciences, University of California, San Francisco. Accessed November 21, 2012. http://www.pascenter.org/documents/State_data_book_on_LTC_2007.pdf.
Harrington, Charlene, Helen Carrillo, Megan Dowdell, Paul P. Tang, and Brandee W. Blank. 2011, October. *Nursing Facilities, Staffing, Residents and Facility Deficiencies, 2005–2010.* San Francisco, California: Department of Social and Behavioral Sciences, University of California-San Francisco. Accessed November 21, 2012. http://aanhr.org/Data/OSCAR%202011%20final.pdf.
Harrington, Charlene, Joseph T. Mullan, and Helen Carrillo. 2004. "State Nursing Home Enforcement Systems." *Journal of Health Politics, Policy, & Law* 29 (1): 43–73.
Harrington, Charlene, James H. Swan, and Helen Carrillo. 2007. "Nurse Staffing Levels and Medicaid Reimbursement Rates in Nursing Facilities." *Health Services Research* 42 (3, Part I): 1105–1129.

Harrington, Charlene, Terence Ng, Mitchell LaPlante, and Stephen Kaye. 2012. "Medicaid Home- and Community-Based Services: Impact of the Affordable Care Act." *Journal of Aging & Social Policy* 24 (2): 169–187.

Hawes, Catherine, Charles D. Phillips, Miriam Rose, Scott Holan, and Michael Sherman. 2003. "A National Survey of Assisted Living Facilities." *The Gerontologist* 43 (6): 875–882.

Hawes, Catherine, Charles D. Phillips, Scott Holan, Michael Sherman, and Linnae L. Hutchison. 2005. "Assisted Living in Rural America: Results from a National Survey." *Journal of Rural Health* 21 (2): 131–139.

Hayward, Jane A. 2013, February 26. *Comments of Rhode Island Health Center Association.* Providence, Rhode Island: Rhode Island Health Center Association. Accessed May 18, 2013. http://www.ohhs.ri.gov/documents/documents13/RIHCA_comments_2_26_13.pdf.

Heberlein, Martha, Tricia Brooks, Joan Alker, Samantha Artiga, and Jessica Stephens. 2013, January. *Getting into Gear for 2014: Findings from a 50-State Survey of Eligibility, Enrollment, Renewal, and Cost-Sharing Policies in Medicaid and CHIP, 2012–2013.* Washington, D.C.: The Henry J. Kaiser Family Foundation. Accessed May 23, 2013. Available at: http://kaiserfamilyfoundation.files.wordpress.com/2013/05/8401.pdf.

Holahan, John. 2001, June. *Restructuring Medicaid Financing: Implications of the NGA Proposal.* Washington, D.C.: The Henry J. Kaiser Family Foundation. Accessed January 12, 2013. http://www.kff.org/medicaid/loader.cfm?url=/commonspot/security/getfile.cfm&PageID=13768.

Holahan John, and Alan Weil. 2003, May 27. "Block Grants Are the Wrong Prescription for Medicaid." *Health Policy Online.* Washington, D.C.: The Urban Institute. Accessed October 28, 2012. http://www.urban.org/UploadedPDF/ 900624_HPOnline_6.pdf.

Holahan, John, and David Liska. 1995, December. *The Impact of the Medigrant Plan on Federal Payments to States.* Washington, D.C.: The Henry J. Kaiser Family Foundation. Accessed November 8, 2012. http://www.kff.org/medicaid/loader.cfm?url=/commonspot/security/getfile.cfm&PageID=14763.

Holahan, John, Matthew Buettgens, Caitlin Carroll, and Stan Dorn. 2012, November. *The Cost and Coverage Implications of the ACA Medicaid Expansion: National and State-by-State Analysis.* Washington, D.C.: The Henry J. Kaiser Family Foundation. Accessed January 9, 2012. http://www.urban.org/UploadedPDF/412707-The-Cost-and-Coverage-Implications-of-the-ACA-Medicaid-Expansion.pdf.

Holahan, John, Matthew Buettgens, Caitlin Carroll, and Victor Chen. 2012, October. *National and State-by-State Impact of the 2012 House Republican Budget Plan for Medicaid.* Washington, D.C.: The Henry J. Kaiser Foundation. Accessed October 28, 2012. http://www.kff.org/medicaid/upload/8185–02.pdf.

Holahan, John, Matthew Buettgens, Victor Chen, Caitlin Carroll, and Emily Lawton. 2011, May. *House Republican Plan: State-by-State Impact of Changes in Medicaid Financing.* Washington, D.C.: The Henry J. Kaiser Foundation. Accessed November 8, 2012. http://www.kff.org/medicaid/upload/8185.pdf.

Holahan, John, and Shanna Rifkin. 2012, February. *ACA Implementation—Monitoring and Tracking: Rhode Island Site Visit Report.* Washington, D.C.: The Urban Institute. Accessed May 16, 2013. http://www.urban.org/UploadedPDF/412502-ACA-Implementation-Monitoring-and-Tracking-Rhode-Island-Site-Visit-Report.pdf.

Holahan, John, and Stacey McMorrow. 2012. "Medicare and Medicaid Spending Trends and the Deficit Debate." *The New England Journal of Medicine* 367 (5): 393–395.

House Republican Study Committee. 2012. *The State Health Flexibility Act.* Accessed November 8, 2012. http://rsc.jordan.house.gov/solutions/statehealth.htm.

Howard, Jhamirah, Terence Ng, and Charlene Harrington. 2011, December. *Medicaid Home and Community-Based Service Programs: Data Update.* Washington, D.C.: The Henry J. Kaiser Family Foundation. Accessed November 12, 2012. http://www.kff.org/medicaid/upload/7720–05.pdf.

Howard, Paul. 2012, September. *How Block Grants Can Make Medicaid Work.* New York, New York: The Manhattan Institute. Accessed May 24, 2013. http://www.manhattan-institute.org/pdf/ir_24.pdf.

Hrebenar, Ronald J., and Clive Thomas. "Most Effective Interest Groups/Organized Interests in the Fifty States." (working paper, Salt Lake City: University of Utah, 1998–2007).

Hurley, Robert E. 2006. "TennCare: A Failure of Politics, Not Policy: A Conversation with Gordon Bonnyman." *Health Affairs* 25 (3): 217–25.

Institute of Medicine. 2002, May 21. *Care without Coverage: Too Little, Too Late.* Washington, D.C.: National Academy Press.

Intrator, Orna, and Vincent Mor. 2004. "Effects of State Medicaid Reimbursement Rates on Hospitalizations from Nursing Homes." *Journal of the American Geriatrics Society* 52 (3): 393–8.

IPRO. 2012, October. *Rhode Island Medicaid Care Program: Annual External Quality Review Technical Report, Report Year 2011.* Lake Success, New York: IPRO. Accessed May 22, 2013. http://www.ohhs.ri.gov/documents/documents13/Aggregate_EQR_Report.pdf.

Jacobson Gretchen, Tricia Neuman, and Anthony Damico. 2012, April 4. *Medicare's Role for Dual Eligible Beneficiaries.* Washington, D.C.: Kaiser Family Foundation. Accessed July 16, 2012. http://kaiserfamilyfoundation.files.wordpress.com/2013/01/8138–02.pdf.

Jick, Todd D. 1979. "Mixing Qualitative and Quantitative Methods: Triangulation in Action." *Administrative Sciences Quarterly,* 24 (4): 602–611.

Johnson, Nicholas, Phil Oliff, and Erica Williams. 2011, February 9. *An Update on State Budget Cuts.* Washington, D.C.: Center on Budget and Policy Priorities. Accessed November 14, 2012. http://www.cbpp.org/files/3–13–08sfp.pdf.

Jones, Adrienne L., Lisa L. Dwyer, Anita R. Bercovitz, and Genevieve W. Strahan. 2009. *The National Nursing Home Survey: 2004 Overview.* National Center for Health Statistics. Vital Health Statistics 13 (167). Accessed December 27, 2012. http://www.cdc.gov/nchs/data/series/sr_13/sr13_167.pdf.

Jones, Alison S., and Parsa S. Sajid. 2010. *A Primer on Health Care Safety Nets.* Princeton, New Jersey: The Robert Wood Johnson Foundation. Accessed December 28, 2012. http://www.rwjf.org/content/dam/supplementary-assets/2010/06/49869.pdf.

Jost, Timothy S., and Sara Rosenbaum. 2012. "The Supreme Court and the Future of Medicaid." *The New England Journal of Medicine* 367 (11): 983–985.

Kaiser Family Foundation. 1996, July 30. *Surveys of Americans on Health Policy: Questionnaire and National Toplines.* Washington, D.C.: The Henry J. Kaiser Family Foundation. Accessed January 9, 2012. http://www.kff.org/kaiserpolls/1166-hlthpol1.cfm.

———. 2001, July. *Medicaid "Mandatory" and "Optional" Eligibility and Benefits.* Washington, D.C.: The Henry J. Kaiser Family Foundation. Accessed January 12, 2013. http://www.kff.org/medicaid/loader.cfm?url=/commonspot/security/getfile.cfm&PageID=13768.

———. 2007, December. *Kaiser Public Opinion Spotlight: The Public's View on Long-Term Care, December.* Accessed July 23, 2008. www.kff.org/spotlight/longterm/upload/Spotlight_Dec07_LongTermCare.pdf.

———. 2011, February. *Medicaid Enrollment: June 2010 Data Snapshot.* Washington, D.C.: The Henry J. Kaiser Family Foundation. Accessed December 31, 2012. http://www.kff.org/medicaid/upload/8050–03.pdf.

———. 2011, May. *Public Opinion on Health Care Issues.* Washington, D.C.: The Henry J. Kaiser Family Foundation. Accessed December 31, 2012. http://www.kff.org/kaiserpolls/upload/8190-F.pdf.

———. 2012a, July. *Health Coverage for Children: The Role of Medicaid and CHIP.* Washington, D.C.: The Henry J. Kaiser Family Foundation. Accessed November 8, 2012. http://www.kff.org/uninsured/upload/7698–06.pdf.

———. 2012b, July. *How Will Medicaid Expansion for Adults Impact Eligibility and Coverage?* Washington, D.C.: The Henry J. Kaiser Family Foundation. Accessed November 16, 2012. http://www.kff.org/medicaid/upload/8338.pdf.

———. 2012c, July. *Health Coverage of Children: The Role of Medicaid and CHIP.* Washington, D.C.: The Henry J. Kaiser Family Foundation. Accessed December 31, 2012. http://www.kff.org/uninsured/upload/7698–06.pdf.

———. 2012, August. *An Historical Review of How States Have Responded to the Availability of Federal Funds for Health Coverage.* Washington, D.C.: The Henry J. Kaiser Family Foundation. Accessed December 30, 2012. http://www.kff.org/medicaid/upload/8349.pdf.

———. 2012, September. *The Uninsured and the Difference Health Insurance Makes.* Washington, D.C.: The Henry J. Kaiser Family Foundation. Accessed December 30, 2012: http://www.kff.org/uninsured/upload/1420–14.pdf.

———. 2012, October. *The Uninsured: A Primer, Key Facts about Americans without Health Insurance.* Washington, D.C.: The Henry J. Kaiser Family Foundation. Accessed December 30, 2012. http://www.kff.org/uninsured/upload/7451–08.pdf.

———. 2013, January 10. *Medicaid Provider Taxes and Federal Deficit Reduction Efforts.* Washington, D.C.: The Henry J. Kaiser Family Foundation. Accessed January 13, 2012. http://www.kff.org/medicaid/quicktake_medicaid_provider_taxes.cfm.

———. 2013, March. *How Much Will Medicaid Cost in the Future and Why: A Look at Federal Projections.* The Henry J. Kaiser Family Foundation. Accessed May 24, 2013. http://kaiserfamilyfoundation.files.wordpress.com/2013/04/8430.pdf.

———. 2013, March 1. *Medicaid: A Primer.* Washington, D.C.: The Henry J. Kaiser Family Foundation. Accessed May 24, 2013. http://kff.org/medicaid/issue-brief/medicaid-a-primer/.

———. 2013, April 30. *Kaiser Health Tracking Poll: April 2013.* Washington, D.C.: The Henry J. Kaiser Family Foundation. Accessed May 25, 2013. http://kff.org/health-reform/poll-finding/kaiser-health-tracking-poll-april-2013/.

———. 2013, May 10. *State Decisions on Health Insurance Exchanges and the Medicaid Expansion, as of May 10, 2013.* The Henry J. Kaiser Family Foundation. Accessed January 13, 2012. http://kff.org/health-reform/state-indicator/state-decisions-for-creating-health-insurance-exchanges-and-expanding-medicaid/.

Kane, Nancy M., Sara J. Singer, Jonathan R. Clark, Kristoff Eeckloo, and Melissa Valentine. 2012. "Strained Local and State Government Finances Among Current Realities that Threaten Public Hospitals' Profitability." *Health Affairs* 31 (8): 1680–9.

Kang, Yu, Hongdao Meng, and Nancy A. Miller. 2011. "Rurality and Nursing Home Quality: Evidence from the 2004 National Nursing Home Survey." *The Gerontologist* 51 (6): 761–73.

Katz, Linda. 2008, November 4. *Rhode Island Global Consumer Choice Compact Medicaid Waiver Proposal.* Providence, Rhode Island: The Poverty Institute.

———. 2009, January 20. *Testimony on H-5112.* Providence, Rhode Island: The Poverty Institute. Accessed November 21, 2010. http://povertyinstitute.org/matriarch/documents/Testimony%20on%20letterhead%20H5112.pdf.

———. 2009, January 21. *Testimony on S-0053*. Providence, Rhode Island: The Poverty Institute. Accessed November 21, 2010. http://povertyinstitute.org/matriarch/documents/Testimony%20on%20letterhead%20S0053.pdf.

———. 2013, March 1. *Re: Comments on Request to Extend the Rhode Island 1115 Research and Demonstration Waiver Project No. 11-W-00242/1*. Providence, Rhode Island: The Economic Progress Institute. Accessed May 8, 2013. http://www.ohhs.ri.gov/documents/documents13/LKatz_EconProgress_3_1_13.pdf.

Katz, Linda, Bill Flynn, and Anne Mulready. 2012, July 1. *Re: Rhode Island Capitated Financial Alignment Demonstration Proposal for Medicare-Medicaid Enrollees*. Providence, Rhode Island: The Economic Progress Institute, Senior Agenda Coalition, Rhode Island Disability Law Center. Accessed May 18, 2013. http://www.financialalignmentproposalcomments.org/default.aspx.

Kaye, Stephen H., Mitchell P. LaPlante, and Charlene Harrington. 2009. "Do Institutional Long-Term Care Services Reduce Medicaid Spending?" *Health Affairs* 28 (1): 262–272.

Kelly, Christopher M., Phoebe S. Liebig, and Lloyd J. Edwards. 2008. "Nursing Home Deficiencies: an Exploratory Study of Interstate Variations in Regulatory Activity." *Journal of Aging and Social Policy* 20 (4): 398–41.

Kingdon, John W. 1995. *Agendas, Alternatives, and Public Policies*, 2nd ed. New York: Harper

Kitchener, Martin, Alice Wong, Micky Willmott, and Charlene Harrington. 2007, February. *Home & Community-Based Services: State-Only Funded Programs*. San Francisco, California: National Center for Personal Assistance Services, University of California-San Francisco. Accessed November 21, 2012. http://www.pascenter.org/state_funded/State-only_Funded_2007_Text.pdf and http://www.pascenter.org/state_funded/State-only_funded_2007_table.pdf.

Kitchener, Martin, Terence Ng, Nancy Miller, and Charlene Harrington. 2006. "Institutional and Community-Based Long-Term Care: A Comparative Estimate of Public Costs." *Journal of Health and Social Policy* 22 (2): 31–50.

Kliff, Sarah. 2013. "Care about Obamacare? Then You Should Really Care About Arkansas." *The Washington Post,* March 18. Accessed May 24, 2013. http://www.washingtonpost.com/blogs/wonkblog/wp/2013/03/18/care-about-obamacare-then-you-should-really-care-about-arkansas/.

———. 2013. "Study: Medicaid Reduces Financial Hardship, Doesn't Quickly Improve Physical Health." *The Washington Post,* May 1. Accessed May 24, 2013. http://www.washingtonpost.com/blogs/wonkblog/wp/2013/05/01/study-medicaid-reduces-financial-hardship-doesnt-quickly-improve-physical-health/.

———. 2013. "Florida Rejects Medicaid Expansion, Leaves 1 Million Uninsured." *The Washington Post,* May 5. Accessed May 24, 2013. http://www.washingtonpost.com/blogs/wonkblog/wp/2013/05/05/florida-rejects-medicaid-expansion-leaves-1-3-million-uninsured/.

Kochera, Andrew, Audrey Straight, and Thomas Guterbock. 2005, May. *Beyond 50.05: A Report to the Nation on Livable Communities; Creating Environments for Successful Aging*. Washington, D.C.: AARP Public Policy Institute. Accessed November 25, 2012. http://assets.aarp.org/rgcenter/il/beyond_50_communities.pdf.

Komisar, Harriet L., Judith Feder, and Judith D. Kasper. 2005. "Unmet Long-Term Care Needs: An Analysis of Medicare-Medicaid Dual Eligibles." *Inquiry* 42 (2): 171–182.

Kronebusch, Karl. 1997. "Medicaid and the Politics of Groups, Recipients, Providers, and Policy Making." *Journal of Health Politics, Policy and Law* 22 (3): 839–78.

Ku, Leighton, and Christine Ferguson. 2011, June. *Medicaid Works: A Review of How Public Insurance Protects the Health and Finances of Children and Other Vulnerable Populations*. Washington, D.C.: George Washington University.

Accessed December 31, 2012. http://www.aucd.org/docs/policy/medicaid/MedicaidWorks.pdf.

Lambrew, Jeanne M. 2005. "Making Medicaid a Block Grant Program: An Analysis of the Implications of Past Proposals. *Milbank Quarterly* 83 (1): 41–63.

Lawless, Julia, and Anthony Ferrier. 2011, June 15. *Hatch Outlines Need for Comprehensive Medicaid Reform.* United States Senate Committee on Finance. Accessed October 26, 2012. http://www.finance.senate.gov/newsroom/ranking/release/?id=310b3b93–25d7–47c7–871a-9832d6a03000.

Leichter, Howard. 2008. "Chapter 8: State Governments: E Pluribus Multa." In *Health Politics and Policy,* edited by James A. Morone, Theodor J. Litman, and Leonard S. Robins, 187–192. Health Politics and Policy, 4th ed. Clifton Park, NY: Delmar Cengage Learning.

Levy, Marc. 2011. "RI Officials Dispute Corbett Nominee's Claims." *Bloomberg Business Week,* February 1. Accessed July 30, 2012. http://www.businessweek.com/ap/financialnews/D9L4NJ2G0.htm.

The Lewin Group. 2008, December. *Administrative and Staffing Recommendations for Implementing the Global Compact.* Falls Church, Virginia: The Lewin Group. Accessed October 26, 2012. http://www.dhs.ri.gov/Portals/0/Uploads/Documents/Public/Reports/Administrative_and_Staffing_Dec_2008.pdf.

The Lewin Group. 2011, December 6. *An Independent Evaluation of Rhode Island's Global Waiver.* Accessed July 30, 2012. http://www.ohhs.ri.gov/documents/documents11/Lewin_report_12_6_11.pdf.

Liberman, Ellen. 2010. "One Year Later, the Global Waiver that Allowed Rhode Island to go its Own Way on Medicaid Has Patients Worrying that Budget Cuts, Not Innovation, Are the Prescription." *Rhode Island Monthly*, June. Accessed: December 6, 2010. http://www.povertyinstitute.org/matriarch/documents/6.24.10%20RI%20Monthly%20Medicaid%20Story.pdf.

Libson, Nancy. 2006. "The Sad State of Affordable Housing for Older People." *Generations* 29 (5): 9–15.

Lillis, Mike. 2008. "State Shortfall Met With Medicaid Cuts Democrats Blast Rhode Island Plan." *The Washington Independent*, September 10. Accessed November 6, 2010. http://washingtonindependent.com/5499/state-shortfall-met-with-medicaid-cuts.

Lindblom, Charles E. 1959. "The Science of 'Muddling Through.'" *Public Administration Review* 19:79–88.

———. 1965. *The Intelligence of Democracy.* New York: Free Press.

The Los Angeles Times. 2009, October. *Los Angeles Times Poll, Study #431: National Survey of Aging.* Accessed February 7, 2012. http://www.latimesinteractive.com/pdfarchive/stat_sheets/la-timespoll431ss.pdf.

MacLaggan, Corrie. 2013. "Texas Legislature Passes Measure To Prevent Medicaid Expansion." *The Huffington Post*, May 26. Accessed May 26, 2013. http://www.huffingtonpost.com/2013/05/27/texas-medicaid_n_3341034.html.

Maigret, M. 2013, January 28. *Comments on the Rhode Island 1115 Extension Request (Project No. 11-W002–42–1).* Providence, Rhode Island: Senior Agenda Coalition. Accessed May 18, 2013. http://www.ohhs.ri.gov/documents/documents13/WrittenPublicComment012813.pdf.

Marcelo, Phillip. 2010. "3 RI Human Service Agencies Fail to Enact Budget Cuts." *The Providence Journal*, December 15.

———. 2011. "Hikes in RIte Care, RIte Share premiums criticized: Health care." *The Providence Journal,* August 26, A2.

Marshall, Lindsey, Vanessa Harbin, Jane Hooker, John Oswald, and Linda Cummings. 2011. "Safety Net Hospital Performance on National Quality of Care Process Measures." *Journal of Healthcare Quality* 34 (2): 21–31.

Mauro, Ellen. 2012, July 23. *Integration of Care and Financing for Medicaid Only and Medicare and Medicaid Eligible: Update to Global Waiver Task Force.* Accessed May 18, 2013. http://www.ohhs.ri.gov/documents/documents12/IntegrateCareInitiative_GWTF_7_23_12.pdf.

McHugh, Meghan, Raymond Kang, and Romana Hasnain-Wynia. 2009. "Understanding the Safety Net: Inpatient Quality of Care Varies Based on How One Defines Safety-Net Hospitals." *Medical Care Research & Review* 66 (5): 590–605.

McKaig, Brian. 2013, February 11. *Testimony on RI Medicaid 1115 Waiver Extension Request.* Providence, Rhode Island: Caregiver Homes of Rhode Island. Accessed May 18, 2013. http://www.ohhs.ri.gov/documents/documents13/BMcKaigWoonsocket.pdf.

McKay, Kevin, and James P. Nyberg. 2009. "For Better Long-Term Care in R.I." *The Providence Journal*, February 9. Accessed November 21, 2010. http://www.projo.com/opinion/contributors/content/CT_nyberg9_02–09–09_AQD0AHO_v13.40052a4.html.

McKeon, Kathleen M. 2013, February 28. *Comments on Rhode Island's Draft 1115 Waiver Extension Request.* Providence, Rhode Island: Diocese of Providence. Accessed May 18, 2013. http://www.ohhs.ri.gov/documents/documents13/KMcKeon_comments_2_28_13.pdf.

MetLife Mature Market Institute. 2009, October. *The 2009 MetLife Market Survey of Nursing Home, Assisted Living, Adult Day Services, and Home Care Costs.* Westport, Connecticut: MetLife Mature Market Institute. Accessed October 28, 2012. http://www.metlife.com/assets/cao/mmi/publications/studies/mmi-market-survey-nursing-home-assisted-living.pdf.

———. 2012, November. *Market Survey of Long-Term Care Costs The 2012 MetLife Market Survey of Nursing Home, Assisted Living, Adult Day Services, and Home Care Costs.* New York, New York: Metlife Mature Market Institute. Accessed November 21, 2012. https://www.metlife.com/assets/cao/mmi/publications/studies/2012/studies/mmi-2012-market-survey-long-term-care-costs.pdf.

Mickus, Maureen, Clare C. Luz, and Andrew Hogan. 2004, April. *Voices from the Front: Recruitment and Retention of Direct Care Workers in Long-Term Care Across Michigan.* Lansing, MI: Michigan State University. Accessed December 5, 2011. www.directcareclearinghouse.org/download/MI_ vocices_from_the_front.pdf.

Miles, Matthew B., and Michael A. Huberman. 1994. *Qualitative Data Analysis: An Extended Sourcebook,* 2nd ed. Thousand Oaks, CA: Sage Publications.

Miller, Edward A. 2002. "State Discretion and Medicaid Program Variation in Long-Term Care: When Is Enough, Enough?" *Journal of Aging & Social Policy* 14 (3–4): 15–35.

———. 2004. "Advancing Comparative State Policy Research: Toward Conceptual Integration and Methodological Expansion." *State & Local Government Review* 36 (4): 25–58.

———. 2005. "State Health Policy Making Theory, Determinants and Methods: A Synthesis." *Social Science and Medicine* 61 (12): 2639–2657.

———. 2006a. "Bureaucratic Policy Making on Trial: Medicaid Nursing Facility Reimbursement, 1988–1998." *Medical Care Research and Review* 63 (2): 189–216.

———. 2006b. "Explaining Incremental and Non-Incremental Change: Medicaid Nursing Facility Reimbursement Policy, 1980–1998." *State Politics & Policy Quarterly* 6 (2): 117–150.

———. 2008. "Federal Administrative and Judicial Oversight of Medicaid: Policy Legacies and Tandem Institutions under the Boren Amendment." *Publius* 28 (2): 315–342.

Miller, Edward A., and David Blanding. 2012. "Pressure Cooker Politics: Partisanship and Symbolism in State Certification of Federal Stimulus Funds." *State Politics & Policy Quarterly* 12 (1): 58–74.

Miller, Edward A., and Jane Banaszak-Holl. 2005. "Cognitive and Normative Determinants of State Policy Making Behavior: Lessons from the Sociological Institutionalism." *Publius: The Journal of Federalism.* 35 (2): 191–216.

Miller, Edward A., and Lili Wang. 2009a. "The Influence of National Policy Change on Subnational Policymaking: Medicaid Nursing Facility Reimbursement in the American States." *Social Science and Medicine* 68 (11): 1926–1934.

———. 2009b. "Maximizing Federal Medicaid Dollars: Nursing Home Provider Tax Adoption, 2000–2004." *Journal of Health Politics, Policy and Law* 34 (6): 899–930.

Miller, Edward A., Lili Wang, Zhanlian Feng, and Vincent Mor. 2012. "Improving Direct Care Compensation in Nursing Homes: Wage Mandate Adoption, 1999–2004." *Journal of Health Politics, Policy and Law* 37 (3): 469–512.

Miller, Edward A., Melissa Clark, and Vincent Mor. 2008, June 6. *The Commonwealth Fund Survey of Long-Term Care Opinion Leaders: Focus Group Report.* Providence, Rhode Island: Center for Gerontology and Health Care Research, Brown University.

Miller, Edward A., Susan Allen, and Vincent Mor. 2009. "Commentary: Navigating the Labyrinth of Long-Term Care: Shoring Up Informal Caregiving in a Home- and Community-Based World." *Journal of Aging and Social Policy* 21 (1): 1–16.

Miller, Edward A., Vincent Mor. 2007. "Trends and Challenges in Building a 21st Century Long-Term Care Workforce." In *Handbook of Long-Term Care Administration and Policy,* edited by C.M. Mara and L. K Olson, 133–156. Boca Raton, FL: Taylor & Francis CRC Press.

———. 2008. "Balancing Regulatory Controls and Incentives: Toward Smarter and More Transparent Oversight in Long-Term Care." *Journal of Health Politics, Policy, and Law* 33 (2): 249–279.

Miller, Edward A., Vincent Mor, David C. Grabowski, and Pedro Gazalo. 2009. "The Devil's in the Details: Trading Policy Goals for Complexity in Medicaid Nursing Home Reimbursement." *Journal of Health Politics, Policy, and Law* 34 (1): 94–135.

Miller, Edward A., Vincent Mor, and Melissa Clark. 2010. "Reforming Long-Term Care in the United States: Findings from a National Survey of Specialists." *The Gerontologist* 50 (2): 238–252.

Miller, Edward A., and William G. Weissert. 2003. "Strategies for Integrating Medicare and Medicaid: Design Features and Incentives." *Medical Care Research & Review* 60 (2): 123–157.

———. 2004. "Managed Care for Medicare-Medicaid Dual Eligibles: Appropriateness, Availability, Payment, and Policy." *Journal of Applied Gerontology* 23 (4): 333–348.

Millman, Jason. 2012. "Debate Brings Attention to States' Medicaid Plans." *Politico,* October 4. Accessed October 28, 2012. http://www.politico.com/news/stories/1012/82782.html.

Mitchell, Alison. 2012, December 18. *Medicaid Disproportionate Share Hospital Payments.* Washington, D.C.: Congressional Research Service. Accessed December 27, 2012. http://www.fas.org/sgp/crs/misc/R42865.pdf.

McDonough, John E., Brian Rosman, Fawn Phelps, and Melissa Shannon. 2006. "The Third Wave of Massachusetts Health Care Access Reform." *Health Affairs* 25 (6): 420–31.

Mobley, Lee, Tzy-Mey Kuo, and Gloria J. Bazzoli. 2011. "Erosion in the Healthcare Safety Net: Impacts on Different Population Groups." *The Open Health Services and Policy Journal* 4: 1–14.

Moe, Terry. 1984. "The New Economics of Organizations." *American Journal of Political Science* 28: 739–77.
Mollica, Robert L. 2009, September. *State Medicaid Reimbursement Policies and Practices in Assisted Living*. Washington, D.C.: National Center for Assisted Living, American Health Care Association. Accessed November 22, 2012. http://www.ahcancal.org/ncal/resources/documents/medicaidassistedlivingreport.pdf.
Mollica, Robert, Enid Kassner, Lina Walker, and Ari Houser. 2009, March. *Taking the Long View: Investing in Medicaid Home and Community-Based Services is Cost-Effective*. Washington, D.C.: AARP. Accessed January 2, 2013. http://assets.aarp.org/rgcenter/il/i26_hcbs.pdf.
Mollica, Robert, Kristin Sims-Kastelein, and Janet O'Keeffe. 2007, November 30. *Resident Care and Assisted Living Compendium: 2007*. Washington, D.C.: U.S. Department of Health and Human Services. Accessed November 22, 2012. http://aspe.hhs.gov/daltcp/reports/2007/07alcom.htm.
Moon, Marilyn. 2012. "Medicare and the Affordable Care Act." *Journal of Aging & Social Policy* 24 (2): 233–247.
Mor, Vincent. 2005. Improving the Quality of Long-term Care with Better Information. *Milbank Quarterly* 83 (3): 333–64.
Mor, Vincent, Andrea Gruneir, Zhanlian Feng, David C. Grabowski, Orna Intrator, and Jacqueline Zinn. 2011. "The Effects of State Policies on Nursing Home Resident Outcomes." *Journal of the American Geriatrics Society* 59 (1): 3–9.
Mor, Vincent, Edward A. Miller, and Melissa Clark. 2010. "The Taste for Regulation in Long-Term Care." *Medical Care Research and Review* 67 (Supp 4): 38S-64S.
Mor, Vincent, Jacqueline Zinn, Joseph Angelelli, Joan M. Teno, and Susan C. Miller. 2004. "Driven to Tiers: Socioeconomic and Racial Disparities in the Quality of Nursing Home Care." *Milbank Quarterly* 82 (2): 227–56.
Mor, Vincent, Jacqueline Zinn, Pedro Gozalo, Zhanlian Feng, Orna Intrator, and David C. Grabowski. 2007. "Prospects for Transferring Nursing Home Residents to the Community." *Health Affairs* 26 (6): 1762–1771.
Mulready, Anne M. 2013, February 28. *Re: Comments on the Medicaid 1115 Waiver Extension Request*. Providence, Rhode Island: Rhode Island Disability Law Center. Accessed May 18, 2013. http://www.ohhs.ri.gov/documents/documents13/RIDisabilityLawCtr_comments.pdf.
Muscumeci, Mary Beth. 2012, July. *A Guide to the Supreme Court's Affordable Care Act Decision*. Washington, D.C.: The Henry J. Kaiser Family Foundation. Accessed November 18, 2012. http://www.kff.org/healthreform/upload/8332.pdf.
Napel, Shelly T., Anne Bulchis, Margaret Trinity, Enrique Martinez-Vidal, Colin McGlynn, and Isabel Friedenzohn. 2009, January. *State of the States, Charting a Course: Preparing for the Future, Learning from the Past*. Washington, D.C.: Academy Health. Accessed November 17, 2012. http://www.statecoverage.org/files/State%20of%20the%20States-2009.pdf.
Nathan, Richard P. 2006a. "There Will Always Be a New Federalism." *Journal of Public Administration Research and Theory* 16 (4): 499–510.
———. 2006b. "Updating Theories of American Federalism." Presented before the Annual Meeting of the American Political Science Association, Philadelphia, PA.
National Academy of Public Administration and National Academy of Social Insurance. 2009. *Administrative Solutions in Health Reform: Report of the Study Panel on Administrative Issues in Expanding Access to Health Care*. Washington, D.C: Authors. Accessed November 14, 2012. http://www.nasi.org/usr_doc/Administrative_Solutions_in_Health_Reform_July_2009.pdf.
National Association of Social Workers. 2009. *Global Medicaid Waiver Application-Rhode Island: Opposition and Comments*. Washington, D.C.: The National

Association of Social Workers. Accessed November 21, 2010. http://www.rinasw.info/globalhouse.pdf.

National Association of State Budget Officers. 2012. *State Expenditure Report: Examining Fiscal 2010–2012 State Spending*. Washington, D.C.: National Association of State Budget Officers. Accessed May 26, 2013. http://www.nasbo.org/sites/default/files/State%20Expenditure%20Report_1.pdf.

National Senior Citizens Law Center. 2011. *Medicaid Payment for Assisted Living: Refusing to Admit Eligible Applicants*. Accessed November 22, 2012. http://medicaidalseries.org/wp-content/uploads/White-Paper-Barriers-to-Admission-Feb-2011.pdf-FINAL.pdf.

Needham, Cynthia. 2009. "All in the Details. 2nd Day of House Committee Hearings (Finance), 1/12/09." *The Providence Journal*, January 13.

Needham, Cynthia, and Katherine Gregg. 2008. "Medicaid Pact Heads to Assembly." *The Providence Journal*, December 23. Accessed November 6, 2010. http://www.projo.com/news/content/MEDICAID_WAIVER_12-23-08_OKCNS0J_v20.3fe5927.html.

———. 2009. "In RI, Sides Line Up Over Governor's Bid to Cap Medicaid Spending." *The Providence Journal*, January 10. Accessed November 21, 2010. http://www.projo.com/news/content/GLOBAL_WAIVER_01-10-09_OCCTODI_v26.3c7ff95.html.

Neighborhood Health Plan of Rhode Island. 2013, February 22. *Re: Rhode Island's Section 1115 Waiver Renewal Application*. Providence, Rhode Island: Neighborhood Health Plan of Rhode Island. Accessed May 18, 2013. http://www.ohhs.ri.gov/documents/documents13/comments_NHPRI_02_22_13.pdf.

Neuman, Patricia, Barbara Lyons, Jennifer Rentas, and Diane Rowland. 2012. "Dx for a Careful Approach to Moving Dual-Eligible Beneficiaries Into Managed Care Plans." *Health Affairs* 31 (6): 1186–94.

New England State Consortium Systems Organization. 2009, December 22. *Value Purchasing for Home and Community Based Services*. Shrewsbury, Massachusetts: New England State Consortium Systems Organization. Accessed November 21, 2010. http://www.eohhs.ri.gov/documents/documentss10/GWTF_mm_12_21_09.pdf.

Ng, Terence, and Charlene Harrington. 2011, October. *State Options that Expand Access to Medicaid Home- and Community-Based Services*. Washington, D.C.: The Henry J. Kaiser Family Foundation. Accessed November 25, 2012. http://www.kff.org/medicaid/upload/8241.pdf.

Ng, Terence, Charlene Harrington, and Jhamirah Howard. 2011, February. *Medicaid Home and Community-Based Service Programs: Data Update*. Washington, D.C.: The Henry J. Kaiser Family Foundation. Accessed November 13, 2012. http://www.kff.org/medicaid/upload/7720–04.pdf.

Ng, Terence, Charlene Harrington, MaryBeth Muscumeci, and Erica Reaves. 2012, December. *Medicaid Home and Community-Based Service Programs: 2009 Data Update*. Washington, D.C.: The Henry J. Kaiser Family Foundation. Accessed December 2, 2012. http://www.kff.org/medicaid/upload/7720–06.pdf.

Nicolella, Elena. 2012, October 22. *Rhode Island's 1115 Research and Demonstration Waiver: The Global Consumer Choice Compact*. Cranston, Rhode Island: Executive Office of Health and Human Services. Accessed May 16, 2013. http://www.ohhs.ri.gov/documents/documents12/GW_presentation_10_22_12.pdf.

———. 2013, January 28. *RI 1115 Waiver Extension Request*. Cranston, Rhode Island: Executive Office of Health and Human Services. Accessed May 16, 2013. http://www.ohhs.ri.gov/documents/documents13/RI_1115_Waiver_Extension_Request_1_28_13.pdf.

Nownes, Anthony J., Clive S. Thomas, and Ronald J. Hrebenar. 2008. "Interest Groups in the States." In *Politics in the American States: A Comparative Analysis*, edited by Virginia Gray and Russell L. Hanson, 9th ed., 98–126. Washington, D.C.: CQ.

Nyberg, Jim. 2013, February 12. *Comments on the Rhode Island 1115 Waiver Extension Request.* Providence, Rhode Island: LeadingAge RI. Accessed May 18, 2013. http://www.ohhs.ri.gov/documents/documents13/JNybergemail.pdf.

Oberlander, Jonathan. 2007. "Health Reform Interrupted: The Unraveling of the Oregon Health Plan." *Health Affairs* 26 (1): 96–105.

———. 2012. "The Future of Obamacare." *The New England Journal of Medicine* 367 (23): 2165–2167.

Office of the Governor. 2008, December 19. *Global Medicaid Waiver Structure.* Providence, Rhode Island: Office of the Governor. Accessed November 6, 2010. http://www.governor.ri.gov/documents/Waiver_Facts.pdf.

Office of the Governor. 2008, December 19. *Rhode Island and Centers for Medicare and Medicaid Services Reach Agreement on Global Medicaid Waiver.* Providence, Rhode Island: Office of the Governor. Accessed November 6, 2010. http://www.lucasgroupinc.com/?cid=73.

Office of U.S. Senator Tom Coburn. 2011, May 19. *Senators Coburn, Burr, Chambliss Introduce Bill to Reform and Strengthen Medicaid.* Washington, D.C.: Office of Tom Coburn, M.D., U.S. Senator from Oklahoma. Accessed May 25, 2013. http://www.coburn.senate.gov/public/index.cfm/2011/5/senators-coburn-burr-chambliss-introduce-bill-to-reform-and-strengthen-medicaid.

Oliff, Phil, Chris Mai, and Vincent Palacios. 2012, June 27. *States Continue to Feel Recession's Impact.* Washington, D.C.: Centers for Budget and Policy Priorities. Accessed October 28, 2012. http://www.cbpp.org/files/2–8-08sfp.pdf.

Oliver, Thomas R. 1991. "Ideas, Entrepreneurship, and the Politics of Health Care Reform." *Stanford Law and Policy Review* 3: 160–180.

Park, Edwin. 2011, June 6. *Medicaid Block Grant or Funding Caps Would Shift Costs to States, Beneficiaries, and Providers.* Washington, D.C.: Center on Budget and Policy Priorities. Accessed November 7, 2012. http://www.cbpp.org/files/1–6-11health2.pdf.

———. 2013, May 8. *Medicaid Per Capita Cap Would Shift Costs to States and Undermine Key Part of Health Reform.* Washington, D.C.: Center on Budget and Policy Priorities. Accessed May 26, 2013. http://www.cbpp.org/files/5–8-13health.pdf.

Park, Edwin, Cindy Mann, Joan Alker, and Melanie Nathanson. 2003, June 5. *NGA Medicaid Task Force Proposal Shifts Fiscal Risks to States and Jeopardizes Health Coverage for Millions: Draft Offers Little Improvement over Flawed Administration Approach.* Washington, D.C.: Center for Budget and Policy Priorities. Accessed January 12, 2013. http://familiesusa2.org/assets/pdfs/CBPP_NGA_report_6–5-03cfa4.pdf.

Park, Edwin, and Judith Soloman. 2011, June 24. *Proposal to Establish Federal Medicaid "Blended Rate" Would Shift Significant Costs to States.* Washington, D.C.: Center on Budget and Policy Priorities. Accessed May 26, 2013. http://www.cbpp.org/files/6–24–11health.pdf.

Park, Edwin, and Matt Broaddus. 2012, March 28. *Draconian Republican Study Committee Budget Would Cut Federal Medicaid Funding Nearly in Half by 2012.* Washington, D.C.: Center on Budget and Policy Priorities. Accessed November 8, 2012. http://www.cbpp.org/files/3–28–12health2.pdf.

———. 2012, April 20. *What If Chairman Ryan's Medicaid Block Grant Had Taken Effect in 2011?* Washington, D.C.: Center on Budget and Policy Priorities. Accessed November 8, 2012. http://www.cbpp.org/files/4–20–12health.pdf.

———. 2012, October 4. *Medicaid Per Capita Cap Would Shift Costs to States and Place Low-Income Beneficiaries at Risk.* Washington, D.C.: Center on Budget and Policy Priorities. Accessed May 26, 2013. http://www.cbpp.org/files/10–4-12health.pdf.

———. 2013, March 26. *Ryan Block Grant Proposal Would Cut Medicaid by Nearly One-Third by 2023 and More After That.* Washington, D.C.: Center on Budget and Policy Priorities. Accessed May 25, 2013. http://www.cbpp.org/files/3–26–13health.pdf.

Patton, Michael Q. 2002. *Qualitative Research & Evaluation Methods.* Thousand Oaks: Sage.

Polzer, Karl. 2011, March. *Assisted Living State Regulatory Review: 2011.* Washington, D.C.: National Center for Assisted Living. Accessed November 25, 2012. http://www.ahcancal.org/ncal/resources/Documents/2011AssistedLivingRegulatoryReview.pdf.

Peoples, Steve. 2008. "Fears Raised by Medicaid Spending Cap." *The Providence Journal*, May 23. Accessed November 6, 2010. http://pqasb.pqarchiver.com/projo/access/1483601171.html?FMT=ABS&FMTS=ABS:FT&date=May+23%2C+2008&author=Steve+Peoples%3BAdelita+Orefice&pub=The+Providence+Journal&edition=&startpage=A.1&desc=Fears+raised+by+Medicaid+spending+cap.

———. 2008. "Budget Savings Plan Not Detailed." *The Providence Journal*, July 21. Accessed July 22, 2008. http://www.projo.com/news/content/GLOBAL_WAIVER_07–21–08_8BASG2O_v17.3958e93.html

———. 2008. "Carcieri Seeks Waiver to Cap Medicaid at $12 billion." *The Providence Journal*, June 30. Accessed July 30, 2008. http://pqasb.pqarchiver.com/projo/access/1521818231.html?FMT=ABS&FMTS=ABS:FT&date=Jul+30%2C+2008&author=Steve+Peoples&pub=The+Providence+Journal&edition=&startpage=A.1&desc=Carcieri+seeks+waiver+to+cap+Medicaid+at+%2412+billion.

———. 2008. "A Lesson From Vermont on Medicaid." *The Providence Journal*, October 5. Accessed November 6, 2010. http://www.projo.com/news/content/VERMONT_MEDICAID_10–05–08_QVBP8GT_v28.160cc7e.html.

———. 2008. "State Gets Federal OK for Medicaid Waiver." *The Providence Journal*, December 20. Accessed November 6, 2010. http://www.projo.com/generalassembly/GLOBAL_WAIVER_12–20–08_ACCN31J_v14.3751ec1.html.

———. 2009. "R.I. Congressional Delegation Opposed Medicaid Waiver Plan." *The Providence Journal*, January 14. Accessed November 21, 2010. http://www.projo.com/news/content/medicaid14x_01–14–09_NMCV67A_v1.624fef.html.

———. 2009. "State Medicaid Waiver Going Through." *The Providence Journal*, January 16. Accessed November 21, 2010. http://www.projo.com/health/content/MEDICAID_WAIVER_01–16–09_23CVUN2_v12.3c7b1b4.html.

———. 2009. "Waiver May Cut Share of Stimulus." *The Providence Journal*, January 29. Accessed November 21, 2010. http://www.projo.com/news/content/MEDICAID_WAIVER_PROBLEM_01–29–09_GCD4ED8_v17.39b02b7.html.

———. 2009. "R.I. May Lack Personnel to Redo Medicaid." *The Providence Journal*, February 2. Accessed November 21, 2010. http://www.povertyinstitute.org/matriarch/documents/2.2.09%20Providence%20Journal%20RI%20may%20lack%20personell.pdf.

———. 2009. "R.I. House Approves Medicaid Oversight." *The Providence Journal*, February 4. Accessed November 21, 2010. http://www.projo.com/health/content/MEDICAID_WAIVER_VOTE_02–04–09_18D6R5M_v13.3e3ae04.html.

———. 2009. "R.I. Medicaid Waiver Clashed with Stimulus." *The Providence Journal*, February 12.

———. 2009. "Plan to Hire Medicaid Consultants Dropped." *The Providence Journal*, March 3. Accessed November 21, 2010. http://www.projo.com/news/content/MEDICAID_CONTRACT_CANCELLED_03-03-09_ANDGQJV_v20.36aa3c2.html.
———. 2009. "Governor Would Cut Dental Coverage for 38,000 Poor Adults." *The Providence Journal*, March 20. Accessed November 21, 2010. http://www.projo.com/news/content/MEDICAID_DENTAL_CUTS_03-20-09_T8DOCQT_v14.29cc36d.html.
———. 2009. "Oversight Legislation Eludes General Assembly." *The Providence Journal*, May 29. Accessed November 21, 2010. http://www.projo.com/health/content/MEDICAID_WAIVER_05-29-09_GJEHIVG_v10.3db4b28.html.
———. 2009. "New Medicaid Rules Aim to Reduce Nursing Home Admissions." *The Providence Journal*, July 9. Accessed November 21, 2010. http://www.projo.com/news/content/NURSING_HOME_RULES_07-09-09_I0EVKBG_v27.3b3c81a.html.
———. 2010. "House Panel Examines Effects of Medicaid Waiver". *The Providence Journal*, January 14. Accessed December 6, 2010. http://www.projo.com/news/content/GLOBAL_WAIVER_01-14-10_I6H3TDK_v9.3988d90.html.
———. 2010. "RI Bars New Home-Health Companies from Operating in Rhode Island." *The Providence Journal*, May 23. Accessed December 6, 2010. http://www.projo.com/news/content/HOME_CARE_MORATORIUM_05-23-10_33IHHFM_v20.17ad2546.html.
Peoples, Steve, and Cynthia Needham. 2008. "House Passes State Budget." *The Providence Journal*, June 19. Accessed November 6, 2010. http://pqasb.pqarchiver.com/projo/access/1497404831.html?FMT=ABS&FMTS=ABS:FT&date=Jun+19%2C+2008&author=Steve+Peoples%3BCYNTHIA+NEEDHAM&pub=The+Providence+Journal&edition=&startpage=A.1&desc=House+passes+state+budget.
———. 2009. "Path Cleared for Medicaid Waiver Plan." *The Providence Journal*, January 15. Accessed November 21, 2010. http://www.projo.com/generalassembly/WAIVER_01-15-09_Q6CVAU1_v21.3df227e.html.
Perry, Michael, Naomi Mulligan, Samantha Artiga, and Jessica Stephens. 2012. *Faces of the Medicaid Expansion: Experiences of Uninsured Adults Who Could Gain Coverage*. Washington, D.C.: The Henry J. Kaiser Family Foundation. Accessed December 31, 2012. http://www.kff.org/medicaid/upload/8385.pdf.
Peterson, Chris. L. 2009, January 14. *Projections of FY2009 Federal SCHIP Allotments Under CHIPRA 2009*. Washington, D.C.: Congressional Research Services. Accessed November 8, 2012. http://assets.opencrs.com/rpts/R40129_20090114.pdf.
PHI. 2005. *The Role of Training in Improving the Recruitment and Retention of Direct-Care Workers in Long-Term Care*. Bronx, NY: PHI. Accessed December 5, 2011. www.directcareclearinghouse.org/ download/WorkforceStrategies3.pdf.
Pollack, Harold. A. 2013. "State Medicaid Policy and Health Reform." *Journal of Health Politics, Policy and Law* 38 (1): 161–163.
Pothas, Anne-Marie, and Andries G. de Wet. 2000. Two Imperatives for Qualitative Research. *Systematic Practice and Action Research* 13 (2): 139–164.
The Poverty Institute. 2008, August 15. *Key Provisions of "The RI Consumer Choice Compact Waiver."* Providence, Rhode Island: The Rhode Island College School of Social Work: The Poverty Institute. Accessed November 6, 2010. http://povertyinstitute.org/matriarch/documents/Summary_of_Waiver_Submission_8.08_on_letterhead.pdf.
Prah, Pamela. M. 2010. "Rhode Island's Medicaid Gamble." *Stateline*, May 11. Accessed: December 6, 2010. http://www.stateline.org/live/details/story?contentId=483799.

Pratt, John. W., and Richard J. Zechkauser, eds. 1985. *Principals and Agents: The Structure of Business*. Boston, MA: Harvard Business School Press.

Proximity. 2012. *State Population Estimates and Projections, 2000–2030: Population Ages 65 Years & Over and Percent of Total Population*. Accessed October 28, 2012. http://proximityone.com/st003065.htm.

Pugh, Tony. 2011. "Rhode Island's Medicaid Funding Experiment Draws Raves, Suspicion." *Saint Paul Pioneer Press*, June 12. Accessed May 20, 2013. Available at: http://www.mcclatchydc.com/2011/05/23/114587/rhode-islands-medicaid-experiment.html.

"Reaction Mixed to Bush's Medicaid Reform Proposal." 2003, February 4. *Kaiser Daily Health Policy Report*. Accessed October 28, 2012. http://www.kaiserhealthnews.org/Daily-Reports/2003/February/04/dr00015855.aspx?p=1.

Reed, Jack, and Sheldon Whitehouse. 2008, September 23. *Letter to HHS Secretary Regarding Rhode Island Medicaid Waiver*.

Reed, Jack, Sheldon Whitehouse, James Langevin, and Patrick Kennedy. 2009, January 13. Letter to Donald Carcieri. Accessed November 21, 2010. http://povertyinstitute.org/matriarch/documents/delegationwaiver_11309.pdf.

Reichard, John. 2008. *Rhode Island Medicaid Plan Arouses Liberal Ire*. New York: The Commonwealth Fund. Accessed November 6, 2010. http://www.commonwealthfund.org/Content/Newsletters/Washington-Health-Policy-in-Review/2008/Sep/Washington-Health-Policy-Week-in-Review—-September-15—2008/Rhode-Island-Medicaid-Plan-Arouses-Liberal-Ire.aspx.

Republican Governors Public Policy Committee. 2011, April 4. *RGA Leadership Supports House GOP Budget; Calls for Medicaid Block Grants*. Washington, D.C.: Republican Governors Association. Accessed January 14, 2013. http://www.rga.org/homepage/rga-leadership-supports-house-gop-budget-calls-for-medicaid-block-grants/.

———. 2011, August 30. *A New Medicaid: A Flexible, Innovative and Accountable Future*. Washington, D.C.: Republican Governors Association. Accessed January 14, 2013. http://www.rga.org/homepage/gop-govs-release-medicaid-reform-report/.

Republican Governors Association. 2011, June 13. *GOP Govs Unveil Medicaid Reform Principles*. Washington, D.C.: Republican Governors Association. Accessed January 14, 2013. http://www.rga.org/homepage/gop-govs-unveil-medicaid-reform-principles/.

Reinhard, Susan C., Enid Kassner, Arl Houser, and Robert Mollica. 2011, September. *State Scorecard on Long-Term Services and Supports for Older Adults, People with Physically Disabilities, and Family Caregivers*. Washington, D.C.: AARP, The Commonwealth Fund, The Scan Foundation. Accessed November 21, 2012. http://assets.aarp.org/rgcenter/ppi/ltc/ltss_scorecard.pdf.

Rivlin, Alice, and Paul Ryan. 2010, November 17. *A Long Term Plan for Medicare and Medicaid*. Accessed November 7, 2012. http://paulryan.house.gov/uploadedfiles/rivlinryan.pdf.

Rhode Island Association of Facilities and Services. 2010, March 22. *RIAFSA Position Paper on the Medicaid Global Waiver*.

Rhode Island Government. 2009, March 9. *Office of Health & Human Services and Department of Human Services Seeking Applications for Members of the RI Global Waiver Implementation Task Force*. Accessed November 21, 2010: www.ri.gov/press/view/8382.

———. 2009, February 26. *Carcieri Names Gary D. Alexander as Secretary of the Executive Office of Health & Human Services*. Accessed November 21, 2010. http://www.ri.gov/press/view/8200.

Rhode Island Health Care Association. 2010, January 5. *DHS Proposed Acuity Based Adjuster*. Warwick, Rhode Island: Rhode Island Health Care Association.

———. 2010, March 29. *Testimony: Acuity Based Payment Adjustment*. Warwick, Rhode Island; Rhode Island Health Care Association.

"Rhode Island's Medicaid Lessons: A Case Study in How Waivers for State Innovations can Work." 2011. *The Wall Street Journal,* March 28. Accessed July 30, 2012. http://online.wsj.com/article/SB10001424052748704893604576198710204114624.html.

"Rhode Island Real Choices: Key Progress to Date." 2011, May 23. Presentation to the Global Waiver External Task Force. Accessed October 26, 2012. http://www.eohhs.ri.gov/documents/documents11/Real_Choices_update_5_23_11.pdf.

Roberts, Janet. 2011. "Rhode Island's Medicaid Experiment Becomes a Talking Point for Budget Cutters." *The New York Times*, May 15. Accessed: May 16, 2011. http://www.nytimes.com/2011/05/16/us/politics/16medicaid.html?nl=us&pagewanted=all.

Robison, Julie, Noreen Shugrue, Martha Porter, Richard H. Fortinsky, and Leslie A. Curry. 2012. "Transition from Home Care to Nursing Home: Unmet Needs in a Home- and Community-Based Program for Older Adults." *Journal of Aging & Social Policy* 24 (3): 251–270.

Romney, Mitt. 2012. *Spending: Smaller, Simpler, Smarter Government.* Accessed October 28, 2012. http://www.mittromney.com/issues/spending.

Rosato, Nancy S., Judith A. Lucas, and Sandra Howell-White. 2005, May. *State Adult Day Health Services Programs: A National Profile (2001–2002).* New Brunswick, New Jersey: Center for Health Policy, Rutgers University. Accessed November 22, 2012. http://www.cshp.rutgers.edu/PDF/StateAdultDayNationalProfile-June%202005.pdf.

Rosenbaum, Sara. 2012. "Threading the Needle—Medicaid and the 113th Congress." *The New England Journal of Medicine.* December 5, 2012. DOI: 10.1056/NEJMp1213901

Rosenbaum, Sara, and Timothy M. Westmoreland. 2012. "The Supreme Court's Surprising Decision on the Medicaid Expansion: How Will the Federal Government and States Proceed?" *Health Affairs* 31 (8): 1663–1672.

Rosenbloom, Sandra. 2009. "Meeting Transportation Needs in an Aging-Friendly Community." *Generations* 33 (2): 33–43.

Rowland, Diane. 1996, March 6. *Testimony before the United States House of Representatives Committee on Commerce on the National Governors Association Proposal on Medicaid.* Washington, D.C.: The Henry J. Kaiser Family Foundation. Accessed January 10, 2013. http://www.kff.onlinemagic.net/health_policy/data/html/kcfm/da.html.

Roy, Avik. 2013, May 2. "Oregon Study: Medicaid 'Had No Significant Effect' on Health Outcomes vs. Being Uninsured." *The Apothecary.* Accessed May 24, 2013. http://www.forbes.com/sites/theapothecary/2013/05/02/oregon-study-medicaid-had-no-significant-effect-on-health-outcomes-vs-being-uninsured/.

———. 201. "Why Block-Granting Medicaid Will Result in Better Health Care for the Poor." *The Apothecary,* September 30. Accessed May 20, 2013. http://www.forbes.com/sites/aroy/2012/09/30/why-block-granting-medicaid-will-result-in-better-health-care-for-the-poor/.

Ryan, Paul. 2011. *The Path to Prosperity: Restoring America's Promise, Fiscal Year 2012* Budget Resolution. Washington, D.C.: House Budget Committee. Accessed October 28, 2012. http://budget.house.gov/uploadedfiles/pathtoprosperityfy2012.pdf.

———. 2012. *The Path to Prosperity: A Blueprint for American Renewal, Fiscal Year 2013* Budget Resolution. Washington, D.C.: House Budget Committee. Accessed October 28, 2012. http://budget.house.gov/uploadedfiles/pathtoprosperity2013.pdf.

———. 2013. *The Path to Prosperity: A Responsible Balanced Budget, Fiscal Year 2014 Budget Resolution*. Washington, D.C.: House Budget Committee. Accessed May 20, 2013. http://budget.house.gov/uploadedfiles/fy14budget.pdf.

Sabatier, Paul. A., and Hank C. Jenkins-Smith, eds. 1993. *Policy Change and Learning: An Advocacy Coalition Approach*. Boulder, CO: Westview Press.

Sabik, Lindsay. M., and Cathy Bradley. 2012. "Differences in Mortality for Surgical Cancer Patients by Insurance and Hospital Safety Net Status." *Medical Care Research and Review*. Published online ahead of print.

The Scan Foundation. 2013, January. *Who Pays for Long-Term Care in the U.S? (Update)*. Long Beach, California: The Scan Foundation. Accessed May 20, 2014. http://www.thescanfoundation.org/sites/thescanfoundation.org/files/who_pays_for_ltc_us_jan_2013_fs.pdf.

Schneider, Saundra. K, and William G. Jacoby. 1996. "Influences on Bureaucratic Policy Initiatives in the American States." *Journal of Public Administration, Research, and Theory* 6 (4): 495–422.

Schneider, Saundra. K., William G. Jacoby, and Jerrell D. Coggburn. 1997. "The Structure of Bureaucratic Decisions in the American States." *Public Administrative Review* 57 (3): 240–249.

Seavey, Dorie, and Abby Marquand. 2011, December. *Caring in America, a Comprehensive Analysis of the Nation's Fastest Growing Jobs: Home Health and Personal Care Aides*. Bronx, New York: Paraprofessional Healthcare Institute. Accessed November 21, 2012. http://phinational.org/sites/phinational.org/files/clearinghouse/caringinamerica-20111212.pdf.

Senate Finance Committee Hearing. 2011, July 14. *Perspectives on Medicaid from Select Governors*. Washington, D.C.: U.S. Government Printing Office.

Senior Agenda Coalition. 2007, February. *Reforming Long-Term Care for Rhode Island: Best Practices from Other States*. Providence, Rhode Island: Senior Agenda Coalition. Accessed October 28, 2012. http://www.rhodestoindependence.org/docs/Reforming%20LTC%20in%20RI.pdf.

Sharma, Leena, and Carol Regan. 2012, June 29. *Re: Rhode Island Capitated Financial Alignment Demonstration Proposal for Medicare-Medicaid Enrollees*. Boston, Massachusetts: Community Catalyst. Accessed May 18, 2013. http://www.financialalignmentproposalcomments.org/default.aspx.

Shirk, Cynthia. 2009, August 26. *The Basics: Medicaid Waivers and Budget Neutrality*. Washington D.C.: The George Washington University. Accessed October 28, 2012. http://www.nhpf.org/library/the-basics/Basics_MedicaidBudgetNeut_08–26–09.pdf.

Shishkin, Phillip. 2008. "States Cut Services for Elderly, Disabled." *Wall Street Journal*, November 20. Accessed January 2, 2013. http://online.wsj.com/article/SB122714130153442755.html.

Smith, David B., Zhanlian Feng, Mary R. Fennell, Jacqueline S. Zinn, and Vincent Mor. 2007. "Separate and Unequal: Racial Segregation and Disparities in Quality across U.S. Nursing Homes." *Health Affairs* 26 (5): 1448–58.

Smith, Kristin, and Reagan Baughman. 2007. "Caring for America's Aging Population: A Profile of the Direct-Care Workforce." *Monthly Labor Review*, September: 20–26.

Smith, Vernon. K., Kathleen Gifford, Eileen Ellis, Robin Rudowitz, and Laura Snyder. 2010, September. *Hoping for Economic Recovery, Preparing for Health Reform: A Look at Medicaid Spending, Coverage and Policy Trends Results from a 50-State Medicaid Budget Survey for State Fiscal Years 2010 and 2011*. Washington, D.C.: The Henry J. Kaiser Family Foundation. Accessed January 3, 2013. http://www.kff.org/medicaid/upload/8105.pdf.

———. 2012, October. *Medicaid Today; Preparing for Tomorrow A Look at State Medicaid Program Spending, Enrollment and Policy Trends: Results from a 50-State Medicaid Budget Survey for State Fiscal Years 2012 and 2013*. Washington, D.C.: The Henry J. Kaiser Family Foundation. Accessed November 14, 2012. http://www.kff.org/medicaid/upload/8380.pdf.

Snyder, Laura, Robin Rudowitz, Rachel Garfield, and Tracy Gordon. 2012, November. *Why Does Medicaid Spending Vary Across States: A Chart Book of Factors Driving State Spending*. Washington, D.C.: The Henry J. Kaiser Family Foundation. Accessed December 31, 2012. http://www.kff.org/medicaid/upload/8378.pdf.

Solomon, Judith. 2008, September 4. *Rhode Island's Medicaid Proposal Would Put Beneficiaries at Risk and Could Undermine the Federal-State Partnerships*. Washington, D.C.: Center on Budget and Policy Priorities. Accessed November 6, 2010. http://www.cbpp.org/files/9–4-08health.pdf.

———. 2009, January. *Rhode Island's Medicaid Waiver: A Bad Deal for the State*. Washington, D.C.: Center on Budget and Policy Priorities. Accessed November 8, 2010. http://povertyinstitute.org/matriarch/documents/CBPP%20Georgetown%20paper.pdf.

Somashekhar, Sandhya. 2013. "In Several States, Medicaid Expansion Remains in Limbo as Time Runs Short. *The Washington Post,* May 2. Accessed May 25, 2013. http://www.washingtonpost.com/national/health-science/in-several-states-medicaid-expansion-remains-in-limbo-as-time-runs-short/2013/05/02/6dafcc02-b1b5–11e2–9a98–4be1688d7d84_story.html.

Sommers, Benjamin D., Katherine Baicker, and Arnold M. Epstein. 2012. "Mortality and Access to Care among Adults after State Medicaid Expansions." *The New England Journal of Medicine* 367 (11): 1025–1034.

Spears, Tina. 2013, February 15. *Comments for Review on the Proposed 1115 Research and Demonstration Waiver.* Cranston, Rhode Island: Rhode Island Parent Information Network. Accessed May 18, 2013. http://www.ohhs.ri.gov/documents/documents13/RIPIN_comments_2_15_13.pdf.

Spillman, Brenda C., Korbin Liu, and Carey McGilliard. 2002, November 25. *Trends in Residential Long-Term Care: Use of Nursing Homes and Assisted Living and Characteristics of Facilities and Residents*. Washington, D.C.: Urban Institute. Accessed November 22, 2012. http://aspe.hhs.gov/daltcp/reports/2002/rltct.pdf.

Stevenson, David G., and David C. Grabowski. 2010. "Sizing Up the Market for Assisted Living." *Health Affairs* 29 (1): 35–43.

Stone, Robyn I. 2004. "The Direct Care Workers: The Third Rail of Home Care Policy." *Annual Review of Public Health* 25: 521–537.

Stone, Robyn I., and Susan C. Reinhard. 2007. "The Place of Assisted Living in Long-Term Care and Related Service Systems." *The Gerontologist* 47 (Special Issue III): 23–32.

Thompson, Frank J. 1998. "Federalism and the Medicaid Challenge." In *Medicaid and Devolution: A View from the States,* edited by F. J. Thompson, and J. J. Dilulio. Washington, D.C.: Brookings Institution.

———. 2011. "The Medicaid Platform: Can the Termites Be Kept at Bay?" *Journal of Health Politics, Policy & Law* 36 (3): 549–554.

———. 2012. *Medicaid Politics: Federalism, Policy Durability, and Health Reform.* Washington, D.C.: Georgetown University Press.

Thompson, Frank J., and Courtney Burke. 2007. "Executive Federalism and Medicaid Demonstration Waivers: Implications for Policy and Democratic Process." *Journal of Health Politics Policy & Law* 32 (6): 971–1004.

———. 2009. "Federalism by Waiver: Medicaid and the Transformation of Long-Term Care." *Publius* 39 (1): 22–46.

Thorpe, Kenneth E. 2011, September. *Estimated Federal Savings Associated with Care Coordination Models for Medicare-Medicaid Dual Eligibles.* Atlanta, GA: Emory University. Accessed July 17, 2012. http://www.ahipcoverage.com/wp-content/uploads/2011/09/Dual-Eligible-Study-September-2011.pdf.

Trapp, Doug. 2008. "Rhode Island seeks Medicaid Overhaul, Cap on Spending." *American Medical News*, November 17. Accessed November 6, 2010. http://www.ama-assn.org/amednews/2008/11/17/gvsa1117.htm.

Trinity, Margaret, Enrique Martinez-Vidal, Isabel Friedenzohn, Amanda Folsom, and Brynnan Cox. 2008, January. *State of the States: Rising to the Challenge.* Washington, D.C.: AcademyHealth. Accessed November 17, 2012. http://www.statecoverage.org/files/SCI%20State%20of%20the%20States%202008.pdf.

Upton, Fred, and Orrin Hatch. 2013, May 1. *Making Medicaid Work: Protect the Vulnerable, Offer Individualized Care, and Reduce Costs.* Washington, D.C.: U.S. House of Representatives Committee on Energy and Commerce, U.S. Senate Committee on Finance. Accessed May 26, 2013. http://energycommerce.house.gov/sites/republicans.energycommerce.house.gov/files/analysis/20130501Medicaid.pdf.

U.S. Bureau of Labor Statistics. 2010. *Selected Occupational Projections Data.* Accessed March 26, 2010. data.bls.gov:8080/oep/servlet/oep.noeted.servlet.ActionServlet? Action=empeduc.

U.S. Department of Health and Human Services. 2013, April 10. *Fiscal Year 2014 Budget in Brief: Strengthening Health and Opportunity for All Americans.* Washington, D.C.: Department of Human Services Accessed May 24, 2013. http://www.hhs.gov/budget/fy2014/fy-2014-budget-in-brief.pdf.

U.S. Government Accountability Office. 2002, July 12. *Medicaid and SCHIP: Recent HHS Approvals of Demonstration Waiver Projects Raise Concerns,* GAO-02–817. Accessed November 13, 2012. http://www.gao.gov/new.items/d02817.pdf.

———. 2003, October. *Medicaid Nursing Home Payments: States' Payment Rates Largely Unaffected by Recent Fiscal Pressures.* Washington, D.C.: U.S. General Accountability Office. Accessed December 27, 2012. http://www.gao.gov/assets/250/240199.pdf.

———. 2007, July 24. *Medicaid Demonstration Waivers: Lack of Opportunity for Public Input During Federal Approval Process Still a Concern,* GAO-07–694R. Accessed November 13, 2012. http://www.gao.gov/assets/100/95034.pdf.

———. 2010, January 29. *Medicaid and CHIP: Enrollment, Benefits, Expenditures, and Other Characteristics of State Premium Assistance Programs.* Accessed May 23, 2013. http://www.gao.gov/new.items/d10258r.pdf.

The Vermont Choices for Care Long-Term Care Plan: Key Program Changes and Questions. 2006, July. Washington, D.C.: The Henry J. Kaiser Family Foundation. Accessed October 28, 2012. http://www.kff.org/medicaid/upload/7540.pdf.

Volsky, Igor. 2011. "Why Rhode Island's Medicaid Waiver Does Not Prove That Block Grants Work." *ThinkProgress,* March 30. Accessed July 30, 2012. http://thinkprogress.org/health/2011/03/30/172007/rhode-island-medicaid/?mobile=nc.

Walker, Jack L. 1969. "The Diffusion of Innovations Among the American States." *American Political Science Review* 63 (3): 880–99.

Walls, Jenna, Kathleen Gifford, Catherine Rudd, Rex O'Rourke, Martha Roherty, Lindsey Copeland, and Wendy Fox-Grage. 2011, January. *Weathering the Storm: The Impact of the Great Recession on Long-Term Services and Supports.* Washington, D.C.: AARP. Accessed November 13, 2012. http://assets.aarp.org/rgcenter/ppi/ltc/CURRENT__Budget_Paper_v9Jan6.pdf.

Walshe, Kieran, and Charlene Harrington. 2001. *The Regulation of Nursing Facilities in the US: An Analysis of the Resources and Performance of State Survey*

Agencies. Birmingham, United Kingdom: Health Services Management Centre, University of Birmingham.
Wardrip, Keith. 2010, March. *Strategies to Meet the Housing Needs of Older Adults*. Washington, D.C.: AARP. Accessed November 22, 2012. http://assets.aarp.org/rgcenter/ppi/liv-com/i38-strategies.pdf.
Watts, Molly O'Mallet, and Katherine Young. 2012, December. *The Medicaid Medically Needy Program: Spending and Enrollment Update*. Washington, D.C.: The Henry J. Kaiser Family Foundation. Accessed January 4, 2012. http://www.kff.org/medicaid/upload/4096.pdf.
Weems, Kerry. 2009, January 16. *Rhode Island Global Consumer Choice Compact Section 1115: Waiver and Expenditure Authority, Waiver List, and Special Terms and Conditions*. Washington, D.C.: Centers for Medicare and Medicaid Services, U.S. Department of Health and Human Services. Accessed October 28, 2012. http://www.eohhs.ri.gov/medicaid/pdf/GlobalWaiverFinal1–09.pdf.
Weissert, Carol S., and William G. Weissert. 2008. "Medicaid Waivers: License to Shape the Future of Fiscal Federalism." In *Intergovernmental Management in the 21st century*, edited by Timothy J. Conlan, and Paul L. Posner, 157–75. Washington, D.C.: Brookings Institution.
Weissert, William G. 1993. "One More Battle Lost to Friendly Fire—Or If You Spend Too Much It's Hard to Save Money." *Medical Care*, 31 (Suppl. 9): 119–121.
Werner, Rachel M., Elizabeth L. Goldman, and Adams R. Dudley. 2008. "Comparison of Change in Quality of Care between Safety-Net and Non-Safety Hospitals." *Journal of the American Medical Association* 299 (18): 2180–2187.
Wiener, Joshua M. 2010. "Long-term Care: Getting on the Agenda and Knowing What to Propose. *Medical Care Research & Review* 67 (4): 126S-140S.
Wiener, Joshua. M., and Jane Tilly. 2002. "Long-Term Care: Can the States Be the Engine of Reform?" In *Federalism & Health Policy,* edited by J. Holohan, A. Weil, and J. M. Wiener, 249–292. Washington, D.C.: The Urban Institute.
Wiener, Joshua. M., Mark P. Freiman, and Davis Brown. 2007, December. *Nursing Home Care Quality: Twenty Years After the Omnibus Budget Reconciliation Act of 1987*. Washington, D.C.: RTI. Accessed December 5, 2011. www.kff.org/medicare/upload/7717.pdf.
Wildavsky, A. 1964. *The Politics of the Budgetary Process*. Boston, MA: Little, Brown.
Williams, Erica, Michael Leachman, and Nicholas Johnson. 2011, July 28. *State Budget Cuts in the New Fiscal Year Are Unnecessarily Harmful*. Washington, D.C.: Center on Budget and Policy Priorities. Accessed November 14, 2012. http://www.cbpp.org/files/7–26–11sfp.pdf.
Williamson, Oliver E. 1981. "The Economics of Organizations: The Transaction Cost Approach." *American Journal of Sociology* 87: 548–577.
Woodcock, Cynthia, Ian Stockwell, Aaron Tripp, and Chuck Milligan. 2011, June 14. *Rebalancing Long-Term Services and Supports: Progress to Date and a Research Agenda for the Future*. Baltimore, Maryland: The Hilltop Institute, University of Maryland-Baltimore County. Accessed November 21, 2012. http://www.hilltopinstitute.org/publications/RebalancingLTSS-ProgressToDateAndResearchAgendaForFuture-June2011.pdf.
Woodcock, Cynthia H., Ian Stockwell, Harriet Komisar, and Aaron Tripp. 2010, February 28. *Rhode Island Real Choices Long-Term Services and Supports Resource Mapping: Final Report*. Baltimore, Maryland: The Hilltop Institute, University of Maryland-Baltimore County. Accessed November 21, 2012. http://www.dhs.ri.gov/Portals/0/Uploads/Documents/Public/Reports/LTSS_Resource_Mapping_Feb_2010.pdf.
Wrigley, W. 2013. "Jan Brewer Vetoes Bills After Vowing Not To Sign Legislation Until State Passes Medicaid Expansion." *The Huffington Post,* May 24. Accessed

May 25, 2013. http://www.huffingtonpost.com/2013/05/24/jan-brewer-vetoes_n_3333631.html.

Wu, Leighton, and Victoria Wachino. 2005, July 7. *The Effect of Increased Cost-Sharing in Medicaid: A Summary of Research Findings*. Washington, D.C.: Center on Budget and Policy Priorities. Accessed October 28, 2012. http://www.cbpp.org/files/5-31-05health2.pdf.

Zimmerman, Sheryl, Ann L. Gruber-Baldini, Phillip D. Sloane, Kevin J. Eckert, Richard J. Hebel, Leslie A. Morgan, Sally C. Sterns, Judith Wildfire, Jay Magaziner, Cory Chen and Thomas Konrad. 2003. "Assisted Living and Nursing Homes: Apples and Oranges?" *The Gerontologist* 43 (Spec. 2): 107–17.

Zuckerman, Stephen, Joshua McFeeters, Peter Cunningham, and Len Nichols. 2004. "Changes in Medicaid Physicians Fees, 1998–2003: Implications for Physician Participation." *Health Affairs*: 374–84. Published electronically June 2004. DOI:10.1377/hlthaff.w4.374.

Index